Lecture Notes of the Institute for Computer Sciences, Social Informatics and Telecommunications Engineering 578

The LNICST series publishes ICST's conferences, symposia and workshops.

LNICST reports state-of-the-art results in areas related to the scope of the Institute. The type of material published includes

- Proceedings (published in time for the respective event)
- Other edited monographs (such as project reports or invited volumes)

LNICST topics span the following areas:

- General Computer Science
- E-Economy
- E-Medicine
- Knowledge Management
- Multimedia
- Operations, Management and Policy
- Social Informatics
- Systems

António Cunha · Anselmo Paiva · Sandra Pereira
Editors

Wireless Mobile Communication and Healthcare

12th EAI International Conference, MobiHealth 2023
Vila Real, Portugal, November 29–30, 2023
Proceedings

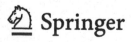
Springer

Editors
António Cunha
University of Trás-os-Montes and Alto Douro
Vila Real, Portugal

Anselmo Paiva ⓘ
Federal University of Maranhão
São Luís, Brazil

Sandra Pereira
University of Trás-os-Montes and Alto Douro
Vila Real, Portugal

ISSN 1867-8211 ISSN 1867-822X (electronic)
Lecture Notes of the Institute for Computer Sciences, Social Informatics
and Telecommunications Engineering
ISBN 978-3-031-60664-9 ISBN 978-3-031-60665-6 (eBook)
https://doi.org/10.1007/978-3-031-60665-6

This Springer imprint is published by the registered company Springer Nature Switzerland AG
The registered company address is: Gewerbestrasse 11, 6330 Cham, Switzerland

If disposing of this product, please recycle the paper.

Preface

We are delighted to introduce the proceedings of the 12th edition of the European Alliance for Innovation (EAI) International Conference on Wireless Mobile Communication and Healthcare (MobiHealth 2023). This conference brought together researchers, developers, and practitioners worldwide who are leveraging and developing wireless communications, mobile computing, and healthcare applications.

The technical program of MobiHealth 2023 consisted of 34 full papers with oral presentation sessions at the main conference track, and 1 Demo paper. Aside from the high-quality technical paper presentations, the technical program also featured two keynote speeches. The two keynote speeches were from Claudio Marroco from Università degli Studi di Cassino e del Lazio Meridionale, Italy, and Víctor Muñoz from Universidad de Málaga, Spain.

Coordination with the steering committee members, Aura Conci and Marcelo Gattass, was essential for the conference's success. We sincerely appreciate their support and guidance. It was also a great pleasure to work with such an excellent organizing committee team for their hard work organizing and supporting the conference.

In particular, the Technical Program Committee, led by our TPC Chairs, Emilio Luque, Jorge Marx Gómez, and TPC Co-Chairs João Rodrigues, Paulo Salgado, Eftim Zdravevski, Francesco Renna, Marta Chinnici, and João Almeida, completed the peer-review process of technical papers and made a high-quality technical program. We are also grateful to all other organizing committee members for their support and to the authors who submitted their papers to the MobiHealth 2023 conference and workshops.

The MobiHealth conference provides a good forum for all researchers, developers, and practitioners to discuss all aspects of science and technology that are relevant to the fields of wireless communications, mobile computing, and healthcare applications. We also expect that future MobiHealth conferences will be as successful and stimulating as indicated by the contributions presented in this volume.

António Cunha
Anselmo Paiva
Sandra Pereira

Organization

Steering Committee

António Cunha   Universidade de Trás-os-Montes e Alto Douro, Portugal

Anselmo Paiva   Universidade Federal do Maranhão, Brazil

Aura Conci   Universidade Federal Fluminense, Brazil

Marcelo Gattass   Pontifícia Universidade Católica do Rio de Janeiro, Brazil

Organizing Committee

General Chair

António Cunha   Universidade de Trás-os-Montes e Alto Douro, Portugal

General Co-chair

Anselmo Paiva   Universidade Federal do Maranhão, Brazil

Technical Program Committee Chairs

Emilio Luque   Autonomous University of Barcelona, Spain

Jorge Marx Gómez   Carl von Ossietzky University of Oldenburg, Germany

Technical Program Committee Co-chairs

João Rodrigues   Universidade do Algarve, Portugal

Paulo Salgado   Universidade de Trás-os-Montes e Alto Douro, Portugal

Eftim Zdravevski   University Ss. Cyril and Methodius, Skopje, Macedonia

Francesco Renna   Universidade do Porto, Portugal

Marta Chinnici   ENEA, Italy
João Dallyson   Universidade Federal do Maranhão, Brazil

Web Chair

António Jorge Gouveia   Universidade de Trás-os-Montes e Alto Douro,
                                  Portugal

Publicity and Social Media Chairs

Miguel Coimbra   Faculdade de Ciências da Universidade do Porto,
                                  Portugal
Pedro Mestre   Universidade de Trás-os-Montes e Alto Douro,
                                  Portugal

Sponsorship and Exhibit Chairs

Joaquim João Sousa   Universidade de Trás-os-Montes e Alto Douro,
                                  Portugal
Emanuel Peres   Universidade de Trás-os-Montes e Alto Douro,
                                  Portugal

Publication Chair

Danilo Leite   Universidade Federal da Paraíba, Brazil

Demo Chairs

Paulo Lopes dos Santos   Universidade do Porto, Portugal
Teresa Perdicoulis   Universidade de Trás-os-Montes e Alto Douro,
                                  Portugal

Posters and PhD Track Chair

Paula Trigueiros   Universidade do Minho, Portugal

Workshops Chair

Paulo Coelho   Instituto Politécnico de Leiria, Portugal

Local Chairs

Sandra Pereira   Universidade de Trás-os-Montes e Alto Douro,
                                Portugal
Cristina Reis   Universidade de Trás-os-Montes e Alto Douro,
                                Portugal

Technical Program Committee

Abbas Aljuboori   University of Information Technology and
                                Communications, Iraq
Alessio Vecchio   University of Pisa, Italy
Alex Gaudio   Carnegie Mellon University, USA
Ali Hassan Sodhro   Kristianstad University, Sweden
Alisson Burrows   University of Minho, Portugal
Ana Maria Mendonça   Universidade do Porto, Portugal
Ana Paula Silva   Polytechnic Institute of Castelo Branco, Portugal
Andre Cavalcante   Federal University of Maranhão, Brazil
André Soares   Federal University of Piauí, Brazil
António Jorge Gouveia   University of Trás-os-Montes e Alto Douro,
                                Portugal
Aykut Karakaya   Zonguldak Bülent Ecevit University, Turkey
Carlos Costa   Polytechnic University of Viseu, Portugal
Carlos Ferreira   Universidade do Porto, Portugal
Catarina Reis   Polytechnic Institute of Leiria, Portugal
Celia Ramos   University of the Algarve, Portugal
Claudio de Souza Baptista   Federal University of Campina Grande, Brazil
Constandinos Mavromoustakis   University of Nicosia, Cyprus
Danilo Leite   Federal University of Paraíba, Brazil
Darlan Quintanilha   Federal University of Maranhão, Brazil
Davi Viana dos Santos   Federal Institute of Maranhão, Brazil
Dibet Garcia Gonzalez   University of Minho, Portugal
E. J. Solteiro Pires   University of Trás-os-Montes e Alto Douro,
                                Portugal
Emanuel Peres   University of Trás-os-Montes e Alto Douro,
                                Portugal
Emmanuel Conchon   University of Limoges, France
Ertugrul Dogruluk   CEiiA, Portugal
Faisal Hussain   University of Engineering and Technology,
                                Pakistan
Fernando Ribeiro   Polytechnic Institute of Castelo Branco, Portugal
Filipe Caldeira   Polytechnic Institute of Viseu, Portugal

Flavio Araujo	Federal University of Piauí, Brazil
Francisco Glaubos Nunes Climaco	Federal University of Maranhão, Brazil
Gabriel Pires	Polytechnic Institute of Tomar, Portugal
Geraldo Braz Junior	Federal University of Maranhão, Brazil
Goranka Stanic	School of Applied Arts and Design, Osijek, Hungary
Henrique Neiva	University of Beira Interior, Portugal
Inês Domingues	Coimbra Institute of Engineering, Portugal
Isabel Bentes	Universidade de Trás-os-Montes e Alto Douro, Portugal
Ivan Ganchev	University of Limerick, Ireland
Jaime Martins	University of the Algarve, Portugal
João Henriques	University of Coimbra, Portugal
João Lanzinha	University of Beira Interior, Portugal
João Otávio Bandeira Diniz	Federal Institute of Maranhão, Brazil
João Pedrosa	University of Porto, Portugal
John Gialelis	University of Patras, Greece
Jonatan Lerga	University of Rijeka, Croatia
Jose Carlos Meireles Metrólho	Polytechnic Institute of Castelo Branco, Portugal
José de Moura Ramos	University of Coruña, Spain
José Lousado	Polytechnic Institute of Viseu, Portugal
José Valente Oliveira	University of the Algarve, Portugal
Kalle Tammemäe	Tallinn University of Technology, Estonia
Kelson Aires	Federal University of Pauí, Brazil
Lio Gonçalves	University of Trás-Os-Montes and Alto Douro, Portugal
Luis Augusto Silva	University of Salamanca, Spain
Luis Jorge Enrique Rivero Cabrejos	Federal Institute of Maranhão, Brazil
Luís Páuda	University of Trás-Os-Montes and Alto Douro, Portugal
Maria Teresa Galvão Dias	University of Porto, Portugal
Miguel Velhote Correia	Universidade do Porto, Portugal
MirHojjat Seyedi	Victoria University, Australia
Oliver Díaz	Universitat de Barcelona, Spain
Ouri Wolfson	University of Illinois, USA
Paula Trigueiros	University of Minho, Portugal
Paulo Lopes dos Santos	University of Porto, Portugal
Paulo Loureiro	Polytechnic of Leiria, Portugal
Paulo Oliveira	University of Trás-os-Montes e Alto Douro, Portugal
Pedro Cardoso	University of the Algarve, Portugal

Contents

Multimedia e-health Data Exchange Services. Signal/Data Processing and Computing For Health Systems

Complex Systems and Optimal Pandemic Control

Medical, Communications
and Networkin

Geometric Perception of the Brain: A Classical Approach Using Image Segmentation

J. Leite[1]([✉]), P. A. Salgado[1], T.-P. Azevedo Perdicoúlis[1],
and P. Lopes dos Santos[2]

[1] Escola de Ciências e Tecnologia, Universidade de Trás-os-Montes e Alto Douro,
Vila Real 5000-811, Portugal
joanaalvesleite@gmail.com, {psal,tazevedo}@utad.pt
[2] Faculdade de Engenharia da Universidade do Porto, Porto 4200-465, Portugal
pjsantos@fe.up.pt

Abstract. This work focuses on the application of image processing techniques to segment and analyze images of brain sections with the aim of facilitating early diagnosis of brain tumors. The aim is to delineate specific regions of the brain, such as the cranial, intracranial, and encephalic regions, for subsequent geometric analysis. The process involves image pre-processing, conversion to polar coordinates, determination of contour points, Fourier Series approximation, and the use of the Least Square Method to obtain accurate representations of the regions. The proposed approach was tested on Magnetic Resonance Images of three different brains, showing its capability to accurately delineating the targeted regions. The results highlight the potential of signal processing techniques for analyzing brain images and provide insights for further research in this area.

Keywords: Medical Imaging · Pre-processing · Image Segmentation · Image Analysis

1 Introduction

Several fields of scientific knowledge have tried to assist medicine and healthcare along the years. Currently, complementary diagnostic tools have become indispensable in modern medicine due to the crucial additional information they offer, which might be unattainable through traditional conventional methods. Medical Imaging is undoubtedly one of the most relevant means in this context and can be analyzed through visualization systems or viewers [1]. While general image processing often emphasises aesthetics or create art, medical image

T-P. A. Perdicoúlis—Supported by FCT - Fundação para a Ciência e a Tecnologia under project UIDB/50014/2020 IDB/00048/2020
P. L. dos Santos—Supported by FCT - Fundação para a Ciência e a Tecnologia under project UIDB/50014/2020.

A. Cunha et al. (Eds.): MobiHealth 2023, LNICST 578, pp. 3–16, 2024.
https://doi.org/10.1007/978-3-031-60665-6_1

processing solely focuses on improving or artistic creativity, medical image is dedicated exclusively to enhancing the interpretability of displayed content. Its objectives include enhancing the image itself to highlight specific features and extracting information either through automated or manual means. The following classification outlines key categories for further exploration:

- Image enhancement: This involves removing image distortions like noise and background irregularities, as well as enhancing image contours and other relevant properties.
- Image segmentation: Its purpose is to demarcate the boundaries or contours of anatomical structures such as organs, vessels, or tumor lesions.
- Quantification: This category involves determining geometric properties of anatomical structures (e.g., perimeter, area, diameter, curvature) or physiological properties like perfusion characteristics or tissue composition.
- Computer-aided detection: The objective is to detect and characterize pathological structures and lesions, such as tumor lesions or vessel obstructions [2].

Medical Imaging, serving as a supplementary diagnostic tool, has evolved beyond mere visualization techniques and in-depth explorations of the human anatomy. This field enables the acquisition of information on the physiology and anatomy of internal organs non-invasively, using a variety of contemporary techniques, such as Magnetic Resonance Imaging (MRI), X-ray, Computed Tomography (CT) and Positron Emission Tomography (PET). These methodologies enable early detection of diseases, better coordination of medical treatments and even better general knowledge of the molecular activity of living organisms [3]. In Neuroscience, research extends beyond studying structure, volume, and morphometry. It also delves into understanding complex human mental processes, like language and consciousness, using tools such as MRI and (Functional MRI) fMRI [4]. These are important tools to support diagnosis, allowing specialists an in-depth study of pathologies of the nervous system and human behavior [5,6].

Medical images capture representations of the human body at various scales, ranging from microscopic to macroscopic. " original:" They come in a wide variety of imaging modalities (e.g. a CT scanner, an ultrasound machine, etc.) and measure a physical property of the human body (e.g. radio-density, the opacity to X-rays). Available in diverse imaging modalities, such as CT scanners or ultrasound machines, they measure specific physical properties of the body, like radio-density or X-ray opacity. Specialized experts, like radiologists, interpret these images for clinical purposes, such as diagnostics, profoundly influencing physicians' decision-making. Computer vision methods have long been employed to automatically analyze medical images. The recent advent of deep learning has replaced many other machine learning methods because it avoids the creation of hand-engineering features, thus removing a critical source of error from the process [7].

The mammalian nervous system consists of two divisions called the Central Nervous System (CNS) and peripheral nervous system (PNS). The CNS is formed by the brain and spinal cord, while the PNS includes nerve cells and receptors outside. When observing an image of the nervous system, we realize that, with rare exceptions, all its structures occur in pairs, one on the left side and the other on the right side, that is, the left side is a specular image of the right side if you divide it into symmetrical halves—bilateral cerebral symmetry [8]. When referring to the CNS, it is common to use the terms white matter and gray matter. These terms arise due to the outermost layer of the brain being of gray color and mainly formed by neurons, while the innermost brain region is of white color, which is due to the myelin that coats these fibers, and consists mainly of nerve fibers (dendrites and axons).

The brain is the organ of the nervous system that is contained in the skull. It is the largest mass of nerve tissue in the body, and contains literally billions of nerve cells. The brain consists of three parts: the brain, the cerebellum and the brainstem [9]. Brain tumors are lesions representing alterations in brain tissues, which can include inflammation, bleeding, infections, or necrosis. These tumors result from the uncontrolled or excessive proliferation of either normal or aberrant cells. Based on their malignancy, tumors can be benign (noncancerous) or malignant (cancerous). Primary tumors can be malignant or benign and originate in the brain, whereas metastatic tumors are malignant, originate from other organs and spread to the brain through the bloodstream. Factors such as growth rate, distinct boundaries, and the ability to spread are considered to distinguish between benign and malignant primary brain tumors. Benign tumors have slow growth and rarely spread, while malignant tumors have rapid growth, are infiltrative and can be fatal [10]. Early detection of malignant tumors is paramount. Hence, technological solutions that can automatically delineate atypical brain regions are particularly valuable during the initial stages of diagnosis.

In this study, we introduce an innovative method for segmenting brain MRI images, which employs a geometric approximation technique based on the Fourier Series (FS), in view to facilitate diagnosis and consequent early detection of brain tumors. Classic approaches of image processing are applied to several images of the horizontal section of brains to perform the segmentation of these images.This procedure targets delineation of specific brain regions like the cranial, intracranial, and encephalic areas for subsequent geometric analysis. For this, image processing and transformation techniques for polar coordinates are used, followed by methods of determination of contours. The contours are approximated using a FS, and the coefficients are determined through a weighted least squares estimator. This estimator takes into account the feasibility of each point belonging to the contour, with lower weights indicating that the point is unlikely to be part of the contour. The main contributions of this paper include:

1. Identifying contour points along with their feasibility assessment.
2. Employing a FS to approximate the contour points.
3. Application of a weighted least squares estimator for the FS estimation, where weights represent the feasibility of the points.

Besides this introduction, this paper is structured as follows: Sect. 2 presents the image pre-processing methods employed to enhance the image quality, defines the coordinate frame and illustrates the conversion from cartesian to polar coordinates and introduces the FS. while Sect. 3 describes the weighted least squares estimator, also explaining how it is used to estimate the contours. Furthermore, the process of determining the contour points and assigning their respective feasibility weights is elaborated upon in this section. In Sect. 4 a comprehensive presentation and discussion of the results is provided. Finally, in Sect. 5, the appropriate conclusions of the study and some directions for future work are presented.

2 Background

2.1 Image Pre-processing Techniques

Image processing involves utilizing several techniques and algorithms to improve analysis and extract meaningful information from digital images. Prior to image analysis, preliminary pre-processing steps are essential. Image enhancement aims to elevate image quality, ultimately to be evaluated by a human observer. In general, it works on the grayscale of the image, transforming it to increase contrast or highlight a particular area of interest [11].

In this project, whether the image has three color channels (RGB), it is converted to gray scale using the following formula for each pixel:

Grayscale Intensity = 0.2989 * Red + 0.5870 * Green + 0.1140 * Blue, with these weightings based on standard coefficients used in the ITU-R BT.601 recommendation, which specifies the luminance values for standard-definition television [12]. Then, a contrast adaptation is also applied to the image. Often, the organization of an image as a pixel matrix form is done in a square symmetry, which is due to the easiness of electronic implementation, whether of acquisition or image visualization systems [11]. Image filtering, prevalent in image processing, aims to bolster image quality, eliminate noise, emphasize key features, and smoothen the image. Within this assignment, a median filter is applied, this filter replaces the values of each pixel in the image by the median of the values of the pixels that are in the neighborhood of that pixel, to make image analysis easier.

2.2 Polar Coordinates

TIn a two-dimensional plane, polar coordinates are denoted as (r, θ) and describe the position of a point in the plane relative to a reference point, where:

$$x = r \cdot cos(\theta) \qquad (1)$$
$$y = r \cdot sin(\theta) \qquad (2)$$

In the cartesian plane, the position of a point is represented by the (x, y) coordinates. To convert these cartesian coordinates (x, y) to polar coordinates (r, θ), only two parameters are needed as given by the following expressions:

$$r = \sqrt{x^2 + y^2} \tag{3}$$
$$\theta = atan2(y, x). \tag{4}$$

In Eq. (3), $atan2(y, x)$ represents the arctangent function of two arguments taking into account the sign of the arguments to determine the correct quadrant of the angle θ. These expressions are used to convert a point in the two-dimensional cartesian plane (x, y) to polar coordinates, where r represents the radial distance from the point to the reference point (usually the origin) and θ is the angle formed between the segment connecting the reference point to the point in question and the positive x-axis, measured counterclockwise.

Initially, it is observed that the regions of the brain have an approximately circular shape, despite having deformations. For this reason, the image, originally in the cartesian coordinates (x, y), is converted to polar coordinates $(radius, angle)$. The center of mass of the image is taken as the origin of the polar coordinates reference frame and is calculated from the values of the pixels and their coordinates X and Y. These coordinates are determined from outside to inside. By converting the cartesian coordinates to polar, it is possible to represent the points of the image in terms of radius and angle, simplifying the analysis process and allowing the application of specific techniques for circular contours.

2.3 Fourier Series

The Fourier Transform is a fundamental tool in both mathematics and engineering, facilitating the analysis of signals within the frequency domain. Applying this transform to images reveals features like textures, edges, straight lines, and periodic patterns, to name a few [13]. The FS decomposes a periodic function with period Θ_0 into a sum of constant and sinusoidal functions with periods $n\Theta_0$, $n = 1, \ldots, \infty$. A sinusoid with period $n\Theta_0$ is denoted as the nth harmonic. FS can also be used to approximate a function $f(x)$ in the interval $x_{min} \leq x \leq x_{max}$. For this purpose, define the periodic function

$$\tilde{f}(x) = \begin{cases} f(x) & x_{min} \leq x \leq x_{max} \\ f(x + k\Theta_0) & x < x_{min} \text{ or } x > x_{max}, \ k = \pm 1, \ldots \end{cases} \tag{5}$$

where $\Theta_0 = x_{max} - x_{min}$ and determine the FS of $\tilde{f}(x)$. If $x_{min} = -\pi$ and $x_{max} = \pi$, then $\Theta_0 = 2\pi$ and the following expression represents $f(x)$ as a FS:

$$f(x) = a_0/2 + \sum (a_n cos(nx) + b_n sin(nx)), \tag{6}$$

where $a_0/2$ is the average value of $f(x)$, a_n and b_n are the coefficients, and n represents the frequency of the sine and cosine terms. The coefficient a_0 , a_n and b_n are determined by integrating $f(X)$ multiplied by the appropriate sine or cosine function over one period (from $-\pi$ to π) and the dividing by π. Expressions (7), (8), and (9) are used to calculate these parameters.

$$a_0 = \frac{1}{2\pi} \int f(x)dx \quad \text{from } -\pi \text{ to } \pi \tag{7}$$

$$a_n = \frac{1}{\pi} \int f(x)\cos(nx)dx \quad \text{from } -\pi \text{ to } \pi \tag{8}$$

$$b_n = \frac{1}{\pi} \int f(x)\sin(nx)dx \quad \text{from } -\pi \text{ to } \pi \tag{9}$$

The sum of these terms, with varying frequencies n, represents an approximation of the original function $f(x)$.

In this work, the FS is used to approximate the points of the outer contour of an image, using a linear combination of sine and cosine functions, in order to obtain a closed oval curve representative of the shape of the image. The objective is to determine the outer contour of an oval-shaped binary image, as well as its ellipse and active points in polar coordinates. To achieve this, we utilize the FS to approximate the image pixels, leading to a mathematically expressed closed oval curve:

$$r = a_0 + \sum_{i=1}^{n}(a_i \cos(i\theta) + b_i \sin(i\theta)), \tag{10}$$

where (r, θ) are the polar coordinates of the pixel. This expression calculates the radius of the pixels based on its angles. The number of terms in the series determines the accuracy of the approximation.

3   Weighted Least Squares Method

The Least Squares Method aims to estimate the parameters of a function by reducing the sum of the squared errors from a set of point measurements associated with that function. Hence, given a set of data points $(\theta_1, r_1), \ldots, (\theta_N, r_N)$, and a function $f(\theta, \alpha)$, where α are the unknown parameters, the least squares method estimates α by

$$\hat{\alpha} = \min_{\alpha} \sum_{i=1}^{N}[r_i - f(\theta_i, \alpha)]^2. \tag{11}$$

Equation (10) can be rewritten as

$$r = \varphi(\theta)\alpha \tag{12}$$

where $\varphi(\theta) = \begin{bmatrix} 1 & \cos\theta & \sin\theta & \ldots & \cos(n\theta) & \sin(n\theta) \end{bmatrix}$ and $\alpha = \begin{bmatrix} a_0 & a_1 & b_1 & \cdots & a_n & b_n \end{bmatrix}^T$. Hence $f(\theta, \alpha)$ is a linear function of α and the Least Squares estimate of α is [14]

$$\hat{\alpha} = \left(\Phi^T \Phi\right)^{-1} \Phi^T Y, \tag{13}$$

where

$$\Phi = \left[\varphi(\theta_1) \cdots \varphi(\theta_N)\right]^T \tag{14}$$

$$Y = \left[r_1 \cdots r_N\right]^T. \tag{15}$$

The Weighted Least Squares Method is an extension of the common Least Square Method, which is used to fit a curve to a data set. The main difference between the two methods is that the Weighted Least Squares Method assigns different weights to the data points based on their reliability [15] or, in this case, their feasibility. It estimates α by [14]

$$\hat{\alpha}_w = \min_\alpha \sum_{i=1}^N \left\{w_i(\theta_i)\left[r_i - f(\theta_i, \alpha)\right]\right\}^2, \tag{16}$$

where w_i, $i = 1, \ldots, N$ are the weights. $\hat{\alpha}_w$ is given by [14]

$$\hat{\alpha}_w = \left(\Phi^T W^2 \Phi\right)^{-1} \Phi^T W^2 Y, \tag{17}$$

where

$$W = \begin{bmatrix} w_1(\theta_1) & \cdots & 0 \\ & \ddots & \\ 0 & \cdots & w_N(\theta_N) \end{bmatrix} \tag{18}$$

The weight of each point (r_i, α_i) is given by

$$w(\theta) = \exp\left[-\frac{\Delta_r^2(\theta)}{Q(\theta)}\right], \tag{19}$$

where $Q(\theta)$ the number of normalized pixels in the direction of θ and

$$\Delta_r(\theta) = r_{max}(\theta) - r_{min}(\theta) - \bar{r}(\theta) \tag{20}$$

with $r_{max}(\theta)$, $r_{min}(\theta)$ and $\bar{r}(\theta)$ being the maximum, minimum and median of the radius in the direction of θ.

The weight assigned to each point considers both the quantity of normalized pixels and the deviation of the difference between the maximum and minimum radii from the median. When the difference between the maximum and minimum radius equals the median, the weight has its maximum value equal to 1. This suggests that the point holds considerable significance in the overall analysis. However, if the difference between the maximum and minimum radius exceeds the median, the weight tends to approach zero. This implies that although these points are not entirely ignored, their contribution to constructing the harmonics is practically negligible in real terms.

3.1   Determination of Contour Points

It was created a function that takes a binary image (BW), the center of mass (CM), the type of mask (tm), and the order of the sinusoidal approximation (p) as inputs. The mask is designed to generate a final result where the interior is transparent and the exterior is opaque. The choice of the sinusoidal approximation order depends on the desired level of accuracy and the specific region to be segmented. Based on our analysis, a second-order FS sufficiently represents the skull. However, the intracranial and cephalic regions necessitate an eighth-order FS for precise modeling. The function returns multiple results, including the mask (M), the harmonic weights for the three lines (inner, middle, and outer) (W), the center of mass (CM), the polar coordinates of the contours (TC, RC), the polar coordinates of the outer boundary of the image (TC, RM), and the polar coordinates of the active points (TR, RR). Initially, the function prioritizes selecting white pixels to avoid processing the entire image unnecessarily. Subsequently, the polar coordinates are calculated using the center of mass, while also determining the radius of the farthest pixel in the desired angular direction. Furthermore, auxiliary variables such as 'a' (angle) and 'Q' (number of pixels found) are assigned for each internal angular value ranging from -179° to 180°.

When applying this function to the image, a graphical representation of its polar coordinates is generated, where the gray color represents the cranial and encephalic parts, while the white color represents the empty areas. Afterwards, the pixels with the maximum radius in the outermost part of the skull are identified for each angle. Next, by assessing the vertical variations, minimum values are ascertained, marking the point where the spherical coordinates graph shifts from gray to white. However, due to potential imperfections in the margins, there may be instances where the maximums and minimums are not precisely located. The presence of a "hole" is indicated if two successive points possess a radius exceeding 1. The weight calculation reduces the contribution of inaccurately determined points, resulting in a more precise representation of the contours.

4   Results

The method was applied to MRI scans of three distinct brains. One image was sourced from the WEB (Fig. 1(a)), while the others were from a dataset obtained from KAGGLE [16], consisting of a collection of cancer-free images (Fig. 1(b) and 1(c)). The objective of the analysis was to accurately assess the geometric characteristics of the brain region in these images. The analysis results are presented below. In the preliminary analysis, it is clear that all three brain regions exhibit a nearly oval shape. Figures 2, 3 and 4 depict the intermediate steps involved

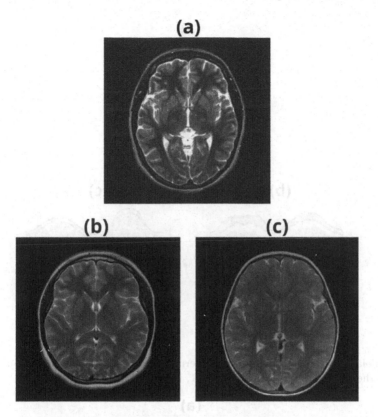

Fig. 1. Original MRI of the brains' horizontal section. (a) Example 1, (b) Example 2 and (c) Example 3.

in contour determination. They display the polar coordinates of the three brain images, highlighting all the determined contours obtained through the proposed method.

Figure 2 provides a visual representation of the outer and inner contours in the cranial region of the three analyzed MRI images. The outer contour is depicted by the black points, while the inner contour represented by the blue points. Additionally, the corresponding contour lines are shown in magenta. The green line represents the median calculated from these sinusoidal curves, which denote the skull's inner and outer contours.

Figure 3 presents an inverted representation for improved analysis, where the gray points have been converted to white and the white points to gray. The figure emphasizes the internal and external contour points of the intracranial regions in the three brains analyzed. The external contours are depicted by

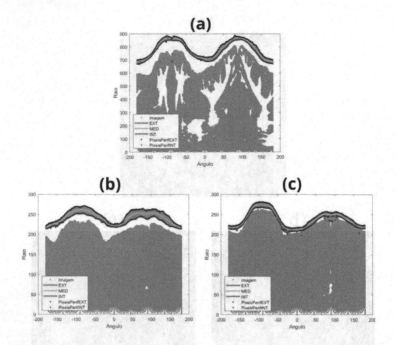

Fig. 2. Polar coordinate image of the external, middle, and internal contours of the skull for the three different images in Fig. 1, respectively, (a), (b) and (c).

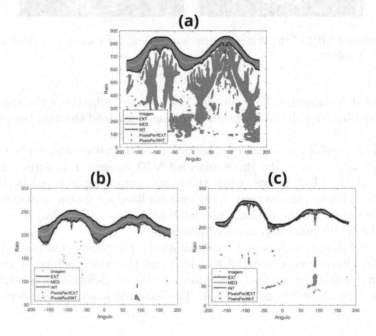

Fig. 3. Polar coordinate image of the outer, middle, and inner contours of the intracranial region for the three different images in Fig. 1, respectively: (a), (b) and (c).

Table 1. Geometric values of close curves.

Curve	Perimeter	Area	Asymmetry V/ H
(cranial) - outer	4997	1999418	8/ 11
(cranial) - middle	4903	1926315	6/ 9
(cranial) - inner	4810	1854696	6/ 10
(intracranial) - outer	4809	1853688	6/ 10
(intracranial) - middle	4567	1674084	11/ 13
(intracranial) - inner	4326	1504656	22/ 26
(encephalic) - outer	4340	1514347	22/ 25

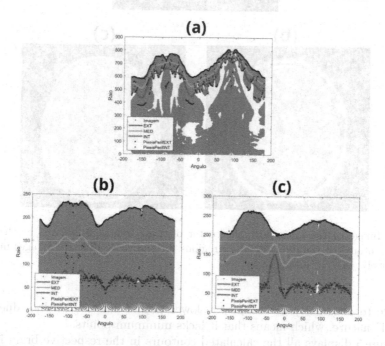

Fig. 4. Polar coordinate image displaying the outer, middle, and inner contours of the brain for the three different images in Fig. 1, respectively: (a), (b) and (c).

black points, while the internal contours are represented by blue points. The respective contours are illustrated by magenta lines. Furthermore, the green line represents the median.

Figure 4 illustrates the points corresponding to the external and internal contours in the encephalic region of the three analyzed brains. Black points represent the outer contour, and the inner contour is denoted by blue points. The respective contour lines are shown in magenta. The green line represents the calculated median of these points. However, in this specific region, it is not

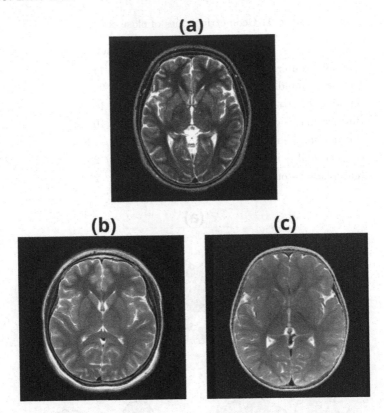

Fig. 5. Image of the brain with the center of mass indicated, as well as the determined contours of the different brain regions for the three different images in Fig. 1, respectively: (a), (b) and (c).

possible to accurately determine the lower points and the median due to its "closed" nature, which means that it lacks minimum points.

Figure 5 displays all the calculated contours in the respective brain images, along with the determined center of mass, which is essential for the calculation of the polar coordinates.

Figure 6 shows the masks constructed for the segmentation of each brain region. Mask 1 corresponds to the skull contour, mask 2 corresponds to the intracranial contour and mask 3 corresponds to the brain contour.

Finally, the values of perimeter, area, and vertical and horizontal asymmetry of each image were calculated, and the results can be found in Table 1. The first three rows of the Table 1 contain the values of the geometric parameters of the skull region, the next three rows represent the parameters of the intracranial region and the last row represents the parameters of the encephalic region. The closed lines of the contours have a length, *Perimeter*, and delimit a region with a certain area, *Area*. The asymmetry factor is a measure of the asymmetry with respect to an axis of symmetry. This factor is determined by averaging the modulus of the difference in distances between symmetrical pixels on the contour

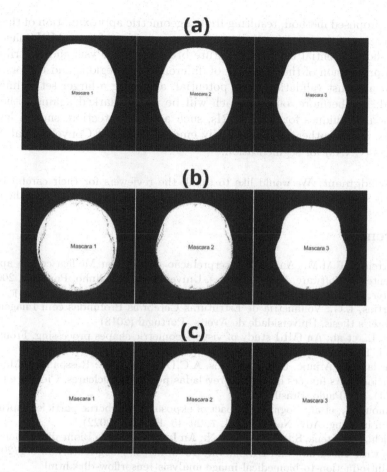

Fig. 6. Generated masks derived from the previously determined contours of the brain regions for the three different images in Fig. 1, respectively: (a), (b) and (c).

and the axis line. In this work, the axes of symmetry are lines containing the centre of mass of the image and the horizontal (H) or vertical (V) orientation. Both perimeter and asymmetry are given in pixels, while area is expressed in square pixels.

5   Conclusion and Future Work

This study demonstrates the feasibility of the use of mathematical models and techniques in the implementation of a method for geometric analysis of medical images, particularly of the brain MRI scans, in view to accurately determine the external and internal contours, as well as some parameters such as the perimeter, area and vertical and horizontal asymmetry of each image. The findings are synthesised in the figures showcasing the identified points of the contours in different brain regions, as well as the calculated contours and corresponding masks for segmentation.

The proposed method, resulting from a geometric approximation of the problem by means of the FS, is a novelty in the segmentation of brain MRI images. The results show potential to improve future brain MRI analysis and contribute to our comprehension of the geometry of different brain regions and tumors. However, for a robust validation of its potential, analyzing a larger set of images is essential. Furthermore, our approach will be bench-marked against other segmentation techniques for brain MRIs, such as edge detection, snakes, level-set methods, among others, or the rapidly emerging field of Convolutional Neural Networks (CNNs) for segmentation.

Acknowledgment. We would like to thank the reviewers for their careful reading and many suggestions that contributed enormously to the improvement of the paper.

References

1. Marreiros, F.M.M.: Análise e Interpretação de Imagem Médica com o apoio de Agentes de Software, Master's thesis, Universidade do Minho, Portugal, 2006
2. Ritter, F., et al.: Medical image analysis. IEEE Pulse **2**(6), 60–70 (2011)
3. Martins, L.G.: Volumetria de Estruturas Cerebrais Profundas com Imagem RM, Master's thesis, Universidade de Aveiro, Portugal (2018)
4. Wei, L., et al.: An fMRI study of visual geometric shapes processing. Front. Neurosci. **17**, 1087488 (2023)
5. Covolan, R., Araujo, D.B.D., Santos, A.C.D., Cendes, F.: Ressonância Magnética Funcional: As funções do cérebro reveladas por spins nucleares. Ciência e Cultura **56**(1). São Paulo, Brasil (2007)
6. Azmoun, S., et al.: Cognitive impact of exposure to airborne particles captured by brain imaging. Adv. Neurotoxicol. **7**, 29–45. Elsevier (2022)
7. Rajchl, M., Ktena, S.I., Pawlowski, N.: An Introduction to Biomedical Image Analysis with Tensorflow and DLTK, July 2018. https://blog.tensorflow.org/2018/07/an-introduction-to-biomedical-image-analysis-tensorflow-dltk.html
8. Bear, M.F., Connors, B.W., Paradiso, M.A.: Neurociências: desvendando o sistema nervoso. Artmed editora (2002)
9. VanPutte, C., Regan, J., Russo, A.: Anatomia e Fisiologia de Seeley- 10ª Edição. McGraw Hill, Brasil (2016)
10. Agostinho, E.T.: Estudo da Evolução de Tumores Cerebrais, Master's thesis, Faculdade de Ciências e Tecnologias da Universdidade do Algarve, Portugal, 2007
11. de Albuquerque, M.P.: Processamento de Imagens: Métodos e Análises, Centro Brasileiro de Pesquisas Físicas MCT, 2000
12. BT, R., et al.: Studio encoding parameters of digital television for standard 4: 3 and wide-screen 16: 9 aspect ratios. International Radio Consultative Committee International Telecommunication Union, Switzerland, CCIR Rep (2011)
13. Pupin, J.R., Silva, K.S., Carbone, V.L.: Introdução às Séries e Transformadas de Fourier e Aplicações no Processamento de Sinais e Imagens. Trabalho (Conclusao de Curso)-Universidade Federal de Sao Carlos, Sao Carlos (2011)
14. Goodwin, G.C.: Dynamic system identification: experiment design and data analysis. Math. Sci. Eng. **136** (1977)
15. Weisberg, S.: Applied Linear Regression, 4th edn. Wiley, Hoboken (2014)
16. Chakrabarty, N.: Brain MRI Images for Brain Tumor Detection (2019). https://www.kaggle.com/datasets/navoneel/brain-mri-images-for-brain-tumor-detection

Determination of Effective Connectivity of Brain Activity in the Resting Brain

Catarina Pião Azevedo[1], Paulo A. Salgado[1], T.-P. Azevedo Perdicoúlis[1], and Paulo Lopes dos Santos[2(✉)]

[1] ECT, UTAD, Vila Real 5000-811, Portugal
{psal,tazevedo}@utad.pt
[2] FEUP, UP, Porto 4200-465, Portugal
pjsantos@fe.up.pt

Abstract. The resting brain has been extensively investigated for low frequency synchrony between brain regions, namely Functional Connectivity. However the other main stream of the brain connectivity analysis that seeks causal interactions between brain regions, Effective Connectivity, has been still little explored. Inherent complexity of brain activities in resting-state, as observed in Blood Oxygenation-Level Dependant fluctuations, calls for exploratory methods for characterizing these causal networks [1].

To determine the structure of the network that causes this dynamics, it is developed a method of identification based on least squares, which assumes knowledge of the signals of brain activity in different regions. As there is no access to functional Magnetic Resonance Imaging, data it is developed a model to obtain the Blood Oxygenation Level Dependent signals and it is implemented a reverse hemo-dynamic function. To assess the performance of the created model Monte Carlo simulations have been used.

Keywords: State-Space Model · Functional Magnetic Resonance Imaging · Monte Carlo Simulation · Effective Connectivity · Independent Component Analysis

1 Introduction

In resting-state functional Magnetic Resonance Imaging (fMRI), a non-invasive neuroimaging technique that uses strong magnetic fields and radio waves to measure changes in blood flow and oxygenation throughout the brain, researchers have observed low-frequency fluctuations of brain activity that are difficult

P. A. Salgado—Supported by FCT - Fundação para a Ciência e a Tecnologia under project UIDB/04033/2020.

T.-P. A. Perdicoúlis—Supported by FCT - Fundação para a Ciência e a Tecnologia under project IDB/00048/2020.

P. L. Santos—Supported by FCT - Fundação para a Ciência e a Tecnologia under project UIDB/50014/2020.

© ICST Institute for Computer Sciences, Social Informatics and Telecommunications Engineering 2024
Published by Springer Nature Switzerland AG 2024. All Rights Reserved
A. Cunha et al. (Eds.): MobiHealth 2023, LNICST 578, pp. 17–32, 2024.
https://doi.org/10.1007/978-3-031-60665-6_2

to explain. Raichle and colleagues proposed the concept of "dark energy" to describe this phenomenon, which refers to the energy associated with these mysterious fluctuations. Interestingly, when the brain transitions from rest to performing a task, the energy of these fluctuations does not increase significantly. By studying the resting brain, researchers hope to gain a better understanding of its intrinsic activity [2].

To unravel the enigma that is the brain's "dark energy", a wide variety of machine learning and signal processing methods and algorithms have been proposed [1]. These methods reveal a low frequency synchrony, Functional Connectivity (FC) [3], within specific networks of brain regions. This issue has been extensively studied, and there are efficient methods to determine these networks. One of these methods is the Independent Component Analysis (ICA) which is a computational technique used to separate a multivariate signal into independent non-Gaussian components. ICA can be used to decompose complex signals, such as those obtained from fMRI, into their underlying neural sources. This allows researchers to identify patterns of neural activity that are not readily apparent in the raw data and can aid in the investigation of brain function and connectivity [4].

However, the other main stream of research in brain connectivity analysis, Effective Connectivity (EC) [3], is the one that we are going to use in this study. Effective Connectivity is introduced to represent the causal influences that each region of the brain exerts over other regions. In fact, there are some aspects of on-going brain activity which cannot be described by inadequate measures of instantaneous coupling, so causal inferences should be employed for better understanding of the neuronal system. Particularly, the activation/deactivation dichotomy of brain areas which can be regularly observed in resting-state Blood Oxygenation-Level Dependant (BOLD) signals, which are a measure of changes in blood oxygenation resulting from neural activity in a brain region and are used to identify active brain regions during specific tasks or activities, should be revisited in a cause and effect view within brain dynamics and structure, rather than evolved patterns of synchrony in brain activity [5]. The low-frequency fluctuations of bold signals reveal a signal transmission dynamics that depends on the structure of the networks connecting different brain regions. The goal is to determine the structure of the network that causes this dynamics.

In this paper, we developed a method of identification based on least squares, which assumes knowledge of the signals of brain activity in different regions of the brain. As fMRI does not directly measure these signals, they are obtained through filters with impulse responses equal to inverse hemo-dynamic functions excited by the BOLD signals, i.e., the signals that are measured by fMRI. This methodology is illustrated in Fig. 1 and Fig. 2. The contributions of this work are: (i) A method of identification based on least squares, which assumes knowledge of the signals of brain activity in different regions, to determine the structure of the network that causes the dynamics. (ii) it is developed a model to obtain the Blood Oxygenation Level Dependent signals and it is implemented a reverse hemo-dynamic function as there is no access to functional Magnetic Resonance Imaging data. (iii) Simulation of the brain activity at rest.

In Sect. 2, we describe the state-space models which are used throughout this paper. In Sect. 3, we demonstrate how the matrix structure can be determined when we have access to the signals from the brain network. As we do not have access to fMRI data, we develop, in Sect. 4, a simulation model that allows for obtaining the BOLD signals. The inverse hemo-dynamic functions to obtain the brain activity signals through BOLD signals are implemented in Sect. 5. In Sect. 6 we illustrate the performance of the developed method using Monte Carlo simulations. Finally, we close with some conclusions and pointing out some directions for future work.

2   State-Space Models

In light of the complexity of observed activity patterns in the resting brain, and in response to questions regarding their generative mechanisms, investigators have developed mathematical models of neuronal communication. Such models allow for inferring, relating, and predicting the dependence of measured communication dynamics on the topology of brain networks [12].

According to recent controversies on different Effective Connectivity detection algorithms in [11] state-space models are used in EC because they can separate the modelling of latent neuronal activity from the hemo-dynamic response function. Additionally, these models allow for a control theory interpretation of causality in connectivity analysis, providing insight into causal interactions in the brain system [1].

Communication models can be roughly classified into three types: dynamical, topological, and information theoretical. Dynamical models aim to capture biophysical mechanisms of signal transformation and transmission, while topological models propose network attributes to explain activity patterns. Information theoretical models use statistical measures to quantify interdependence, direction, and causality between nodes.

2.1   Dynamic Models and Measures

Dynamical models also differ in terms of the spatiotemporal scales of phenomena that they seek to explain. The choice of the explanatory scale impacts the precise communication dynamics that the model produces, as well as the scale of collective dynamics that can emerge. The general form of a deterministic dynamical model at an arbitrary scale is given by [13]

$$\frac{dx}{dt} = f(x, A, u, \beta). \tag{1}$$

Here, x encodes the state variables that are used to describe the state of the network, A encodes the underlying connectivity matrix, and u encodes the input variables. The functional form of f is set by the requirements (i.e., the expected utility) of the model. Finally, β encodes other parameters of the model, independent of the connectivity strength A. The β parameters can be phenomenological, thereby allowing for an exploration of the whole phase space of possible behaviours; alternatively, the β parameters can be determined from experiments in more data-driven models [13].

The use of temporal precedence and lead-lag relationships is also a basis for alternative definitions of causality. Notably, this relationship can be used to measure the causal effect between neural masses coupled according to the structural connectome [14].

2.2   Topological Models and Measures

It has been believed that long routes in a network are metabolically costly and result in slower signal propagation [18]. Therefore, shortest paths are often used to infer the efficiency of communication between two regions. However, relying solely on shortest paths has been questioned for three reasons. First, networks that depend solely on shortest paths are vulnerable to targeted attacks. Second, investing solely in shortest paths means that alternative routes are underutilized and this is not optimal. Third, routing a signal by the shortest path would require biologically implausible knowledge of the global network structure [15].

By denoting the adjacency matrix by A, we can define the communicability between node i and node j as the weighted sum of all walks starting at node i and ending at node j [16]

$$G_{ji} = \sum_{k=0}^{\infty} c_k (A^k)_{ji}, \tag{2}$$

where A^k denotes the k-th power of matrix A, and c_k are the coefficients chosen to ensure convergence of the series and to give less weight to longer paths. If all entries of A are non-negative (which is often the case in communicability), the resulting values of G_{ji} are also non-negative and real.

2.3   Information Theoretic Models and Measures

Information theory and statistical mechanics have been used to develop measures of information transfer in brain networks such as transfer entropy and Granger causality [19]. These measures rely on the fact that the propagation of signals through the brain networks generates time-dependent activity patterns that can be measured as time series. Entropic measures of communication aim to identify statistical relationships between these time series, in order to infer the amount and direction of information transfer between different brain regions.

A central concept in information theory is the Shannon entropy [17], which quantifies the uncertainty in a discrete random variable I that follows the probability distribution $p(i)$. It is defined as $H(I) = -\sum_i p(i)log(p(i))$. Another measure of statistical interdependence between two random variables I and J

is their mutual information, $M_{IJ} = \sum p(i,j) \dfrac{log(p(i,j))}{log(p(i)), log(p(j))}$, where $p(i,j)$ is their joint distribution and $p(i)$ and $p(j)$ are their marginal distributions. However, since mutual information is symmetric, it does not capture the direction of information flow between two processes or sequences of random variables [17].

Transfer entropy takes into account the transition probability between different states, which can be the result of a stochastic dynamic process and obtained from the time series of activities of brain regions through imaging techniques. To measure the direction of information transfer between processes I and J, the notion of mutual information is generalized to the mutual information rate. The transfer entropy between processes I and J is given by [17]

$$T_{J \to I} = \sum p(i_{n+1}, i_n^k, j_n^l) log \frac{p(i_{n+1}|i_n^k, j_n^l)}{p(i_{n+1}|i_n^k)} \tag{3}$$

The processes I and J are assumed to be stationary Markov processes of order k and l, respectively. The quantity i_n^k, j_n^l denotes the state of process $I(J)$ at time n, while $p(i_{n+1}|i_n^k)$ denotes the transition probability to state i_{n+1} at time $n+1$, given knowledge of the previous k states. Similarly, $p(j_{n+1}|j_n^l)$ is the transition probability for process J. The quantity $p(i_{n+1}|i_n^k, j_n^l)$ is the same as $p(i_{n+1}|i_n^k)$ if the process J does not influence the process I.

3   Identification of Networks in the Resting Brain

It is important to notice that in this procedure, it is assumed that the hemo-dynamic response functions of different regions in the brain are known. These functions describe how neural activity in a particular brain region is converted into changes in blood flow and oxygenation, which are measured by fMRI signals. The hemo-dynamic response functions are used to model the relationship between brain activity and fMRI signals, and thus estimate the matrix A that relates brain activity to observed fMRI signals. It is important to have a good understanding of the hemo-dynamic response functions in order to properly model brain activity and obtain accurate estimates of matrix A.

According to [1], the brain activity measurement system at rest using functional magnetic resonance imaging (fMRI) can be described by the following linear time-invariant (LTI) state model:

$$z(t+1) = A_0 z(t) + q_0(t) \tag{4}$$

$$x_m(t) = \begin{bmatrix} z_m \\ z_m(t-1) \\ z_m(t-L+1) \end{bmatrix} \tag{5}$$

$$y_m(t) = c_m x_m(t) + r_m(t), m = 1, ..., M \tag{6}$$

The signals $y_m(t)$ represent the BOLD signals in the m brain regions that are measured by fMRI, while $q_0(t)$ and $r_m(t)$ are noise signals ($q_0(t)$ is process noise and $r_m(t)$ is measurement noise, both of which are assumed to be Gaussian white noise). The goal is to estimate the matrix A_0 that defines the causal network structure of the resting brain based on the measurements of $y_m(t)$, $m = 1, \ldots, M$.

The row vectors c_m are formed by samples of hemo-dynamic response functions $h(t)$. It is important to note that, according to Eq. (4), each signal $y_m(t)$ is the convolution of $z_m(t)$ with a hemo-dynamic response function $h_m(t)$. This means that, as illustrated in Fig. 1, each signal $y_m(t)$ can be viewed as the output of a linear time-invariant (LTI) system excited by the signal $z_m(t)$. In Eqs. (4)–(6), it is assumed that these systems have finite impulse responses (FIR systems), i.e., that $c_m(t) = h_m(t)$ for $t = 0, \ldots, L$ and $c_m(t) = 0$ for $t > L$. However, existing studies on hemo-dynamic response functions conclude that these are impulse responses of LTI systems with infinite impulse responses, with orders significantly smaller than those of the FIR approximations [7]. Therefore, assuming FIR systems unreasonably increases the dimension of the model. Since the resting brain model is described by a state-space model, it makes sense to describe the convolution of the state variables with hemo-dynamic response functions as state-space models as well. This implies that the brain activity measurement system represented in Fig. 1 can be described by a state-space model of lower order than the model in Eqs. (4)–(6) assumed in [1]. In this context, $y_m(t)$ and $z_m(t)$, $m = 1, \ldots, M$, are related by state-space models of order n_m with $n_m \ll L$:

$$w_m(t+1) = A_m w_m(t) + B_m z_m(t) + q_m(t) \tag{7}$$

$$y_m(t) = C_m w_m(t) + D_m z_m(t) + r_m(t) \tag{8}$$

With $w_m(t) \in \mathbb{R}^{n_m}$, $A_m \in \mathbb{R}^{n_m \times n_m}$, $B_m \in \mathbb{R}^{n_m}$, $C_m \in \mathbb{R}^{1 \times n_m}$, and $D_m \in \mathbb{R}$ for $m = 1, \ldots, M$, combining Eqs. (4), (7), and (8) yields the following state-space model:

$$x(t+1) = A_x(t) + q(t) \tag{9}$$

$$y(t) = C_x(t) + r(t) \tag{10}$$

where

$$x(t) = \begin{bmatrix} z(t) \\ w_1(t) \\ w_2(t) \\ \vdots \\ w_M(t) \end{bmatrix} \tag{11}$$

$$y(t) = \begin{bmatrix} y_1(t) \\ y_2(t) \\ \vdots \\ w_M(t) \end{bmatrix} \tag{12}$$

$$A_x = \begin{bmatrix} a_1 & \cdots & a_M & 0_{M \times n_1} & \cdots & 0_{M \times n_M} \\ B_1 & \cdots & 0_{n_1} & A_1 & \cdots & 0_{n_1 \times n_M} \\ 0_{n_2} & \cdots & 0_{n_2} & 0_{n_2 \times n_1} & \cdots & 0_{n_2 \times n_M} \\ \vdots & \ddots & \vdots & \vdots & \ddots & \vdots \\ 0_{n_M} & \cdots & B_M & 0_{n_M \times n_1} & \cdots & A_M \end{bmatrix} \tag{13}$$

$$C_x = \begin{bmatrix} D_1 & 0 & \cdots & C_1 & \cdots & 0_{1 \times n_M} \\ 0 & D_2 & \cdots & 0_{1 \times n_1} & \cdots & 0_{1 \times n_M} \\ \vdots & \vdots & \ddots & \vdots & \ddots & \vdots \\ 0 & 0 & \cdots & 0_{1 \times n_1} & \cdots & C_M \end{bmatrix} \tag{14}$$

$a_i \in \mathbb{R}^M, i = 1, \ldots, M$ are the columns of $A_0 \in \mathbb{R}^{M \times M}$, $x(t) \in \mathbb{R}^{n_x}, y(t) \in \mathbb{R}^M, A_m \in \mathbb{R}^{n_m \times n_m}, B_m \in \mathbb{R}^{n_m}, C_m \in \mathbb{R}^{1 \times n_m}, D_m \in \mathbb{R}, m = 1, \ldots, M$, where $A \in \mathbb{R}^{n_x \times n_x}$ and $C \in \mathbb{R}^{M \times n_x}$, with $n_x = M + n_1 + \cdots + n_M$. If the system (9)–(10) is observable, then it can be identified by any algorithm that estimates models in state space; The problem is that these methods produce data-driven models, i.e., realizations determined by the data, different from those we intend to estimate and that are described by equations (9)–(14). Despite the orders of the models that relate $y_m(t)$ with $z_m(t)$ having been significantly reduced, the number of parameters remains very large.

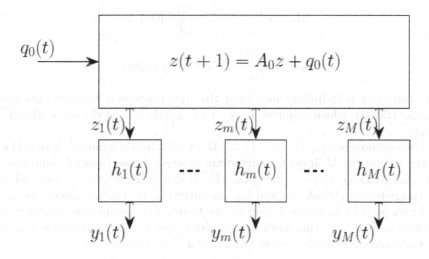

Fig. 1. The brain activity measurement system at rest using fMRI

4 Simulation Model of Resting Brain Activity and Functional Magnetic Resonance

4.1 Resting Brain Model

According to [1], the activity of a resting brain can be described by the state model:

$$z[k+1] = A_0 z[k] + q_0[k] \tag{15}$$

where $z(t) = [z_1(t), \ldots, z_M(t)]^T \in \mathbb{R}^M$, $q_0(t) \in \mathbb{R}^M$, and $A_0 \in \mathbb{R}^{M \times M}$. The components $z_m(t)$, $m = 1, \ldots, L$ are signals in different regions of the brain resulting from this activity, and the components of $q_0(t)$ are stimuli for brain activity. This is a sampled model of the continuous-time model:

$$\dot{z}(t) = A_c z(t) + q_c(t) \tag{16}$$

which models an underlying continuous system. The model (15) represents (16) at sampling instants. That is,

$$z[k] = z(kT_s) \tag{17}$$

where T_s is the sampling period. The relationship between (15) and (16) is well known and is given by the following equations:

$$A_0 = e^{A c T_s} \Leftrightarrow Ac = \frac{1}{T_s} \ln(A_0) \tag{18}$$

$$q_0[k] = \int_{kT_s}^{(k+1)T_s} e^{A(t-\tau)} q_c(\tau) d\tau. \tag{19}$$

The state $z(t)$ is indirectly measured through functional magnetic resonance imaging (fMRI), which acquires a vector of signals $y(t)$ of the same dimension as $z(t)$.

The components $y_m(t)$, $m = 1, \ldots, M$ of $y(t)$ are designated by BOLD and are the outputs of M linear time-invariant systems whose impulse responses are the hemo-dynamic response functions. Each system is excited by one and only one component $z_m(t)$ of $z(t)$ and has an output $y_m(t)$ that indirectly measures the brain activity in the m region of the brain. The continuous system is represented in Fig. 1. In this work, we consider that the hemo-dynamic response functions are equal to the canonical function [7,8] given by:

$$h_c(t) = K \left(\frac{t^5 e^{-t}}{5!} - \frac{1}{6} \frac{t^{15} e^{-t}}{15!} \right). \tag{20}$$

After applying the Laplace Transform, we obtain the transfer function

$$H_c(s) = K \frac{6(s+1)^{10} - 1}{6(s+1)^{16}}. \tag{21}$$

The objective of the simulation is to obtain

$$y[k] = \begin{bmatrix} y_1[k] \\ \vdots \\ y_M[k] \end{bmatrix}, \quad k = 1, \ldots, N, \tag{22}$$

that is, $y(kT_s)$ for $k = 1, \ldots, N$. Since the output signal is discrete-time with sampling period T_s, one might think that to perform the simulation it would be sufficient to generate a realization of white noise for the input $q_0[k]$, simulate the continuous-time system (15), discretize the transfer functions $H_m(s)$, $m = 1, \ldots, M$, and simulate the discrete-time systems, taking the signals $z_m[k]$ as inputs. However, for this procedure to be possible, it is necessary to postulate the evolution of the signals $z_m(t)$ between the sampling instants. Existing sampling methods typically assume that in these time intervals, the signals remain constant (ZOH) or are piecewise linear. These assumptions are not suitable for this problem since the components of $q_c(t)$ are not persistent signals.

4.2   Brain Activity Stimuli

Brain activity stimuli can be seen as sequences of impulses with random amplitudes that occur at random instants. To simulate these stimuli, we divide the sampling intervals into N_s parts and consider that the probability of an impulse with random amplitude and duration T_s/N_s occurring in each sub-interval is p. That is, the presence of an impulse in each of these sub-intervals follows a Bernoulli distribution. The number of impulses in each sampling interval follows a binomial distribution. Therefore, the average number of impulses in each sampling interval is given by

$$N_i = pN_s. \tag{23}$$

If we fix N_i (the average number of impulses in each sampling interval), we can calculate p through

$$p = \frac{N_i}{N_s}. \tag{24}$$

Given T_s, the sampling period, N_s, the number of divisions of each sampling interval, and p, the probability of an impulse occurring in each sub-interval, the probability of an impulse existing at each instant kT_s/N_s is then given by

$$q_c(t) = B \times U, \tag{25}$$

where B is a random variable with Bernoulli distribution $B(p)$ and U is a random variable with Gaussian distribution $N(0, \sigma^2)$.

5 Inverse Hemo-Dynamic Models

The identification of the system (9)–(14) by a subspace state identification method presents the following problems:

1. It is a stochastic identification problem and the estimated model can be non-minimum phase.
2. It is a high-order model with a large number of parameters.
3. The estimated realization is determined by the data and needs to be converted to that of the model (9)–(14).

These three coupled problems make it very difficult to obtain estimates of A_0 with acceptable precision unless some *a priori* knowledge about the hemo-dynamic response function is used. However, this can be estimated using fMRI [6]. Therefore, it makes sense for this work to consider that the different hemo-dynamic response functions $h_m(t)$ are known. Many studies consider this function to be equal to a canonical function [7,8] given by Eq. (20).

The function $h_c(t)/K$ is the impulse response of the LTI system with transfer function:

$$H_c(s) = K \frac{6(s+1)^{10} - 1}{6(s+1)^{16}}. \tag{26}$$

In this work, we consider $h_m(t) = h_c(t)$, where $h_c(t)$ is the impulse response of the discretization $H_c(s)$ with $K_m = K$ randomly generated. That is, $y_m(t)$ is the output of a system with transfer function $K_m H_c(z)$ excited by $z_m(t)$, where $H_c(z)$ is the discretization of $H_c(s)$. The state variables $z_m(t)$, $m = 1, \ldots, M$, can be reconstructed, $\hat{z}_m(t)$, from $y_m(t)$ through simulation of the inverse systems of $K_m H_c(z)$, denoted by $H_m^i(z)$. Once $\hat{z}(t)$, $t = 1, \ldots, N$, is known, A_0 can be also estimated through

$$\hat{A}_0 = \hat{Z}_2^\dagger \hat{Z}_1, \tag{27}$$

where

$$\hat{Z}_1 = \left(\hat{z}(1) \cdots \hat{z}(N-1) \right), \tag{28}$$

$$\hat{Z}_2 = \left(\hat{z}(2) \cdots \hat{z}(N) \right), \tag{29}$$

The main difficulty of this approach lies in the computation of the inverse model because, on one hand, the transfer function is not proper and, on the other hand, although $H_c(s)$ is an inversely stable transfer function, the same does not hold for its corresponding continuous-time transfer function, $H_c(z)$.

The whole procedure is illustrated in Fig. 2.

Due to the large difference between the degrees of the numerator and denominator of the transfer function $H_c(s)$, it is convenient to determine the system in discrete time. The difference between the degrees of the numerator and denominator of the discrete transfer function $H_c(z)$ is one unit. Since we can only invert proper and strictly proper transfer functions (where the degree of the

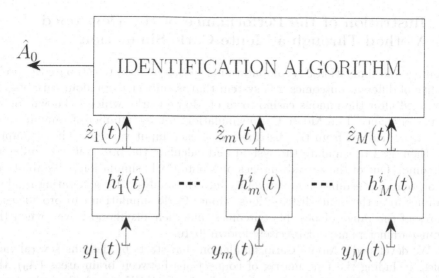

Fig. 2. The brain activity excitation signals are obtained from measurements at rest using the inverse fMRI signals

denominator is greater than or equal to the degree of the numerator), we need to multiply $H_c(z)$ by z before determining the inverse model. Multiplying $H_c(z)$ by z is equivalent to advancing the system output by one sampling period, so when we calculate $z_m(t)$ using the inverse model, this signal will be delayed by one sampling period. As mentioned earlier, there is still another difficulty, which is that the discrete versions of $H_c(s)$ are not inversely stable. Since the outputs $y_m(t)$ are stationary stochastic processes, we can maintain their spectral density by reflecting the unstable zeros of $H_c(z)$ inside the unit circle with a gain adjustment. Therefore, if we have

$$H_c(z) = (z - z_i)H_{cr}(z) \tag{30}$$

with $|z_i| > 1$, then

$$H_c^{min}(z) = \frac{(z - 1/\bar{z}_i)(1 - z_i)}{1 - 1/\bar{z}_i}H_{cr}(z) \tag{31}$$

where $\bar{z}_i$ is the complex conjugate of z_i, has frequency response with the same magnitude

$$|H_c^{min}(e^{jw})| = |H_c(e^{jw})|. \tag{32}$$

If two systems with transfer functions $H_c(z)$ and $H^{min}(z)$ are excited by the same stochastic process, then their outputs, although different, have the same spectral density. Therefore, by reflecting the unstable zeros of $H_c(z)$ inside the unit circle, we do not alter the spectral density of the signals $y_m(t)$, $m = 1, \ldots, M$.

6   Ilustration of the Performance of the Developed Method Through a Monte Carlo Simulation

Monte Carlo simulation is a computational technique used to estimate the probability of different outcomes in a system that is subject to random variables. It is named after the famous casino town of Monte Carlo, which is known for its games of chance. In a Monte Carlo simulation, a large number of random samples are generated from the distribution of each input variable. These samples are then used to simulate the system and calculate the probability of different outcomes. One of the key advantages of Monte Carlo simulation is its ability to incorporate uncertainty and variability into the analysis. By generating random samples from the input distributions, Monte Carlo simulation can provide estimates of the range of possible outcomes and their likelihoods, even when the input parameters are not precisely known [9, 10].

We developed a Monte Carlo simulation that starts by defining several variables, including the true matrix of connections between brain areas (A_0), the sampling rate (T_s), the number of samples in the fMRI signal (N_s), the interval between samples in the fMRI signal (N_i), the number of brain areas (M), the number of points in the simulated brain activity signal (N), the number of Monte Carlo runs (N_{mc}), the noise standard deviation (σ), and the vector of the gains of the hemo-dynamic responses of each brain area (H).

Next, the simulation initializes a matrix to store the Monte Carlo results $(\hat{A}_{2,mc})$ and enters a Monte Carlo simulation loop. Within the loop, the code generates a simulated brain activity signal called q_c, simulates the fMRI signal called y, and estimates matrix A using the $\hat{Z}_{e_{mc}}$ matrix. The estimated matrix is then stored in the $\hat{A}_{2,mc}$ tensor. The equation for estimating A is given by

$$\hat{A} = \hat{Z}_{e_{mc}}(:, 2 : end) / \hat{Z}_{e_{mc}}(:, 1 : end - 1), \tag{33}$$

where $Z_{e_{mc}}$ is an $M \times N$ matrix representing the simulated fMRI signals for each brain area in each Monte Carlo run. The $\hat{A}$ matrix is an estimate of the state matrix A, which represents the dynamics of connections between brain areas.

The simulation creates histograms for each element of the estimated A matrix, calculates the standard deviation of each element of the estimated A matrix, and the mean and standard deviation of the estimated A matrices.

In a histogram, the variability of different parameters is represented by the distribution of values along the histogram bars. Each bar represents a range of values, and the height of the bar indicates the frequency or count of occurrences within that range.

When creating a histogram, we can observe the variability of different parameters through the dispersion or spread of values along the bars. If a parameter has lower variability, the values will be more concentrated around a central value, and the corresponding bars will be taller. On the other hand, if a parameter has higher variability, the values will be more dispersed, and the corresponding bars will be shorter, indicating a lower frequency in each range.

The following parameters were used:

$$A_0 = \begin{bmatrix} 0.7 & 0.31 & 0 & 0 & -0.46 \\ 0 & 0.7 & 0 & 0 & 0 \\ 0 & 0 & 0.7 & 0.55 & 0 \\ -0.38 & 0 & 0 & 0.7 & 0 \\ 0 & 0 & 0 & 0 & 0.7 \end{bmatrix},$$ (34)

$$T_s = 1,$$ (35)

$$N_s = 10,$$ (36)

$$N_i = 1,$$ (37)

$$N = 1000,$$ (38)

$$N_{mc} = 100,$$ (39)

$$\sigma = 0.1,$$ (40)

$$H^T = \begin{bmatrix} 1.9005 & 0.9101 & 1.8404 & 1.3685 & 0.9977 \end{bmatrix}.$$ (41)

The equations involved in these calculations are

$$\sigma_{ij} = \text{std}(\hat{A}_{ij}),$$ (42)

where σ_{ij} is the standard deviation of the (i,j) element of the estimated A matrix and $\hat{A}_{ij}$ is the (i,j) element of the estimated A matrix.

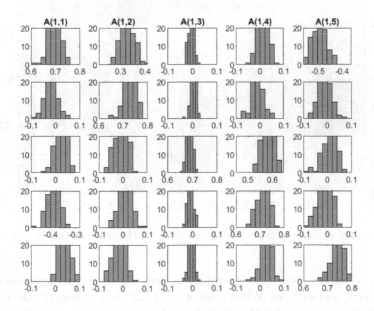

Fig. 3. Visualization of the distribution of the estimated values for each element of matrix A and comparison with the true value

$$\bar{A} = \text{mean}(\hat{A}_{mc}), \tag{43}$$

where $\bar{A}$ is the mean of the estimated A matrices and $\hat{A}_{mc}$ is the estimated A matrix for each Monte Carlo run. Also

$$\sigma_A = \text{std}(\hat{A}_{mc}) \tag{44}$$

where σ_A is the standard deviation of the estimated A matrices and $\hat{A}_{mc}$ is the estimated A matrix for each Monte Carlo run.

These equations are used to evaluate the reliability and stability of the A matrix estimation, as well as to evaluate the influence of different parameters on the estimation accuracy. They also help to understand the uncertainty in the A matrix estimation and provide useful information for the analysis of brain connections in fMRI signals.

Finally, the simulation displays the results and the mean value of the state matrix in a color scale, represented in Fig. 4.

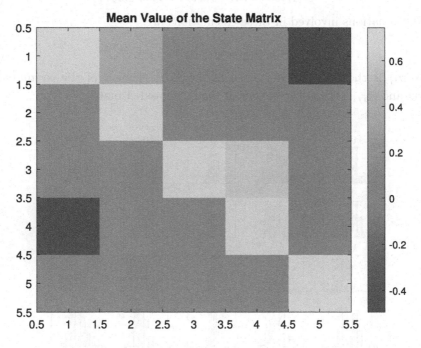

Fig. 4. Display of the results and the mean value of the state matrix in a color scale

Color scales are used to assign colors to data values in visualizations such as plots, images, and surfaces. When using a colormap, we can observe the variation in variability among different parameters through the intensity or hue of the colors assigned to them. Generally, darker colors represent lower values or lower variability, while lighter colors represent higher values or greater variability. In this color scale, the colors range from dark blue to yellow, with light blue and green in between. The colors are assigned to a range of values in a dataset, with dark blue being the lowest value and yellow being the highest. More specifically, the color scale assigns the color dark blue to the minimum value in the dataset, and transitions through shades of light blue and green as values increase, before transitioning to shades of orange and yellow for the maximum value. The exact mapping of colors to values is nonlinear, which means that the perceived change in color is not constant as the values increase.

The performance of a Monte Carlo simulation depends on several factors, including the number of simulations, the complexity of the system being modelled, and the efficiency of the simulation algorithm. In general, increasing the number of Monte Carlo runs can improve the accuracy and reliability of the simulation results. Nonetheless we can state, through the analysis of Figs. 2 and 3, that the performance of our simulation is satisfactory because despite displaying variations in the average value of the state matrix they are not very significant (as most of the color scale is the same tone of blue, which corresponds to the same value).

7   Conclusions and Future Works

The determination of effective connectivity of brain activity in the resting state is a complex process that requires the use of sophisticated mathematical models and simulations. State-space models and inverse hemo-dynamic models have proven to be powerful tools for analyzing resting state fMRI data, allowing for the identification of key brain regions and their effective connections. The use of Monte Carlo simulations has further demonstrated the accuracy and reliability of these methods. Hence, through the development of a simulation model of resting brain activity and fMRI, we have been able to evaluate the performance of these methods and gain important insights into the functional organization of the brain. The findings have significant implications for understanding the neural mechanisms underlying brain function and for developing new diagnostic and therapeutic approaches for neurological and psychiatric disorders. Overall, the determination of effective connectivity of brain activity in the resting state holds great promise for advancing our understanding of the brain and improving human health.

One potential avenue for future research is the investigation of other mathematical models, such as deep learning algorithms, that may provide a more comprehensive understanding of the brain's functional organization. Additionally, the integration of multiple imaging modalities, such as fMRI, EEG, and MEG, could provide a more complete picture of the brain's effective connectivity. Also, a comparison with other methods available in the literature needs to be undertaken.

Acknowledgments. We would like to express our gratitude to the reviewers whose valuable suggestions greatly helped to improve this manuscript.

References

1. Bakhtiari, S.K., Hossein-Zadeh, G.A.: Subspace-based identification algorithm for characterizing causal networks in resting brain. NeuroImage **60**(2), 1236–1249 (2012). ISSN: 1053–8119. https://doi.org/10.1016/j.neuroimage.2011.12.075
2. Zhang, D., Raichle, M.E.: Disease and the brain's dark energy. Nat. Rev. Neurol. **6**, 15–28 (2010). https://doi.org/10.1038/nrneurol.2009.198. PMID: 20057496
3. Friston, K.J.: Functional and effective connectivity in neuroimaging: a synthesis. Hum. Brain Mapp. **2**, 56–78 (1994)
4. Tharwat, A.: Independent component analysis: an introduction. Appl. Comput. Inform. **17**(2), 222–249 (2018). https://doi.org/10.1016/j.aci.2018.08.006
5. He, B.J., Raichle, M.E.: The fMRI signal, slow cortical potential and consciousness. Trends Cogn. Sci. **13**, 302–390 (2009)
6. Friston, K.J.: Bayesian estimation of Dynamical systems: an application to fMRI. Neuroimage **16**, 513–30 (2002)
7. MLindquist, M.A., Loh, J.M., Atlas, L.Y., Wager, T.D.: Modeling the hemodynamic response function in fMRI: efficiency, bias and mis-modeling. NeuroImage **45**, S187–S198 (2009)
8. Henson, R., Friston, K.J.: Convolution models for fMRI. Statistical parametric mapping: the analysis of function brain images, pp. 178–192 (2007)
9. Muralidhar, K.: Encyclopedia of Information Systems. 1ạ edição. Academic Press, Cambridge (2002)
10. Harrison, R.L.: Introduction to Monte Carlo simulation. In: AIP Conference Proceedings, vol. 1204, pp. 17–21 (2010)
11. Friston, K.J.: Dynamic causal modeling and Granger causality Comments on: the identification of interacting networks in the brain using fMRI: model selection, causality and deconvolution. Neuroimage **58**, 303–305 (2011)
12. Srivastava, P., et al.: Models of communication and control for brain networks: distinctions, convergence, and future outlook. Netw. Neurosci. **4**, 1122–1159 (2020)
13. Breakspear, M.: Dynamic models of large-scale brain activity. Nat. Neurosci. **20** (2017)
14. Stam, C.J., van Straaten, E.C.W.: Go with the flow: use of a directed phase lag index (DPLI) to characterize patterns of phase relations in a large-scale model of brain dynamics. Neuroimage **62**, 1415–1428 (2012)
15. Avena-Koenigsberger, A., Misic, B., Sporns, O.: The physics of communicability in complex networks. Nat. Rev. Neurosci. **19**, 17–33 (2018)
16. Estrada, E., Hatano, N., Benzi, M.: Communication dynamics in complex brain networks. Phys. Rep. **514**, 89–119 (2012)
17. Schreiber, T.: Measuring information transfer. Phys. Rev. Lett. **85**, 461 (2000)
18. Bullmore, E., Sporns, O.: The economy of brain network organization. Nat. Rev. Neurosci. **13**, 336–349 (2012)
19. Valdes-Sosa, P.A., Roebroeck, A., Daunizeau, J., Friston, K.: Effective connectivity: influence, causality and biophysical modelling. Neuroimage **58**, 339–361 (2011)

Evanescent Wave Filtering for Ultrasound RF-Data Compression

Edgar M. G. Dorausch[1]([✉]), Moritz Herzog[3], Cornelius Kühnöl[1], Daniel Swist[1], Tönnis Trittler[2], Julian Kober[2], and Gerhard Fettweis[1]

[1] Department of Electrical Engineering, Vodafone Chair Mobile Communications Systems, Technische Universität Dresden, Dresden, Germany
edgar.dorausch@tu-dresden.de

[2] Else Kröner Fresenius Center for Digital Health, Technische Universität Dresden, Dresden, Germany

[3] Department of Medicine I, University Hospital Dresden, Dresden, Germany

Abstract. Multistatic imaging techniques, such as Synthetic Aperture Ultrasound (SAU) or Plane Wave Imaging (PWI), offer several advantages in terms of image quality for diagnostic ultrasound imaging. However, the vast amount of data generated by these methods can be challenging to process and store. To address this issue, various compression techniques have been developed. In this work, we propose a compression method based on a physical approach utilizing evanescent wave components in the radio frequency (RF) data.

The basic idea behind our approach is to eliminate the higher frequencies in the data that are no longer necessary, due to the limited spatial sampling frequency. By doing so, we can reduce the amount of data without sacrificing noticeable amounts of image quality, as shown by simulation results. An additional advantage of our approach is that no decompression steps have to be conducted if the image reconstruction algorithm operates in the spatial frequency-domain.

Keywords: diagnostic ultrasound · multistatic-imaging · radio-frequency-data-compression · evanescent-wave-filtering · spatial-frequency-filtering · Fourier-based data-compression

1 Introduction

In the past decades, the paradigm of multistatic imaging like *synthetic aperture ultrasound* (SAU) or *plane wave imaging* (PWI) has steadily gained importance in the field of diagnostic ultrasound imaging. In contrast to classical beamforming methods - which aim to generate sound beams that are as focused as possible - SAU methods use wide-angle transmission. Through multiple transmissions of the wide-angled sound signals at different positions, an overall image can be generated through downstream calculation steps (usually performed by a computing backend), where, in contrast to the classic beamforming methods, the resulting

A. Cunha et al. (Eds.): MobiHealth 2023, LNICST 578, pp. 33–44, 2024.
https://doi.org/10.1007/978-3-031-60665-6_3

image is focused in each image point [7]. PWI, on the other hand, comprises the successive transmissions of ultrasonic plane waves [11]. The reflected signal is captured by the full receiving array (similar to SAU) and processed the by the computing backend.

The use of such multistatic methods is accompanied by high amounts of *radio-frequency* (RF) data generated by the sensor array. The resulting high data rates are a challenge for not only the computing backend, but also for the electronics built into the transducer and the connection to the computing backend [1]. For this reason, minimizing the data rates can simplify the system design, reduce energy consumption, and contribute to an increase in refresh rates.

In this work we will present a new data-compression method utilizing the effect of *evanescent waves*. In Sect. 2, we will reference related compression methods. Section 3 gives a short explanation of the concept of evanescent waves. Our compression method is described in Sect. 4. The according decompression method will be described in Sect. 5. The proposed method is evaluated, using simulation-generated data, in Sect. 6. Our results are shortly concluded in Sect. 7.

2   Related Work

The task of compressing raw acoustic measurement data has been investigated for several use-cases and several approaches. In most cases, compression is performed for each received time trace independently. Examples of this category include:

- the exploitation of different dynamic ranges for different depth levels using *linear predictive coding* (LPC) to achieve a lossless compression [12]
- the detection of changes in the time signal above predefined thresholds and storage of the according data samples and their positions resulting in a lossy reconstruction of the signal [3]
- converting the signal using *discrete wavelet transform* (DWT) or *discrete cosine transform* (DCT) and omitting small coefficients [9]
- projecting the time traces on a specially designed lower dimensional base consisting of phase-shifted window functions [8]

Compression methods utilizing multiple time traces are also subject to research. In this context, the following methods have already been published:

- the reduction of dynamic range by only storing differences between neighboring time traces [9]
- the RF-frame compression using the MPEG video codec [13]

However, to our best knowledge no one has explicitly utilized evanescent waves as physical properties of the received signal to compress the RF data. We furthermore want to highlight, that this type of compression is different from simple band-pass filtering, since it incorporates the spatio-temporal relationship of the received pressure signal. Thus, evanescent wave-based compression approaches are more complex to realize.

3   Evanescent Waves

The occurrence of evanescent waves in the recordings of an acoustic receiving array can be analyzed by utilizing the linear wave equation. Specifically, in the monofrequency case, the reflected wave field can be described by the Helmholtz equation as follows:

$$\left[\nabla^2 + k_0^2\right] \tilde{p}_{ref}(x, y, z, k_0) = \tilde{q}(x, y, z, k_0) \tag{1}$$

with $k_0 = \frac{2\pi f}{c_0}$ being the temporal frequency f, rescaled by the mean speed of sound c_0, which is usually assumed to be $1540\,\mathrm{ms}^{-1}$. p_{ref} is the reflected sound pressure field and q is a source term which is usually - in the case of a reflected wave field - the product of an incident sound pressure field and a reflectance function.

It is assumed that the receiving array is one dimensional, elongated at the x dimension and all array elements having a constant $z = 0$, as illustrated in Fig. 1. Hence the signal $\tilde{s}_{rx}(x, k_0)$, measured by the array at position x, can be approximated to be the reflected wave field with z and y set to zero:

$$\tilde{s}_{rx}(x, k_0) = \tilde{p}_{ref}(x, 0, 0, k_0) \tag{2}$$

By using a Green's function satisfying the Sommerfeld radiation boundary condition [15], the Eq. 1 can be solved for the measured signal by the array:

$$\tilde{s}_{rx}(x, k_0) = \left(q(x, y, z, k_0) *_{x,y,z} \frac{e^{jk_0\sqrt{x^2+y^2+z^2}}}{\sqrt{x^2 + y^2 + z^2}} \right)\Bigg|_{y,z=0} \tag{3}$$

$$= \iiint\limits_{x',y',z' \in \mathbb{R}} \tilde{q}(x', y', z', k_0) \frac{e^{jk_0\sqrt{(x-x')^2+y'^2+z'^2}}}{\sqrt{(x - x')^2 + y'^2 + z'^2}} dz'dy'dx' \tag{4}$$

This equation can further be simplified by performing a Fourier transform with respect to x. Using Weyl's identity [2] it can be shown that:

$$\tilde{S}_{rx}(k_x, k_0) = \int\limits_{x \in \mathbb{R}} \tilde{s}_{rx}(x, k_0) e^{-jxk_x} dx \tag{5}$$

$$= \iint\limits_{y',z' \in \mathbb{R}} \tilde{Q}(k_x, y', z', k_0) \frac{e^{j\sqrt{y'^2+z'^2}\sqrt{k_0^2-k_x^2}}}{\sqrt{k_0^2 - k_x^2}} dz'dy' \tag{6}$$

It can be seen that for any $|k_x| > |k_0|$ the square root term $\sqrt{k_0^2 - k_x^2}$ results in a positive purely imaginary value. Hence, the complex unit in the exponential cancels out, yielding to a decaying real-valued exponential. Due to this effect S_{rx} values for $|k_x| > |k_0|$ tend to be close to zero and hence are called *evanescent waves*.

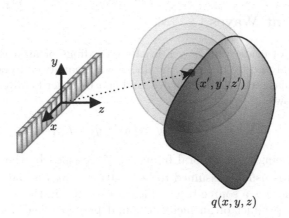

$$q(x, y, z)$$

Fig. 1. Illustration of the receiver array, the source term q and the Green's function originating from every point from q. (Color figure online)

4   The Compression Algorithm

The following section describes our new compression algorithm. First, we describe the compression in the k_x-k_0-domain. Then, this compression procedure is transferred to the k_x-t-domain to generate an efficient compression scheme.

The compression method operates on the RF frames in k_x-k_0-space. The measurement system only provides temporal frequency information within the bounds of $k_0 \in [-\frac{\pi f_s}{c_0}, \frac{\pi f_s}{c_0}]$, with f_s being the systems sampling frequency. Similarly, the spatial frequency information can only be measured within the bounds of $k_x \in [-\frac{\pi}{p}, \frac{\pi}{p}]$, where p is denoting the array pitch. However, since the signal $s(x, t)$, recorded by the receiver array, is purely real, it underlies the symmetry properties of real signals in the Fourier-domain, i.e.: $\tilde{S}(k_x, k_0) = \tilde{S}^*(-k_x, -k_0)$ where $\tilde{S}^*$ is the complex conjugate of $\tilde{S}$. Hence, only half the k_x-k_0-space datapoints needs to be stored, in order to fully reconstruct the signal in the x-t-space. For this reason only positive $k_x >= 0$ will be used for further analysis. The according RF-frames are illustrated in Fig. 2.

The first step for compressing the data is to perform a cyclic shift of half the size of the RF-frame ($\frac{\pi f_s}{c_0}$) in the k_0-dimension of the RF-frame region with k_x greater than a threshold value: $k_x \geq k_x^{\mathrm{thr}}$. This threshold defines a line in the k_0-direction that is contained by the same amounts in the evanescent and non-evanescent regions. Hence, the line is at the k_x-value where k_x is exactly the half of the maximal temporal frequency of the RF-frame, i.e.:

$$k_x^{\mathrm{thr}} = \frac{k_0^{\mathrm{max}}}{2} = \frac{\pi f_s}{2c_0} \tag{7}$$

Due to the evanescent waves, RF values on the lines in the k_0-direction with the same distance to k_x^{thr} have a nearly disjoint support and thus are orthogonal. Therefore, if these corresponding signal values are added, they can be separated again at a later stage. This makes it possible to pack all data for $k_x \geq k_x^{\text{thr}}$ into the low-frequency regions. The aforementioned steps are illustrated in Fig. 2a).

This process can be efficiently replicated in the k_x-t-domain. If the compression process is transformed into the time domain, the cyclic shift becomes a scalar multiplication of the complex phase term:

$$\exp\left(jt\frac{\pi f_s}{c_0}\right) \tag{8}$$

Due to the linearity of the Fourier transform, all further steps remain the same as in the frequency procedure as shown in Fig. 2b).

To describe the algorithm used in digital processing, it is assumed that the RF-data is a matrix. Let $D_{n,m}$ ($n = 0, \ldots, N-1$ and $m = 0, \ldots, M-1$) be this $N \times M$ matrix, holding the received signal values in the x-t-domain. Every column represents the N-dimensional signal-vector for a single receiving element and every row represents the M-dimensional full array measurement for a time point t. To transform the RF-data matrix $D_{n,m}$ from the x-t-domain into the k_x-t-domain efficiently, a *fast Fourier transform* (FFT) can be used. However, since only positive k_x are required for the algorithm, data processing can be further speed-up by using a *real-valued fast Fourier transform* (rFFT) [16] instead of a regular FFT. The rFFT operation transforms the M real-valued traces into $M/2 + 1$ or $(M + 1)/2$ complex-valued traces depending if M is even or odd. Moreover, the threshold-value k_x^{thr} will be represented by a threshold-index τ, defined by:

$$\tau = \left\lceil \frac{k_x^{\text{thr}}}{\Delta k_x} \right\rceil = \left\lceil \frac{p \cdot f_s}{4c_0} M \right\rceil \tag{9}$$

where Δk_x is the width of a FFT bin, given by $\Delta k_x = \frac{2\pi}{p \cdot M}$. In the discretized setting, the temporal phase-shift-term from Eq. 8 can be expressed by $\exp(j\pi n) = (-1)^n$, which alternatingly changes the sign for each increment in n. Overall, the compression algorithm comprises two main steps:

(C1) **Transforming RF Data into (positive) frequency-domain:**

$$\tilde{D}_{n,l} = \text{rFFT}_m \left[D_{n,m}\right]_l \tag{10}$$

$$\tilde{D}_{n,m} \in \mathbb{C}^{N \times L} \text{ with } L = \begin{cases} M/2 + 1, M \text{ is even} \\ (M+1)/2, M \text{ is odd} \end{cases}$$

(C2) **Add the phase-shifted high-frequency time traces to their corresponding low-frequency traces:**

$$\tilde{D}_{n,l}^{\text{comp}} = \begin{cases} \tilde{D}_{n,l}, l < 2\tau - L \\ \tilde{D}_{n,l} + (-1)^n \tilde{D}_{n,2\tau-l}, \text{otherwise.} \end{cases} \tag{11}$$

$$\tilde{D}_{n,l}^{\text{comp}} \in \mathbb{C}^{N \times \tau}$$

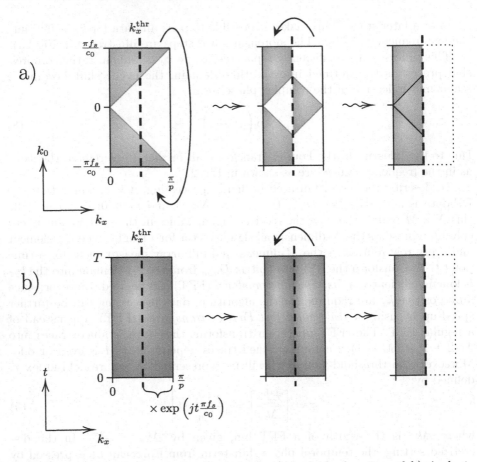

Fig. 2. Illustration of the compression steps in a): in k_x-k_0-domain and b): in k_x-t-domain. The blue-shaded regions of the RF-frames shown in a) are non-evanescent wave components. (Color figure online)

Since there are no data dependencies between different time points the algorithm can be very efficiently used for data stream processing. The incoming M real-valued time signals will be transformed into τ complex valued time signals - hence, the algorithm returns 2τ real-valued time signals. The overall compression ratio CR (the ratio of the original data size A_{orig} and the compressed data size A_{orig}) is purely dependent on the system parameters and can be approximated by the ratio of the maximal spatial frequency $k_x^{\mathrm{max}} = \frac{\pi}{p}$ and the threshold-frequency k_x^{thr}:

$$CR \approx \frac{A_{\mathrm{orig}}}{A_{\mathrm{compr}}} = \frac{k_x^{\mathrm{max}}}{k_x^{\mathrm{thr}}} = \frac{2c_0}{p \cdot f_s} \tag{12}$$

Since the presented compression algorithm has a very simple structure, it also allows hardware-related implementations, e.g. by means of field programmable gate arrays (FPGA). Figure 3 shows the schematic structure of the compression as a block diagram.

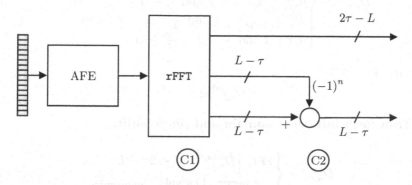

Fig. 3. Block diagram. Sensory data is digitalized by the *analog frontend* (AFE) and directly processed by the compression steps.

5   The Decompression Algorithm

If image reconstruction uses a k-space based method [4,10], it can be used without the further decompression steps by directly adapting its k-space coordinate transformations. However, to use the RF data for time- and space-based image reconstruction methods the data must be decompressed again. For this purpose, the compressed data $\tilde{D}_{n,l}^{\text{comp}}$ must be transformed into the k_x-k_0-domain by another Fourier transformation. Afterwards, the signals added in step (C2) of the compression must be separated and rearranged again. In the next steps, an inverse Fourier transformation in the time dimension, a phase correction, and an inverse Fourier transformation in the spatial dimension must be performed.

The decompression algorithm can be described by the following steps:

(D1) **Transforming the compressed data into the k_x-k_0-domain:**

$$\tilde{D}_{k,l}^{\text{freq}} = \text{FFT}_n \left[\tilde{D}_{n,l}^{\text{comp}} \right]_k \tag{13}$$

$$\tilde{D}_{k,l}^{\text{freq}} \in \mathbb{C}^{N \times \tau}$$

(D2) **Reordering data:**

$$\tilde{D}_{k,l}^{\text{reord}} = \begin{cases} \tilde{D}_{k,l}^{\text{freq}}, l < 2\tau - L \\ \tilde{D}_{k,l}^{\text{freq}}, 2\tau - L \leq l < \tau \text{ and } \frac{N}{2} - |k - \frac{N}{2}| \geq \alpha l \\ 0, 2\tau - L \leq l < \tau \text{ and } \frac{N}{2} - |k - \frac{N}{2}| < \alpha l \\ \tilde{D}_{k,2\tau-l-1}^{\text{freq}}, \tau \leq l \text{ and } \frac{N}{2} - |k - \frac{N}{2}| < \alpha l \\ 0, \tau \leq l \text{ and } \frac{N}{2} - |k - \frac{N}{2}| \geq \alpha l \end{cases} \tag{14}$$

with $\alpha = \frac{N \cdot c_0}{M \cdot p \cdot f_s}$

$$\tilde{D}_{n,l}^{\text{reord}} \in \mathbb{C}^{N \times L}$$

(D3) **Transform into time domain and phase shift:**

$$\tilde{D}_{n,l}^{\text{time}} = \begin{cases} \text{FFT}_n \left[\tilde{D}_{n,l}^{\text{reord}} \right]_k, l < 2\tau - L \\ (-1)^n \text{FFT}_n \left[\tilde{D}_{n,l}^{\text{reord}} \right]_k, \text{otherwise.} \end{cases} \tag{15}$$

(D4) **Transform into space domain:**

$$\hat{D}_{n,m} = \text{irFFT}_l \left[\tilde{D}_{n,m}^{\text{comp}} \right]_m \tag{16}$$

$$\hat{D}_{n,m} \in \mathbb{R}^{N \times M}$$

6   Simulation Results

Since evanescent waves are only exponentially attenuated - but not completely eliminated - artifacts can result from the compression process. To estimate the extent of the compression artifacts, the compression method was tested with data generated by the Field II [5,6] simulation. The simulated data has been generated for a virtual cyst phantom compromising five hypoechoic cyst regions, five highly scattering hyperechoic regions and five point targets - all located in a background medium with Gaussian reflectivity-strength distribution. The virtual ultrasound probe mimics the properties of the GE M5Sc-D ultrasound probe, which has a center frequency of 2.8 MHz, a fractional bandwidth of 90%, a pitch of 0.23 mm, 80 elements in azimuth direction, an elevation focus of 77 mm. In total, our algorithm achieves a compression ratio of 1.49 with these parameter settings. The simulation is run with a sampling frequency of 9 MHz. The virtual probe uses the *Coherent Plane-Wave Compounding* (CPWC) [11] transmission and reconstruction scheme implemented by the UltraSound ToolBox [14] for MATLAB.

A comparison based on the RF-data has been conducted using the *signal-to-noise-ratio* (SNR), and the *peak-signal-to-noise-ratio* PSNR metric. A central building block for both of these metrics is the *root-mean-square-error* (RMSE) defined by:

$$\text{RMSE} = \sqrt{\frac{1}{NM} \sum\sum (\hat{D}_{n,m} - D_{n,m})^2} \qquad (17)$$

which gives rise to the following definitions:

$$\text{SNR} = 20 \log_{10} \left(\frac{\sigma_D}{RMSE} \right) \text{[dB]} \qquad (18)$$

$$\text{PSNR} = 20 \log_{10} \left(\frac{D^{\max}}{RMSE} \right) \text{[dB]} \qquad (19)$$

where σ_D is the standard deviation of the original RF-data frame $D_{n,m}$ and $D^{\max}$ is the maximal absolute value of $D_{n,m}$. We have measured a RMSE-to-σ_D-ratio of 10.2% which translates to a SNR of 19.8 dB. Moreover, a RMSE-to-$D^{\max}$-ratio of 0.9% was measured, which corresponds to a PSNR of 41.2 dB.

In order to evaluate the effect of compression artifacts on the reconstructed images, comparison studies have been conducted here as well. Images have been generated by the *delay-and-sum* (DAS) implementation of the UltraSound Tool-Box using the original data, as well as compressed and decompressed data. The reconstructed images have been normalized by their maximum value, log-compressed and clipped to a range from -60 dB to 0 dB. Figure 4 shows the according reconstruction results, as well as their (signed) difference. In order to provide a concise quantification for the image quality, the *structural similarity index* (SSIM) [17] was used to assess the difference of the image reconstructed using the original RF-data and the image reconstructed using the compressed and decompressed RF-data. Given two images A and B, the SSIM is defined by:

$$\text{SSIM} = \frac{(2\mu_A\mu_B + c_1)(2\sigma_{AB} + c_2)}{(\mu_A^2 + \mu_B^2 + c_1)(\sigma_A^2 + \sigma_B^2 + c_2)} \qquad (20)$$

with μ_A and μ_B being the mean values of A and B, σ_A^2 and σ_B^2 is the variance of A and B and σ_{AB} is the covariance of A and B. The variable L represents the dynamic range which is set to 60 dB in our case. Furthermore, we set c_1 and c_2 to $(0.01L)^2$ and $(0.02L)^2$ respectively. Th SSIM ranges from 0 to 1, where a SSIM of 1 indicates maximal similarity of A and B, i.e. $A = B$. An overall SSIM of 99.8% was obtained by comparing - indicating that only minor artifacts are produced by the compression.

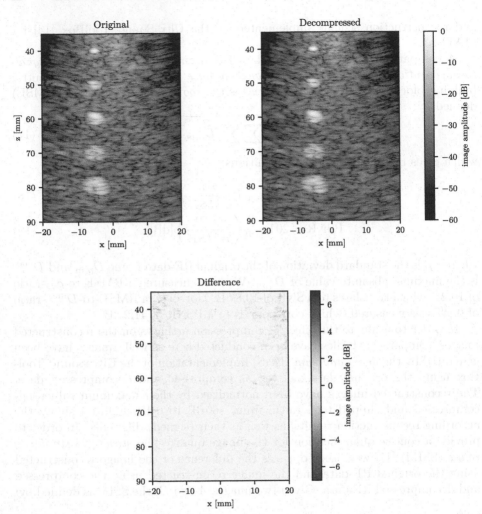

Fig. 4. Plot of the reconstructed image, using the original RF-data ("Original"), a reconstructed image, using compressed and decompressed RF-data ("Decompressed") and the difference of both images ("Difference")

7   Conclusion

We were able to propose a method that makes it possible to compress data from a receiving array by means of a spatial Fourier transformation. This can lead to savings in bandwidth when transmitting the RF data from the ultrasound probe to the computing-backend. Such savings could presumably result in more faster, more stable and more energy efficient connections of the ultrasound probe and the computing backend - especially for wireless data transmission. If a k-space based algorithm is used for the subsequent reconstruction, no further decompression step has to be performed. Otherwise, decompression as shown in this work, is possible. Using simulatively generated data, it could be shown that the artifacts generated by the compression have no noticeable effect on the image quality.

Our proposed algorithm can presumably be implemented very efficiently on an FPGA in terms of its execution time and the required hardware resources. Benchmarks of specific implementations on FPGA hardware could therefore be the subject of further research. In addition, only one simulation model was used in this study to evaluate the algorithm. More extensive testing of the algorithm using in-vivo data is also of interest for further investigations.

Acknowledgement. This work was supported by the German Federal Ministry of Education and Research (BMBF) as part of the project "MEDGE" under grant 16ME0531.

References

1. Boni, E., Yu, A.C.H., Freear, S., Jensen, J.A., Tortoli, P.: Ultrasound open platforms for next-generation imaging technique development. IEEE Transa. Ultrason. Ferroelectr. Freq. Control **65**(7), 1078–1092 (2018). https://doi.org/10.1109/TUFFC.2018.2844560, https://ieeexplore.ieee.org/document/8374071/

2. Chew, W.C.: Planarly Layered Media. In: Waves and Fields in Inhomogenous Media. IEEE (2009). https://doi.org/10.1109/9780470547052.ch2, http://ieeexplore.ieee.org/search/srchabstract.jsp?arnumber=5271009

3. Freitas, M.D.A., Jimenez, M.R., Benincaza, H., Von Der Weid, J.P.: A new lossy compression algorithm for ultrasound signals. In: 2008 IEEE Ultrasonics Symposium, pp. 1885–1888. IEEE, Beijing, China, November 2008. https://doi.org/10.1109/ULTSYM.2008.0464, http://ieeexplore.ieee.org/document/4803348/

4. Garcia, D., Tarnec, L.L., Muth, S., Montagnon, E., Porée, J., Cloutier, G.: Stolt's f-k migration for plane wave ultrasound imaging. IEEE Trans. Ultrason. Ferroelectr. Freq. Control **60**(9), 1853–1867 (2013). https://doi.org/10.1109/TUFFC.2013.2771

5. Jensen, J., Svendsen, N.: Calculation of pressure fields from arbitrarily shaped, apodized, and excited ultrasound transducers. IIEEE Trans. Ultrason. Ferroelectr. Freq. Control **39**(2), 262–267 (1992). https://doi.org/10.1109/58.139123, conference Name: IEEE Transactions on Ultrasonics, Ferroelectrics, and Frequency Control

6. Jensen, J.A.: Field: a program for simulating ultrasound systems: 10th Nordic-Baltic conference on biomedical imaging. Med. Biol. Eng. Comput. **34**(sup. 1), 351–353 (1997)

7. Jensen, J.A., Nikolov, S.I., Gammelmark, K.L., Pedersen, M.H.: Synthetic aperture ultrasound imaging. Ultrasonics **44**, e5–e15 (2006). https://doi.org/10.1016/j.ultras.2006.07.017, https://linkinghub.elsevier.com/retrieve/pii/S0041624X06003374

8. Kleparnik, P., Zemcik, P., Jaros, J.: Efficient lossy compression of ultrasound data. In: 2017 IEEE International Symposium on Signal Processing and Information Technology (ISSPIT), pp. 232–237. IEEE, Bilbao, December 2017. https://doi.org/10.1109/ISSPIT.2017.8388647, https://ieeexplore.ieee.org/document/8388647/

9. Liu, R.: Data compression in ultrasound computed tomography. PhD Thesis, Karlsruhe Institute of Technology (2011). http://digbib.ubka.uni-karlsruhe.de/volltexte/1000023057
10. Moghimirad, E., Villagomez Hoyos, C.A., Mahloojifar, A., Mohammadzadeh Asl, B., Jensen, J.A.: Synthetic aperture ultrasound fourier beamformation using virtual sources. IEEE Trans. Ultrason. Ferroelectr. Freq. Control **63**(12), 2018–2030 (2016). https://doi.org/10.1109/TUFFC.2016.2606878, https://ieeexplore.ieee.org/document/7562394/
11. Montaldo, G., Tanter, M., Bercoff, J., Benech, N., Fink, M.: Coherent plane-wave compounding for very high frame rate ultrasonography and transient elastography. IEEE Trans. Ultrason. Ferroelectr. Freq. Control **56**(3), 489–506 (2009). https://doi.org/10.1109/TUFFC.2009.1067, http://ieeexplore.ieee.org/document/4816058/
12. Pesavento, A., Burow, V., Ermert, H.: Compression of ultrasonic RF data, vol. 2, pp. 1471–1474. IEEE, Toronto, Ont., Canada (1997). https://doi.org/10.1109/ULTSYM.1997.661854, http://ieeexplore.ieee.org/document/661854/
13. Cheng, P.-W., Shen, C-C., Li, P.C.: Ultrasound RF channel data compression for implementation of a software-based array imaging system. In: 2011 IEEE International Ultrasonics Symposium, pp. 1423–1426. IEEE, Orlando, FL, USA, October 2011. https://doi.org/10.1109/ULTSYM.2011.0352, http://ieeexplore.ieee.org/document/6293721/
14. Rodriguez-Molares, A., et al.: The ultrasound toolbox. In: 2017 IEEE International Ultrasonics Symposium (IUS), pp. 1–4. IEEE, Washington, DC, September 2017. https://doi.org/10.1109/ULTSYM.2017.8092389, https://ieeexplore.ieee.org/document/8092389/
15. Sommerfeld, A.: Eigenfunctions and Eigen Values. In: Pure and Applied Mathematics, vol. 1, pp. 166–235. Elsevier (1949). https://doi.org/10.1016/S0079-8169(08)60771-0, https://linkinghub.elsevier.com/retrieve/pii/S0079816908607710
16. Sorensen, H., Jones, D., Heideman, M., Burrus, C.: Real-valued fast Fourier transform algorithms. IEEE Trans. Acoustics Speech Signal Process. **35**(6), 849–863 (1987). https://doi.org/10.1109/TASSP.1987.1165220, http://ieeexplore.ieee.org/document/1165220/
17. Wang, Z., Bovik, A., Sheikh, H., Simoncelli, E.: Image quality assessment: from error visibility to structural similarity. IEEE Trans. Image Process. **13**(4), 600–612 (2004). https://doi.org/10.1109/TIP.2003.819861, conference Name: IEEE Transactions on Image Processing

SpinalTracking: An Application to Help Track Spinal Deformities

Estephane Mendes Nascimento[✉], João Dallyson S. de Almeida,
Geraldo Braz Júnior, and Aristófanes Correa Silva

Federal University of Maranhão - UFMA, Applied Computing Group - NCA/UFMA,
São Luís, Brazil
estephane.mn@discente.ufma.br

Abstract. The human vertebral column (HVC) comprises specialized
tissues and structures that allow it to support body weight with an extensive range of movement and protect the spinal cord, which is essential
for routine activities. HVC deformities are highly prevalent in individuals
over 65, affecting between 32% and 68% of this population, and represent
a public health problem with a profound impact on society. Physicians
evaluate and monitor HVC deformities in practice by physical examination and analyzing imaging tests. In this context, the SpinalTracking App
was developed to enable specialists to manually or automatically measure
the Cobb angle in X-ray images of the spine of patients with scoliosis,
using image processing and deep learning techniques. The measurements
provided by the app are stored so that treatment can be monitored. The
application obtained a Pearson correlation of 0.94 and 0.92 for the calculation made with the manual measurement functionalities and an average
correlation of 0.74 for the automatic calculation. This demonstrated the
potential use of SpinalTracking as a tool for measuring and controlling
the evolution of each patient's scoliosis deviation.

Keywords: SpinalTracking · Mobile App · Cobb angle · Scoliosis

1 Introduction

The spine is a critical mechanism for balancing and supporting the body. The
three essential functions of the spine are to absorb load, allow movement, and
protect the spinal cord. The anatomy of the spine is perfectly adapted to provide
these functions. The spine consists of seven cervical vertebrae, twelve thoracic
vertebrae, five lumbar vertebrae, five fused sacral vertebrae, and three to four
coccygeal segments, also fused. The spine seen from the front, in the frontal
plane, is generally straight and symmetrical. In the sagittal plane, there are four
physiological curves. These are anteriorly convex curves (lordosis) in the cervical
and lumbar regions and posteriorly convex curves (kyphosis) in the thoracic
and sacrococcygeal regions. The mechanical explanation for these physiological
curves would be that they allow for greater flexibility and an increased capacity

© ICST Institute for Computer Sciences, Social Informatics and Telecommunications Engineering 2024
Published by Springer Nature Switzerland AG 2024. All Rights Reserved
A. Cunha et al. (Eds.): MobiHealth 2023, LNICST 578, pp. 45–58, 2024.
https://doi.org/10.1007/978-3-031-60665-6_4

to absorb loads while the intervertebral joints adequately maintain strength and stability [13].

Scoliosis affects between 2–3% of the population [2]. In scoliotic spine, the number and segmentation of the vertebrae are the same as in the normal spine. However, the column is no longer straight in the frontal plane. Instead, they are lateral curves, typically right convex in the thoracic region and left convex in the thoracolumbar and lumbar region [18]. This postural deviation is diagnosed by checking image exams by measuring the Cobb angle. The curve is measured using the position of the end/transitional vertebrae. The end vertebra are the upper and lowermost vertebrae which are the least displaced from the midline and the most severely tilted. A line is drawn along the superior (top) endplate of the top end vertebra, and a second line is drawn along the inferior (bottom) end plate of the bottom end vertebra. The angle formed by these two lines (or the lines drawn perpendicular to them) is the Cobb angle [17]. Treatment is related to the degree of deviation that the deformity may present in relation to the normal formation of the spine, and can be corrected or mitigated through treatments such as physiotherapy sessions, use of braces or, in more serious cases, surgical correction.

Given the need for health professionals to work in locations with different infrastructures, the creation of applications for mobile devices aimed at the health area can be considered a tool to help specialists carry out examinations and obtain a diagnosis for each patient. Based on this perspective, this study aimed to develop an application to measure the Cobb angle in X-ray spine images. This method is used to measure the magnitude of spinal deformities and monitor the development of the problem.

The app has three functions for measuring Cobb's angle, the first by obtaining the inclination of the smartphone, captured by the phone's accelerometer, a function developed based on analysis of measurements made in works such as [6, 16], the other by manipulating lines in an image provided by the user and the last by automatic calculation using deep learning and image processing techniques. This application stands out because it combines three functions in just one application, allows patients to be registered, and stores the measurement data for each patient, enabling the development of the deformity to be monitored using the stored exams. The application can also be used in Portuguese or English, depending on the language settings of the device used by the user.

2   Related Work

Several applications are designed to calculate the Cobb angle using X-ray images, including Scodiac, Scoliogauge, and Tiltmeter. Scodiac was developed to measure deformities of the spine and trunk, calculate the Cobb angle and vertebral rotation. The Scoliogauge, available on the App Store, was evaluated by [6], comparing the measurement made by the Scoliogauge with that of the standard scoliometer, concluding that the measurements showed corresponding results. The Tiltmeter, also developed for the iPhone and evaluated by [16], collects the inclination of the device using the accelerometer. When the specialist positions the smartphone on the X-ray, the inclination captured calculates the Cobb angle on the upper and lower vertebrae chosen. The assessment carried out on the Tiltmeter depends on the direct intervention of the specialist.

Many studies have been conducted to calculate Cobb's angle automatically by providing the X-ray image and obtaining the angles found. In [7], the vertebrae were located, and then the landmarks were detected, consisting of passing the X-ray to the vertebrae detection network and then calculating the landmarks using a DenseNet, followed by the calculation of the angles. The work in [4] details the steps involved in segmenting the X-ray image, recognizing the corners of each vertebra, and then calculating the Cobb angle.

A three-step method was proposed in [8]. The first finds the centroids of each vertebra using Centroid-Net, the second applies M-net to find the inclination of each vertebra, and finally, the Cobb angle is calculated. In [5] two networks were used. The first focused on segmenting the spine, and the second was developed to extract the center line of the spine using the results of the first network, with post-processing to estimate the Cobb angles. The method developed in [11] was used as the basis for the automatic calculation functionality developed in the App proposed in this study.

In summary, SpinalTracking stands out from other available applications as it combines three methods for calculating the Cobb angle in a single app: through accelerometer data, manual line marking, and automatic measurement. Additionally, it enables the storage of examination results, allowing professionals to track the progression of each patient's deformity.

3   Materials and Method

The specialist usually measures the Cobb angle using an X-ray of the spine, choosing the vertebrae that delimit the curvature to be measured and drawing two lines, one passing through the upper limit of the upper vertebra and the other through the lower limit of the lower vertebra. A goniometer is usually used to calculate the angle formed by the lines and thus obtain the Cobb angle. The result of this measurement is used to monitor the progression or containment of the deformity. However, it is only sometimes convenient to keep the X-rays for analysis by a specialist, as the examination may deteriorate or be lost over time. As a result, the use of applications that make it possible to store the image of the examinations carried out is becoming increasingly indispensable.

The SpinalTracking app was developed to provide specialists with a more practical way of measuring Cobb's angle, which has three measurement functions: by tilting the cell phone positioned on the x-ray (function 1), by marking the upper and lower vertebrae on the scan provided to the App (function 2) and automatic marking (function 3). All measurements are stored in the App, so it is possible to track each patient's history.

Functionalities 1 and 2 were developed based on the traditional examination method, requiring the specialist to analyze and choose the vertebrae to be used for the measurement. For functionality 3, simply sending the x-ray to the application is enough to calculate the angles.

3.1   Measurement by Tilting the Cell Phone on the X-Ray Image

Considering the conventional measurement, functionality 1 simulates the marking of lines by positioning the handset on the vertebrae selected in the x-ray examination. This mode allows the calculation to be based on the inclination of the cell phone about the x-ray. The data obtained from the accelerometer integrated within the phone is utilized to attain the measurement, and the Cobb angle is calculated by utilizing the inclinations obtained. Figure 1 shows the screens for measuring and checking the saved result.

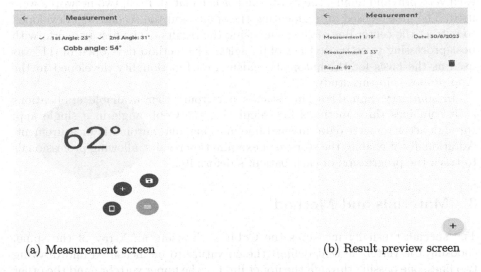

(a) Measurement screen   (b) Result preview screen

Fig. 1. Screens for measuring the Cobb angle by capturing the inclination of the cell phone in relation to the X-ray.

3.2   Measurement Through the Vertebrae Markings on the X-Ray

This method has the same procedure as traditional measurement: the professional makes the markings on the x-ray image provided to the application, and the calculation is made by the application using the Cobb method, followed by the storage of both the image and the measurement result. Figure 2a shows the marking made with the lines on the exam provided, Fig. 2b shows the saved exam in reduced form, and Fig. 2c shows the saved exam expanded.

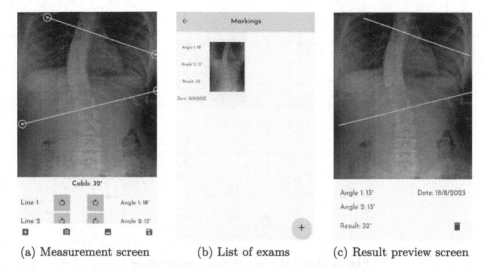

(a) Measurement screen   (b) List of exams   (c) Result preview screen

Fig. 2. Cobb angle measurement screens by demarcating the vertebrae in the X-ray provided to the application.

3.3 Automated Measurement

The development of the automatic measurement was divided into two stages: searching for automatic calculation methods and creating the API that processes the X-ray.

Firstly, some methods developed to estimate Cobb angles were analyzed. The method proposed in [11] was used as a basis among the works found. This method was chosen because it is feasible to implement in the API and has good results for the estimated angles.

The method uses image processing and deep learning techniques to calculate Cobb angles, consisting of:

Segmentation: A network based on the U-net [14] was used to segment the spine's vertebrae. The network takes a 128×256 resized x-ray image as input and uses 3×3 convolution layers with an ELU [3] activation function and dropout. Four hundred eighty-one images from the [19] database were used for training, with augmentation being performed for 200 epochs, using Tversky loss [15] as the loss function. Figure 3 shows the network architecture and operations.

Post-processing: The mask resulting from the segmentation goes through the noise removal process. At this stage, morphological transformations were used to remove some noise. The Watershed [1] method was used to delimit the structures present in the mask, followed by calculating the areas of these elements to check and remove components that had an area smaller than the threshold used.

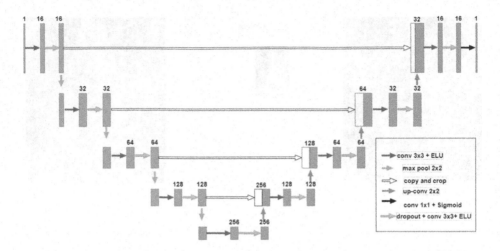

Fig. 3. Modified U-net network architecture

Calculation of Cobb's Angle: To calculate the Cobb angle, the centroids of each vertebra are found with regionprops algorithm through the centroids property, then the contours finding perimeter and fit minimum bounding rectangle, and finally, the four corners of each vertebra, extracting points on the top and bottom endplates. The four corners of each vertebra in the post-processed mask (endplates) and the centroids are used as input for the Cobb angle calculation algorithm. Finally, the result is three angles, corresponding to the PT (proximal thoracic), MT (main thoracic), and TL/L (thoracolumbar or lumbar) regions, the vertebrae that are the apex and the location of the angles.

To calculate each of the angles, the inclinations found for the selected upper and lower vertebrae are used, employing the following calculation:

$$|arctan(slopesup) - arctan(slopeinf)| \tag{1}$$

For the post-processing and Cobb angle calculation steps, the scripts were initially implemented in Matlab [12] and transcribed into Python using the necessary libraries for later implementation in the API. The steps described are shown in Fig. 4.

The method is designed to interpret standing anteroposterior radiographs and is available at [10].

The API was developed to process and analyze the image the App will send in the automatic calculation exam. The application performs the following sequence of actions: it receives the x-ray image sent by the App, processes it, and returns to the application the segmented image with the markings of the vertebrae selected by the method, as well as the value of each angle calculated. The process in question is shown in Fig. 5.

The screens corresponding to sending the x-ray and storing the markings and angles obtained as a result of the automatic calculation are shown in Fig. 6.

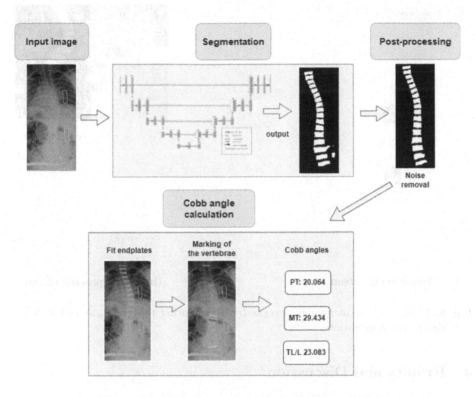

Fig. 4. Steps of the automatic calculation method.

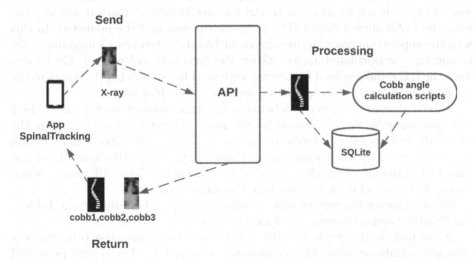

Fig. 5. Steps for sending, processing and returning the X-ray image via the API.

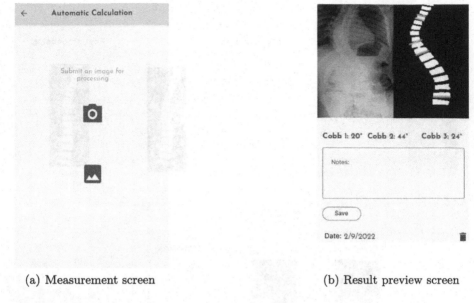

(a) Measurement screen   (b) Result preview screen

Fig. 6. Cobb angle measurement screens by demarcating the vertebrae in the X-ray provided to the application.

4   Results and Discussion

Tests were conducted to assess the efficacy of each function. The accelerometer data and line markings were measured using images with the vertebrae marked and the Cobb angle calculated by an expert. The tests carried out at this stage were done with few images due to the low availability of marked images, and with the Cobb angle calculated to compare the real and the predicted. In this way, the application made the measurement based on the expert's markings, only comparing the calculated angles. About the automatic calculation, 128 images from the [19] database used for testing were used by submitting the X-ray to the application to compare the predicted angle with the real one.

Table 1 shows the comparison between the measurement made by the expert and that made by the application for the measurement functionality, using the tilt of the cell phone in relation to the X-ray image. The Application column shows the result of the measurement made by the App, the Manual column shows the value of the angle calculated by the expert. The Difference column shows the degree of difference between the measurements.

Figure 7 shows the scatter plot, constructed using the results from Table 1. An R^2 of 0.9 and a Pearson correlation of 0.94 were achieved.

According to the study by [18], the difference between the two exams is clinically significant when the measurements exceed 5º. The results presented indicate that, of the nine images analyzed, five are within the acceptable variation

Table 1. Comparison between app and expert measurement using mobile phone tilt.

Images	Application	Manual	Difference
Image 1	41º	49º	8°
Image 2	41º	48º	7°
Image 3	36º	32º	4°
Image 4	83º	80º	3°
Image 5	72º	70º	2°
Image 6	50º	63º	13°
Image 7	66º	63º	3°
Image 8	37º	35º	2°
Image 9	17º	9º	8°

limit, while the other four are slightly above, except image 6, which showed a significant variation between measurements.

The variation between measurements taken with the app and those of the specialist may have occurred due to variations in tilt during the positioning of the mobile device on the X-ray image or during the capture of the device's tilt, as the accelerometer data is constantly changing.

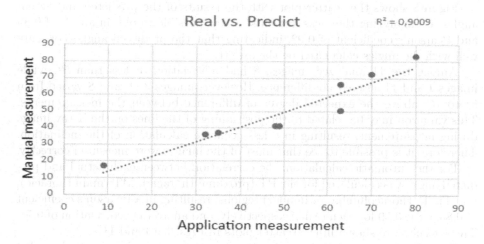

Fig. 7. Scatter plot of the results of the measurement functionality through the inclination of the cell phone about the X-ray image.

Table 2 contains the test results for the measurement by marking the vertebrae on the x-ray. The Application column shows the degree of Cobb's angle obtained by marking lines on the images supplied to the application. The manual column shows the results of the measurements made by the expert with a pen and goniometer to calculate the angle mentioned, and the Difference column shows the degree of difference between the measurements.

Table 2. Comparison between the app's measurement and the specialist is use of the markings of the vertebrae on the X-ray.

Images	Application	Manual	Difference
Image 1	48º	48º	0º
Image 2	28º	32º	4º
Image 3	60º	70º	10º
Image 4	60º	80º	20º
Image 5	36º	40º	4º
Image 6	15º	12º	3º
Image 7	10º	9º	1º
Image 8	80º	63º	17º
Image 9	18º	16º	2º
Image 10	48º	49º	1º
Image 11	63º	63º	0º

Figure 8 shows the scatter plot with the results of the predicted and actual angles. By analyzing the measurements, it was possible to obtain an R^2 of 0.86 and Pearson's coefficient of 0.92, indicating that the predicted angles correlate well with the angles calculated by the expert.

Among the 11 analyzed images, 8 had a variation of less than 5º, while images 1 and 11 showed no difference. However, images 3, 4, and 8 varied from 5° to 15° above the expected degree of difference between the measurements. This variation may be related to the positioning of the lines on the X-ray image during measurement, resulting in a less accurate calculation of the inclination. Therefore, it is possible to see that most of the images were measured correctly.

For the automatic calculation, the correlation between each actual and predicted angle was calculated for the PT (proximal thoracic), MT (main thoracic), and TL/L (thoracolumbar or lumbar) regions, resulting in a Pearson's coefficient of 0.83, 0.81, 0.59 for each region respectively, and an average correlation of 0.74. These results are shown in the scatter plots in Figs. 9, 10 and 11.

To measure the level of dispersion between the predicted and actual results, the standard deviation was calculated, resulting in 3.59 for PT (proximal thoracic), 9.38 for MT (main thoracic) and 11.76 for TL/L (thoracolumbar or lumbar) angles, indicating that there is still a considerable difference between some measurements, which can be seen in the number of measurements that were above and below the 5º of variation considered between measurements. Of the 128 images measured for PT, 40 were above the limit, and 88 were within the limit. For MT, 89 images were above, and 39 were within the limit. Finally, 105

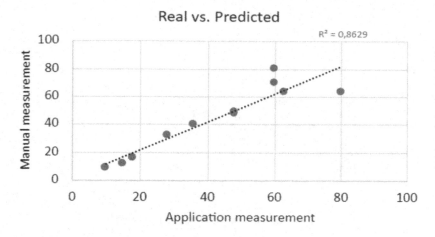

Fig. 8. Scatter plot with application and expert measurement results.

images were above and 23 within the limit for TL. Therefore, there was a smaller difference between the measurements taken for PT compared to MT and TL.

The difference in the number of correct measurements compared to the angle calculated by the specialist for PT, MT, and TL may have occurred due to the choice of vertebrae by the method to perform the Cobb angle calculation, given that the vertebrae used are not fixed and are selected based on their inclination and position.

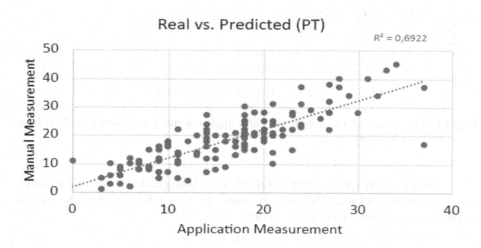

Fig. 9. Test results of the automatic Cobb angle calculation feature for PT (proximal thoracic).

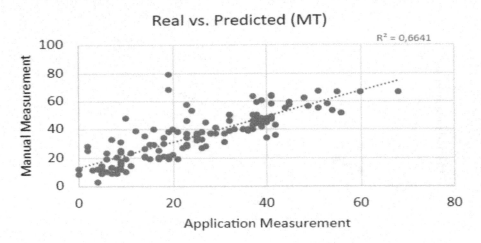

Fig. 10. Test results of the automatic Cobb angle calculation feature for MT (main thoracic).

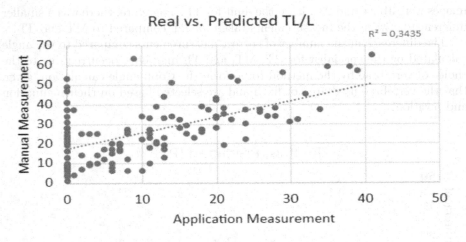

Fig. 11. Test results of the automatic Cobb angle calculation feature for TL/L (thoracolumbar or lumbar).

As shown, good results were obtained, even though there were some significant differences between the measurements. It is therefore possible to use the application in everyday clinical practice.

5   Conclusion

Three functionalities have been developed to calculate the Cobb angle: two manual ones, which require the intervention of an expert, and an automatic one that allows the calculation of three angles using image processing and deep learning techniques. The application stands out from other applications because it combines the two manual functionalities offered separately and provides an automatic method for conducting measurements, enabling an objective assessment by the specialist. In addition, by storing the exams, the professional will be able to monitor the progress of each patient's treatment. The limited number of X-ray images with the calculated Cobb angle restricted the ability to perform more tests; nonetheless, the tests demonstrated that the application can be used in clinical practice.

Furthermore, in future work, we intend to develop a method to calculate the Cobb angle automatically, also based on segmenting the spine in X-ray images as an initial step and then using a regression network to measure the Cobb angle, using approaches such as that presented in [9], whose method obtained good results.

Acknowledgement(s). The authors acknowledge the Coordenação de Aperfeiçoamento de Pessoal de Nível Superior (CAPES) - Finance Code 001, Brazil, Conselho Nacional de Desenvolvimento Científico e Tecnológico (CNPq), Brazil, and Fundação de Amparo à Pesquisa e ao Desenvolvimento Científico e Tecnológico do Maranhão (FAPEMA), Brazil, for the financial support.

References

1. Beucher, S.: Use of watersheds in contour detection. In: Proceedings of the International Workshop on Image Processing, September 1979, pp. 17–21 (1979)
2. Center, S.C.: Scoliosis Facts and Figures (2022). https://www.spinecorrectioncenter.com/scoliosis-facts-and-figures. Accessed 18 Aug 2023
3. Clevert, D.A., Unterthiner, T., Hochreiter, S.: Fast and accurate deep network learning by exponential linear units (ELUS) (2015). arXiv preprint arXiv:1511.07289
4. Cui, J.L., Gao, D.D., Shen, S.J., Wang, L.Z., Zhao, Y.: Cobb angle measurement method of scoliosis based on u-net network (2021)
5. Dubost, F., et al.: Automated estimation of the spinal curvature via spine centerline extraction with ensembles of cascaded neural networks. In: Cai, Y., Wang, L., Audette, M., Zheng, G., Li, S. (eds.) CSI 2019. LNCS, vol. 11963, pp. 88–94. Springer, Cham (2020). https://doi.org/10.1007/978-3-030-39752-4_10
6. Franko, O.I., Bray, C., Newton, P.O.: Validation of a scoliometer smartphone app to assess scoliosis. J. Pediatr. Orthop. **32**(8), e72–e75 (2012)
7. Khanal, B., Dahal, L., Adhikari, P., Khanal, B.: Automatic cobb angle detection using vertebra detector and vertebra corners regression. In: Cai, Y., Wang, L., Audette, M., Zheng, G., Li, S. (eds.) CSI 2019. LNCS, vol. 11963, pp. 81–87. Springer, Cham (2020). https://doi.org/10.1007/978-3-030-39752-4_9
8. Kim, K.C., Yun, H.S., Kim, S., Seo, J.K.: Automation of spine curve assessment in frontal radiographs using deep learning of vertebral-tilt vector. IEEE Access **8**, 84618–84630 (2020)
9. Liang, Y., Lv, J., Li, D., Yang, X., Wang, Z., Li, Q.: Accurate cobb angle estimation on scoliosis x-ray images via deeply-coupled two-stage network with differentiable cropping and random perturbation. IEEE J. Biomed. Health Inform. **27**(3), 1488–1499 (2022)

10. Maguire, D.: Darraghmaguire (2020). https://github.com/darraghmaguire/automatic-scoliosis-assessment. Accessed 18 Aug 2023
11. Maguire, D.: Scoliosis Tools (2020). https://www.scoliosistools.com/. Accessed 18 Aug 2023
12. MathWorks: Matlab (2023). https://www.mathworks.com/products/matlab.html. Accessed 18 Aug 2023
13. Pudles, E., Defino, H.L.: A coluna vertebral: conceitos básicos. Artmed Editora (2014)
14. Ronneberger, O., Fischer, P., Brox, T.: U-Net: convolutional networks for biomedical image segmentation. In: Navab, N., Hornegger, J., Wells, W.M., Frangi, A.F. (eds.) MICCAI 2015. LNCS, vol. 9351, pp. 234–241. Springer, Cham (2015). https://doi.org/10.1007/978-3-319-24574-4_28
15. Salehi, S.S.M., Erdogmus, D., Gholipour, A.: Tversky loss function for image segmentation using 3D fully convolutional deep networks. In: Wang, Q., Shi, Y., Suk, H.-I., Suzuki, K. (eds.) MLMI 2017. LNCS, vol. 10541, pp. 379–387. Springer, Cham (2017). https://doi.org/10.1007/978-3-319-67389-9_44
16. Shaw, M., Adam, C.J., Izatt, M.T., Licina, P., Askin, G.N.: Use of the iphone for cobb angle measurement in scoliosis. Eur. Spine J. **21**, 1062–1068 (2012)
17. Strauss, A.: The Truth About Adult Scoliosis: What You Need to Know About History, Treatment Options, and How to Prevent Progression. Hudson Valley Scoliosis (2018)
18. Vavruch, L.: Adolescent Idiopathic Scoliosis: A Deformity in Three Dimensions, vol. 1635. Linköping University Electronic Press, Sweden (2018)
19. Wu, H., Bailey, C., Rasoulinejad, P., Li, S.: Automatic landmark estimation for adolescent idiopathic scoliosis assessment using BoostNet. In: Descoteaux, M., Maier-Hein, L., Franz, A., Jannin, P., Collins, D.L., Duchesne, S. (eds.) MICCAI 2017. LNCS, vol. 10433, pp. 127–135. Springer, Cham (2017). https://doi.org/10.1007/978-3-319-66182-7_15

Optimising Wheelchair Path Planning

B. Ribeiro[1], Paulo A. Salgado[1], T.-P. Azevedo Perdicoúlis[1], and Paulo Lopes dos Santos[2(✉)]

[1] ECT, UTAD, Vila Real 5000-811, Portugal
al74565@alunos.utad.pt, {psal,tazevedo}@utad.pt
[2] FEUP, UP, Porto 4200-465, Portugal
pjsantos@fe.up.pt

Abstract. This article addresses the problem of wheelchair path planning. In particular, to minimize the length of the trajectory within an environment containing a variable number of obstacles. The positions and quantities of these obstacles are pre-determined. To tackle this challenge, we present a methodology that integrates optimisation techniques and heuristic algorithms to find trajectories both optimal and collision-free. The effectiveness of this methodology is illustrated through a practical example, demonstrating how it successfully generates a collision-free trajectory, even when a large number of obstacles is present in the workspace. In the future, we intend to continue investigating the same problem, taking into account energy consumption as well as time minimisation.

Keywords: Energy · Optimisation · Robotics · Wheelchair path planning · Obstacle avoidance

1 Introduction

Efficient and safe navigation in wheelchair mobility is a paramount concern for individuals with mobility impairments. In this article, we delve into the realm of Optimizing Wheelchair Path Planning, exploring advanced strategies and technologies aimed at enhancing the quality of life for wheelchair users. By addressing the intricate challenges of path planning in an environment populated with a variable number of obstacles, we aim to empower individuals with greater independence and accessibility while minimizing trajectory length and ensuring a smooth and obstacle-free journey. Minimizing the wheelchair trajectory length offers several significant benefits for individuals with mobility impairments and their caregivers. Namely:

P. A. Salgado—Supported by FCT - Fundação para a Ciência e a Tecnologia under project UIDB/04033/2020.
T.-P. Azevedo Perdicoúlis—Supported by FCT - Fundação para a Ciência e a Tecnologia under project IDB/00048/2020.
P. L. dos Santos—Supported by FCT - Fundação para a Ciência e a Tecnologia under project UIDB/50014/2020.

A. Cunha et al. (Eds.): MobiHealth 2023, LNICST 578, pp. 59–72, 2024.
https://doi.org/10.1007/978-3-031-60665-6_5

Efficiency—A shorter path allows wheelchair users to reach their destination more quickly and with less effort. This can be particularly crucial in emergencies or time-sensitive situations. Reduced Fatigue—A shorter trajectory means less physical exertion for the wheelchair user, which can reduce fatigue and discomfort, enhancing his overall comfort and well-being during transit. Extended Battery Life—Electric wheelchairs and mobility devices typically rely on batteries. By minimizing the trajectory length, less power is consumed during each journey, leading to an extended battery life and reducing the frequency of recharging. Improved Safety—Shorter paths often translate to reduced exposure to potential hazards and obstacles, thereby enhancing safety during mobility. This is especially important in environments with complex layouts or high traffic. Enhanced Independence—An optimized trajectory empowers wheelchair users with a greater sense of independence and autonomy, as they can navigate their environment more efficiently without relying as heavily on assistance from others. Increased Accessibility—In public spaces, shorter paths can contribute to increased accessibility for wheelchair users. By reducing the need for lengthy detours or workarounds, it promotes equitable access to facilities and services. Time Savings—Minimizing trajectory length saves time, which can be vital in daily life, whether it's for work, appointments, or leisure activities. It allows wheelchair users to allocate their time more effectively and engage in a wider range of activities. Cost Savings—For those using motorized wheelchairs or other mobility devices, less wear and tear on the equipment can lead to reduced maintenance and replacement costs over time. Enhanced Quality of Life—Ultimately, optimizing wheelchair path planning contributes to an improved overall quality of life for individuals with mobility impairments. It reduces the physical and logistical challenges they face daily, allowing them to focus on pursuing their goals and enjoying a fuller, more active life.

To achieve the goal of minimizing distance, various strategies can be employed. These strategies encompass advanced Navigation Algorithms such as Dijkstra's [4,12,14,16], A-star [9,12,14], Probabilistic Roadmaps (PRM) [1] or Rapidly-exploring Random Trees (RRT) [1,11], which are used to discover the shortest path while navigating around obstacles. Both Dijkstra's and A-star are categorized as grid-based algorithms. Grid-based algorithms partition the environment into a grid structure and employ search techniques within this grid. These algorithms are particularly well-suited for discrete, grid-like environments but may not exhibit the same level of efficiency in continuous spaces.

Conversely, RPM and RRT are sampling-based approaches. These methods use random sampling to explore the configuration space and establish connections between sampled points to construct a path. While these techniques can be highly efficient, they typically yield sub-optimal, non-repetitive solutions. Moreover, they often encounter difficulties in situations that necessitate navigating through narrow gaps or passages within the configuration space.

More recently, machine learning algorithms, exemplified by reinforcement learning in [6], and deep learning in [8], have found applications in wheelchair path planning. These methods are capable of learning from data and adapting to diverse environments. Deep learning techniques excel at capturing intricate and non-linear relationships between sensory inputs and desired paths. However, they usually demand a substantial amount of labeled training data, which can be both costly and time-consuming to amass and annotate. Additionally, deep learning models do not offer assurances regarding the optimality or safety of the generated paths or decisions, as their decisions are rooted in statistical patterns learned from data.

In contrast, reinforcement learning provides a versatile and adaptive approach to obstacle avoidance, enabling robots to acquire effective avoidance strategies through interaction with their surroundings. Nevertheless, it can be computationally intensive, and the design of the reward function and training process play pivotal roles in determining the success of the model.

Additionally to theses strategies, effective hardware designs are crucial, which entails incorporating electronic sensors capable of continuously monitoring the system's state. A central computing unit, such as a microcontroller or a microprocessor, can implement intelligent control strategies to optimise the path, reduce waste, and adapt the wheelchair behaviour to environmental conditions during the task execution [5]. Some systems involve human input to guide the path planning process. Users can interact with a graphical interface or joystick to navigate the wheelchair, with the system assisting in avoiding obstacles [4].

In this article, a motion planning approach to minimize the trajectory's length of a wheelchair in an environment populated with circular obstacles is proposed [10]. The wheelchair moves in like a Bratenberg vehicle using an algorithm that efficiently identifies feasible trajectories without any collisions. The study tests the proposed strategies using a wheelchair equipped with two DC motors or servomotors. The primary objective is to develop and assess a trajectory planning system with dual functionality: (i) to avoid obstacles within the workspace, (ii) to optimise the trajectory length. To accomplish this, the direct and inverse kinematic models were constructed.

During a simple movement with constant actuation, the wheelchair follows a semicircular trajectory, where the curvature radius and center coordinates are determined by the rotation amplitude of the two driving wheels. If the right wheel undergoes a greater displacement (larger rotation amplitude) than the left wheel, the wheelchair moves along a circular path in the opposite direction of the clockwise motion. When both wheels have equal amplitudes of movement, the wheelchair travels in a straight line, equivalent to an infinite curvature radius. While executing these basic movements, the wheelchair can initiate from any starting point, take an arbitrary initial direction, and reach any point in space through a curved circular path, eventually reaching the desired endpoint. However, it lacks the freedom to control the arrival angle. It is evident that this basic movement is not the most efficient way to travel from the initial to the final point. In practice, a trajectory consists of multiple basic movements, each with reduced amplitude and a narrow time window.

To enable a broader range of motion between two points, we introduce an inverse model featuring three distinct points, which includes an intermediate time moment that requires determination. This methodology guarantees a trajectory characterized by reduced curvature, shorter travel distance, and the capability to manage the desired final orientation. This model is the basis of the proposed optimization strategy, and further details can be found in Sects. 2, 3.1, and 3.2.

The optimisation of this differential drive—the wheelchair—trajectory is an NP-complex problem for which there are no fully capable methods that can simultaneously find the shortest path and avoid obstacles. The Particle Swarm Optimization (PSO) algorithm possesses characteristics that make it a potential method to solve the optimization problem with near-optimal perspectives. The PSO algorithm is inspired by the social behavior of birds flocking or fish schooling. It was first introduced by James Kennedy and Russell Eberhart in 1995 [3, 7]. PSO is a type of meta-heuristic algorithm, which means that it is not based on explicit mathematical models but rather on probabilistic methods to explore and find optimal solutions in complex search spaces.

The base algorithm and its variants are among the most popular and capable methods for solving various optimization problems in high-dimensional spaces, where traditional methods may struggle due to the high dimensionality and non-linearity of the search space, in various fields, including engineering, robotics, finance, and data mining [2]. However, to use it in the path optimisation problem requires some modifications to make it convergent and adequately explore the solution space.

The proposed path planning algorithm initiates by generating a set of random trajectories. To each trajectory it is assigned a cost equal to its length, and it incurs a penalty from a barrier function if it intersects with an obstacle. These trajectories are then updated following the PSO framework, meaning they all endeavor to approach the best trajectory encountered so far while simultaneously exploring new regions within the workspace. The algorithm halts after a specified number of iterations or upon detecting convergence in the best trajectory.

The method we present can be seen as an hybrid, combining aspects of both sampling-based and reinforcement learning approaches. It exhibits sampling-based characteristics as the trajectories are randomly generated and subsequently updated in a stochastic manner. Additionally, it embraces reinforcement learning principles because the cost associated with the trajectories acts as feedback, akin to a reward, directing the exploration of new areas within the workspace. A Matlab R2022 program was developed to implement the proposed method and provide a way to test, simulate, and validate the results.

Besides this introduction, this paper is structured as follows: The direct kine-matic mode is presented in Sect. 2, followed by the inverse kinematic models—the one-step and the two-step—in Sect. 3. Section 4 outlines the PSO algorithm and explains how it is used to determine the optimal solution for the trajectory. The case study that illustrates the methodology is presented in Sect. 5, as well as the discussion of the obtained results. Finally, the main conclusions and the work outlook are presented in Sect. 6.

2   Direct Kinematic Model

The wheelchair's position and orientation are determined by its coordinates and steering angle, representing its direction relative to a reference direction, typi-cally the OX axis. At a specific discrete time instant t_i, the wheelchair is located at position P_i and oriented at an angle ϕ_i. Its movement is influenced by the uniform motion of its wheels, with amplitudes $\Delta S_{R,i}$ and $\Delta S_{L,i}$ for the right and left wheels, respectively. As it moves, the wheelchair follows a semi-circular trajectory to reach position P_{i+1} while aligning itself with a direction ϕ_{i+1}. Figure 1 illustrates the counterclockwise trajectory and the main geometric vari-ables involved.

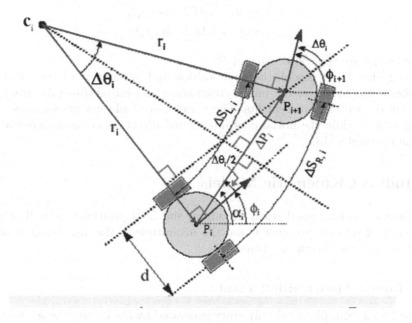

Fig. 1. Movement in the counterclockwise direction

In the time interval between t_i and t_{i+1}, the wheelchair executes circular motion, with its center at c_i, transitioning from point from point P_i to point

P_{i+1}. The parameters that describe this movement include the angle of rotation and the radius of curvature, which are given by:

$$\Delta\theta_i = \frac{\Delta S_{R,i} - \Delta S_{L,i}}{d}, \tag{1}$$

$$r_i = \frac{d}{2} \cdot \frac{\Delta S_{L,i} + \Delta S_{R,i}}{\Delta S_{L,i} - \Delta S_{R,i}} = \frac{1}{2} \cdot \frac{v_{L,i} + v_{R,i}}{\Delta\theta_i/\Delta t}, \tag{2}$$

where d is the length of the axle. The linear velocities of the right and left wheels are denoted as $v_{R,i} = \frac{\Delta S_{R,i}}{\Delta t}$ and $v_{L,i} = \frac{\Delta S_{L,i}}{\Delta t}$, respectively. Δt indicates the time interval of the movement. The distance between P_i and P_{i+1} is $|\Delta P_i| = 2r_i \sin\left(\frac{\Delta\theta_i}{2}\right)$. Additionally, the angular direction at P_{i+1} is given by: $\phi_{i+1} = \phi_i + \Delta\theta_i$, where ϕ_i is the steering angle at position P_i. The displacement vector ΔP_i of the wheelchair forms an angle with the horizontal equal to $\Delta\theta_i$, and the phase angle α_i, representing the angle of the displacement vector, is given by:

$$\alpha_i = \phi_i + \frac{\Delta\theta_i}{2}. \tag{3}$$

Finally, the Cartesian coordinates of the endpoint P_{i+1} are given by:

$$x_{i+1} = x_i + |\Delta P_i| \cdot \cos(\alpha_i), \tag{4}$$

$$y_{i+1} = y_i + |\Delta P_i| \cdot \sin(\alpha_i), \tag{5}$$

where (x_i, y_i) are the coordinates of P_i.

Using this direct model, the new position and orientation of the robot can be determined based on the initial coordinates and initial direction, using the values of the wheel displacements. The wheelchair displacements serve as internal variables, while the initial coordinates and direction are considered as the external variables [13].

3   Indirect Kinematic Models

The inverse model is used when the initial and final positions, as well as their respective directions, are known and the magnitude of the displacement of the two wheels is not known in advance.

3.1   Inverse Model with 2–Point

Figure 2 is an example of the trajectory generated by the inverse model, with the positions P_i and P_{i+1} known *a priori*, along with the starting angles ϕ_i and α_i. The angle α_i represents the orientation of the wheelchair's displacement vector relative to the horizontal and it is given by:

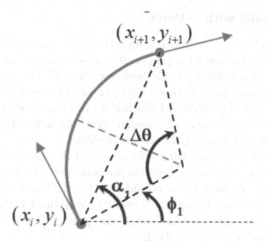

Fig. 2. Clockwise movement

$$\alpha_i = \tan^{-1}\left(\frac{\Delta y_i}{\Delta x_i}\right), \tag{6}$$

where Δx_i and Δy_i are the increments in the (x, y) coordinates. The curvature angle of the trajectory is calculated by:

$$\Delta\theta_i = 2(\alpha_i - \phi_i) \tag{7}$$

corresponding to the radius:

$$r_i = \frac{|\Delta P_i|}{2\sin(\alpha_i - \phi_i)}, \tag{8}$$

where $|\Delta P_i| = \sqrt{(x_{i+1} - x_i)^2 + (y_{i+1} - y_i)^2}$. To execute this movement, the wheelchair's wheels must move by:

$$\Delta S_i = \frac{|\Delta P_i|}{\sin(\alpha_i - \phi_i)} = \frac{|\Delta P_i|}{\sin(\frac{\Delta\phi_i}{2})}. \tag{9}$$

The arrival angle ϕ_{i+1} is determined by Eq. (4), which, combined with Eq. (5), results into:

$$\phi_{i+1} = 2 \times \alpha_i - \phi_i, \tag{10}$$

making it a dependent variable. As a consequence, it is not possible to reach the final point with a different desired direction.

3.2 Inverse Model with 3–Point

The previous model does not allow reaching the final point with a desired angle. Hence, a 3-point inverse model is proposed, introducing an intermediate point, P_2, to achieve the final point in the desired direction. The inverse 3–point model determines the optimal path between two points, P_1 and P_3, passing through an intermediate point, P_2, while calculating its position and the corresponding tangent angle to the trajectory. This model, given its flexibility, will be applied to the wheelchair's trajectory optimisation problem.

The goal of the 3–point inverse model is to find the most efficient trajectory, minimising the distance traveled. For this purpose, the coordinates and orientation of the points P_1, P_2, and P_3 are considered. Point P_2 acts as an intermediary point along the trajectory. Using the 3–point inverse model, one can determine the ideal coordinates and trajectory angle for point $P2$, resulting in the best path between P_1 and P_3 (see Fig. 3) [13].

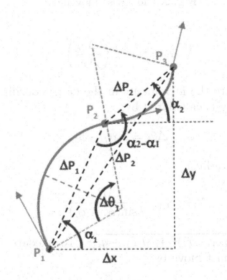

Fig. 3. Movement of the inverse model with three points

Through a geometric analysis and considering the direct model from Sect. 2, applying (10) twice and for $i = 1$ and $i = 2$, it follows that:

$$\phi_3 = 2(\alpha_2 - \alpha_1) + \phi_1. \tag{11}$$

Similarly, we have $\phi_2 = 2\alpha_1 - \phi_1$, or in alternative:

$$\phi_2 = 2\alpha_2 - \phi_3. \tag{12}$$

By combining the displacement vectors from P_1 to P_2 and from P_2 to P_3, it results in:

$$\begin{cases} x_3 = x_1 + |\Delta P_1|.cos(\alpha_1) + |\Delta P_2|.cos(\alpha_2), \\ y_3 = y_1 + |\Delta P_1|.sin(\alpha_1) + |\Delta P_2|.sin(\alpha_2). \end{cases} \tag{13}$$

Hence, the system is constrained by the following three equations:

$$\begin{cases} \Delta x = |\Delta P_1|.cos(\alpha_1) + \Delta P_2|.cos(\alpha_2), \\ \Delta y = |\Delta P_1|.sin(\alpha_1) + \Delta P_2|.sin(\alpha_2), \\ \Delta\phi = \phi_3 - \phi_1 = 2(\alpha_2 - \alpha_1), \end{cases} \tag{14}$$

where the unknowns are $\Delta P_1, \Delta P_2, \alpha_1, \alpha_2$, resulting in one degree of freedom. After some algebraic manipulations, we obtain:

$$\Delta P_1 = \frac{\Delta x \times sin(\alpha_2) - \Delta y \times cos(\alpha_2)}{sin(\phi_m)}, \tag{15}$$

$$\Delta P_2 = \frac{\Delta x \times sin(\phi_m - \alpha_2) + \Delta y \times cos(\phi_m - \alpha_2)}{sin(\phi_m)}, \tag{16}$$

where $\phi_m = \alpha_2 - \alpha_1 = \frac{\Delta\phi}{2}$. Assuming $|\Delta P_1| = |\Delta P_2|$, we find:

$$\alpha_2 = \tan^{-1}\left(\frac{\Delta y}{\Delta x}\right) + \frac{1}{2}\phi_m. \tag{17}$$

By substituting this result into Eq. (12), the angle ϕ_2 can be calculated. With the above direct model, it becomes possible to determine the position of point P_2, thus solving the problem.

4   Particle Swarm Optimization Algorithm

The PSO algorithm is an optimisation technique inspired by the social behavior of animals, such as insect swarms, bird flocks, or fish schools. It was proposed by Eberhart and Kennedy in 1995 [7]. PSO works by simulating the social behavior of these animals to find solutions of complex problems. It does this by generating a population of particles, each of which represents a potential solution to the problem. The particles then move through the search space, updating their positions based on their own best-known solution. PSO is particularly well-suited for problems with complex search spaces and multiple optima. It has been applied in a variety of fields, including engineering, computer science, and economics [15].

In the context of path optimization, PSO can be used to find the shortest and safest path between two points, taking into account obstacles. Each particle represents a potential path, with a cost determined by its length and its minimum distance to an obstacle, given by.

$$V = L + \exp(-5D) \tag{18}$$

where:

- V is the cost of the particle
- L is the length of the path
- D is the minimum distance of the path to an obstacle

If the trajectory crosses an obstacle, D is negative and the cost is exponentially increased. This is because the algorithm is trying to discourage trajectories from crossing obstacles. Therefore, the second term of the cost function, $\exp(-5D)$, acts as a barrier function. It penalizes paths that cross obstacles, making it less likely that they will be selected as the best solution.

Each particle X_i is made up of N points with coordinates $x_{i1}, \ldots, x_{iN}$ in the workspace, i.e.

$$X_i = \begin{bmatrix} x_{i1} \ldots x_{iN} \end{bmatrix}^T \in \mathbb{R}^{N \times 2} \tag{19}$$

with $x_{ij} \in \mathbb{R}^2$. If one or more of the points change, the particle moves to a new position. The speed of the trajectory is determined by the difference between the old and the new positions, divided by the number of steps. The algorithm works by iteratively updating the position of each particle based on its current position and the best position it has found so far. The algorithm terminates when a stopping criterion is met, and the solution is the path with the smallest cost. In each iteration, denoted as t, the ith particle is at position $X_i(t)$ and moves with a velocity

$$V_i(t) = \begin{bmatrix} v_{i1}(t) \, v_{i2}(t) \ldots v_{iN}(t) \end{bmatrix}^T \in \mathbb{R}^{N \times 2} \tag{20}$$

The optimum position ever reached by X_i up to iteration t is:

$$P_i(t) = \begin{bmatrix} p_{i1}(t) \, p_{i2}(t) \ldots p_{iN}(t) \end{bmatrix}^T \tag{21}$$

The particle moves around the working space of possible paths, updating its position based on the current position and the best path they have found so far. In each iteration, its position is updated by:

$$X_i(t+1) = X_i(t) + V_i(t+1). \tag{22}$$

where speed $V_i(t+1)$ is given by

$$V_i(t+1) = V_i(t) + C(P_i(t) - X_i(t)) \tag{23}$$

with C being a diagonal matrix defined as:

$$C = \begin{bmatrix} c_1 & 0 & \cdots & 0 \\ 0 & c_2 & \cdots & 0 \\ \vdots & \vdots & \ddots & \vdots \\ 0 & 0 & \cdots & c_N \end{bmatrix} \otimes I_2 R \tag{24}$$

where R is a diagonal matrix whose elements are random numbers uniformly distributed in the interval $[0, 1]$. The individual best position is updated as follows:

$$P_i(t+1) = \begin{cases} X_i(t+1), \text{ if } V(X_i(t+1)) < V(P_i(t)) \\ P_i(t), \qquad \text{otherwise} \end{cases} \tag{25}$$

where $V(X(t))$ is the cost of the trajectory $X(t)$. The PSO algorithm terminates when a stopping criterion is met, such as a maximum number of iterations or when a satisfactory solution is found. The solution is the trajectory with the smallest cost.

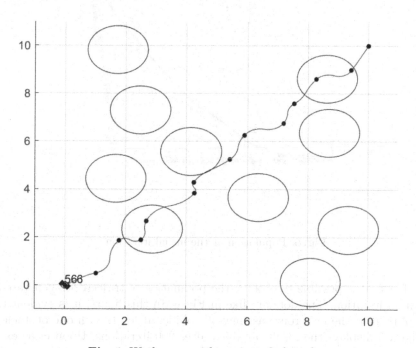

Fig. 4. Workspace with generated obstacles

5   Case Study

A simulation was performed in Matlab to test the methods mentioned above. Initially, the obstacles are generated. The wheelchair knows the number and position of each object before starting the movement. A set of (non-optimized) trajectories is generated, where the wheelchair may collide with the objects. Then, applying the 3–point method and the PSO algorithm, after several iterations, a route in which the robot moves to the destination point without any collision is obtained.

In Fig. 4, the workspace is shown with 10 objects, represented by the circles, that the robot must navigate around. The dots are the successive points used to generated the trajectory by the 3D inverse model. This is an example of a densely populated workspace. By using the method mentioned above, the wheelchair determines a trajectory without collisions to the desired destination point.

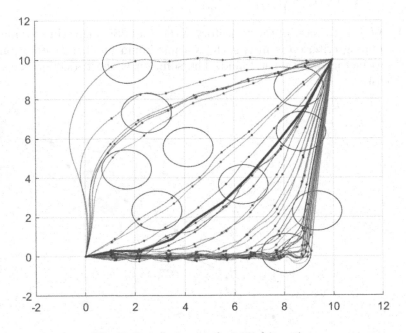

Fig. 5. Population at the initial iteration

In Fig. 5, it is possible to observe the population of trajectories generated in the initial iteration. The dots are like in Fig. 4. In this figure, it is evident that none of them is the best route as they all collide, at least, with one obstacle.

Figure 6 displays the result obtained after 200 iterations. Upon close examination, it can be seen that the robot has successfully determined a trajectory that avoids collisions (indicated by the solid red line). With a higher number of iterations, even better results could be achieved.

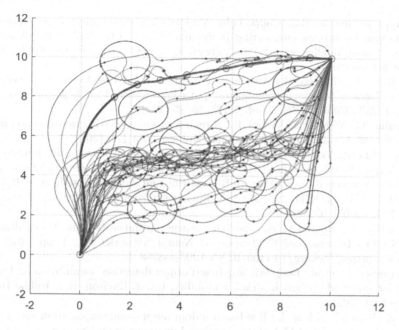

Fig. 6. Population after 200 iterations

6   Conclusions

In this work, the best trajectory was calculated for a autonomous wheelchair in a space populated with 10 objects. The objects are randomly generated at the beginning of the simulation, and the wheelchair has prior knowledge of the workspace topology. By using the 3–Point Kinematic Model and the PSO algorithm, the robot can determine and follow a feasible trajectory, i.e., reach the initial position to the final position (both predefined), without colliding with any obstacles. It was observed that with a larger number of iterations, even more satisfactory results can be achieved. As for energy and travel time optimisation, conclusive results were not possible to obtain, and it will be a matter for future improvements, thus giving continuation to this work.

Acknowledgements. The authors would like to thank the reviewers for their valuable suggestions.

References

1. Ajay, M., Srinivas, P., Netam, L.: Smart wheelchair. AI and IoT-Based Intelligent Automation in Robotics, pp. 271–284 (2021)
2. Alam, M.N.: Particle swarm optimization: algorithm and its codes in MATLAB. ResearchGate **8**(1), 10 (2016)

3. Gomes de Almeida, B.S., Coppo Leite, V.: Particle swarm optimization: a powerful technique for solving engineering problems. In: Ser, J.D., Villar, E., Osaba, E. (eds.) Swarm Intelligence—Recent Advances, New Perspectives and Applications. IntechOpen (2019)

4. Arai, K., Mardiyanto, R.: Autonomous control of eye based electric wheel chair with obstacle avoidance and shortest path finding based on Dijkstra algorithm. Int. J. Adv. Comput. Sci. Appl. **2**(12), 19–25 (2011)

5. Carabin, G., Wehrle, E., Vidoni, R.: A review on energy-saving optimization methods for robotic and automatic systems. Robotics **6**(4), 39 (2017)

6. Chatzidimitriadis, S., Sirlantzis, K.: Deep reinforcement learning for autonomous navigation in robotic wheelchairs. In: El Yacoubi, M., Granger, E., Yuen, P.C., Pal, U., Vincent, N. (eds.) Pattern Recognition and Artificial Intelligence. ICPRAI 2022. LNCS, vol. 13364, pp. 271–282. Springer, Cham (2022). https://doi.org/10.1007/978-3-031-09282-4_23

7. Kennedy, J., Eberhart, R.: Particle swarm optimization. In: Proceedings of ICNN'95 - International Conference on Neural Networks, vol. 4, pp. 1942–1948 (1995). https://doi.org/10.1109/ICNN.1995.488968

8. Lecrosnier, L., et al.: Deep learning-based object detection, localisation and tracking for smart wheelchair healthcare mobility. Int. J. Environ. Res. Public Health **18**(1), 91 (2021)

9. Li, Z., Xiong, Y., Zhou, L.: Ros-based indoor autonomous exploration and navigation wheelchair. In: 2017 10th International Symposium on Computational Intelligence and Design (ISCID), vol. 2, pp. 132–135. IEEE (2017)

10. Liu, S., Sun, D.: Minimizing energy consumption of wheeled mobile robots via optimal motion planning. IEEE/ASME **19**(2), 401–414 (2014)

11. Moon, C.B., Chung, W.: Kinodynamic planner dual-tree RRT (DT-RRT) for two-wheeled mobile robots using the rapidly exploring random tree. IEEE Trans. Ind. Electron. **62**(2), 1080–1090 (2014)

12. Randria, I., Khelifa, M.M.B., Bouchouicha, M., Abellard, P.: A comparative study of six basic approaches for path planning towards an autonomous navigation. In: IECON 2007-33rd Annual Conference of the IEEE Industrial Electronics Society, pp. 2730–2735. IEEE (2007)

13. Salgado, P.: Robótica: Cinemática e planeamento de trajetórias. UTAD (2020)

14. Sariff, N., Buniyamin, N.: An overview of autonomous mobile robot path planning algorithms. In: 2006 4th Student Conference on Research and Development, pp. 183–188. IEEE (2006)

15. Wang, D., Tan, D., Liu, L.: Particle swarm optimization algorithm: an overview. Soft Comput. **22**, 387–408 (2018)

16. Zhang, Z., Zhao, Z.: A multiple mobile robots path planning algorithm based on a-star and Dijkstra algorithm. Int. J. Smart Home **8**(3), 75–86 (2014)

eDEM-CONNECT: An Ontology-Based Chatbot for Family Caregivers of People with Dementia

Maurice Boiting[1]([✉]), Niklas Tschorn[1], Sumaiya Suravee[2], Kristina Yordanova[2], Margareta Halek[3], Franziska A. Jagoda[3], Stefan Lüdtke[4], and Anja Burmann[1]

[1] Fraunhofer Institute for Software and Systems Engineering ISST, 44147 Dortmund, Germany
{maurice.boiting,niklas.tschorn,anja.burmann}@isst.fraunhofer.de
[2] Institute for Data Science, Universität Greifswald, 17489 Greifswald, Germany
{sumaiya.suravee,kristina.yordanova}@uni-greifswald.de
[3] School of Nursing Science, Faculty of Health, Universiät Witten/Herdecke, 58453 Witten, Germany
{margareta.halek,franziska.jagoda}@uni-wh.de
[4] Institute for Visual and Analytic Computing, Universät Rostock, 18059 Rostock, Germany
stefan.luedtke@uni-rostock.de

Abstract. Home care of people with dementia (PwD) is mainly organized and carried out by non-professional family caregivers, who struggle to interpret the needs of PwD correctly and are confronted with the challenging behavior of their relatives. Although support services for family caregivers are widespread in Germany, they are rarely used due to the fact that information is poorly organized and relatives are faced with a flood of disorganized, outdated, and confusing content. Due to the technical development of chatbot technologies (*ChatGPT*), chatbots gain more and more relevance. Based on the new technological possibilities, we developed an online communication and service platform with an integrated chatbot within the *eDEM-CONNECT* project, with the aim of making structured and easily understandable information accessible for family caregivers. This work focuses on the development of a chatbot pipeline that has broad domain knowledge through a provided ontology on the topic of agitation of PwD. This allows the chatbot to provide relevant and peer-reviewed information to family members. In our approach, a patient history is first taken based on several diagnostic questions so that relevant information can be output in a later step. For this purpose, we demonstrate that agitations in natural language can be correctly recognized by the used *BERT model* and that our developed chatbot is able to select further diagnostic questions based on the predictions of a *Markov logic network*.

Keywords: chatbot · ontology · home care · natural language processing · transformer models · Markov logic network

M. Boiting and N. Tschorn—contributed equally to this work.

A. Cunha et al. (Eds.): MobiHealth 2023, LNICST 578, pp. 73–91, 2024.
https://doi.org/10.1007/978-3-031-60665-6_6

1   Introduction

The home care of people with dementia (PwD) is mostly organized and executed by their relatives. According to the German Ageing Survey (DEAS) 04/2022 [13], there are about 1.8 million people with dementia and a total of 1.4 million caregiving relatives of PwD in Germany in 2022 [9]. The main challenge for family caregivers in this context is the confrontation with agitation and challenging behavior [27]. Relatives are often no professional caregivers and struggle to recognize the needs of PwD correctly. PwD often express their needs in actions [18] that are misinterpreted as aggressive behavior [23]. The challenging behavior often results in an increasingly unstable relationship between the PwD and their caregiving relatives and therefore mostly leads to the PwD moving to a retirement home [8].

Help services for family caregivers are widespread in Germany but rarely used [16] due to the sheer amount of these services and regarding the fact that the information on them is mostly very poorly organized. Most users first contact occurs via an online search engine like Google. In such a case, the information is commonly presented unsorted and might even contain sources that contradict each other. Unhelpful and confusing content like outdated information or local law differences due to Germany's federal state system can not be filtered out. Caregivers have often expressed their need to understand the changing behavior of the PwD, emphasizing that, in their belief, the family home was the best place for the PwD to stay [19]. Therefore, there is a strong demand for user-centered, tailored and up to date information in the domain of familycare of PwD.

Studies have shown the potential that chatbots can provide in the area of home care of PwD. They offer constant availability and intuitive usability, especially for elderly people who tend to have a lower affinity towards current technology [17,28]. Nonetheless, chatbots that address such topics are still in their infancy and users are challenged when trying to solve more complex problems with these bots [22].

In recent years, chatbot technology has gained an increased amount of attention in the technological and scientific field. More and more schematic tasks, typically performed by humans (like telephone services), are now outsourced to chatbots [24]. Due to its rising popularity in recent years, chatbot technology has improved as well, enabling the bots to handle increasingly complex tasks [24]. New use cases keep occurring and raise the need for new, more advanced and problem-specific chatbot technology. Easy tasks might just require a simple question-answer pattern, while more complex tasks require a set of multiple questions, the need to store the conversation context during the runtime of the bot or the domain knowledge of complex thematical landscapes. Designing such technology for more advanced user scenarios to be addressed by chatbots is a relevant question in the current chatbot development and scientific research [5].

In the *eDEM-CONNECT* project we developed a chatbot-based online communication and service platform. For intelligent interactions of the chatbot with caregiving relatives, we present a new approach based on a transformer model for understanding user input and a *Markov logic network (MLN)* to be able to react intelligently to these user concerns through reasoning.

The goal of this project was to provide structured information for family caregivers on dementia and agitation, empowering them to confront their everyday challenges with their relatives. In contrast to the unstructured nature of search engines, the information should be presented in an easy to understand and user-friendly form. Besides information on dementia and agitation itself, the platform provides information on local care facilities, which can be categorized and searched based on their offered services. The user can utilize the chatbot to navigate through the website and also communicate directly with the bot to find the exact help texts and instructions he needs in a given situation. To ensure the quality and correctness of the provided information, the chatbot uses an expert-validated ontology as its knowledge base, in contrast to other chatbots that only operate on raw dialog data. This is crucial due to the fact that false information in a health-critical domain like this one can possibly cause great harm.

In this paper, we present the results of the project *eDEM-CONNECT* and discuss whether a chatbot is able to offer a helpful user interface and functionality in this specific context. The chatbot is operated in German language and provides curated and purposeful information instead of the more chaotic results of search engines. It offers an intuitive and easy to use interface, even for elderly users with low technical affinity. We examine how effectively the chatbot is capable to identify the domain-specific concepts and user intents and discuss the potential for further development and technical limitations.

2   Related Work

A chatbot is a computer program designed to hold an intelligent conversation between a human user and the bot itself [1]. The most simple chatbots come in the form of decision trees, while more complex chatbots are able to have open conversations with the user. They rely on full-text search engines, searching for specific keywords to identify the users' intents [1,2].

A current milestone in the development of chatbot technology is the project *ChatGPT* by OpenAI. It features a non-topic-specific chatbot that is able to react and chat about a wide variety of subjects and is even able to perform creative tasks like generating a speech on a given topic. *ChatGPT* was launched in November 2022 and had already reached a number of 100 million active users in January 2023, only two months after its release [7,14].

In the medicine domain, the diagnostic app *Ada Health* enables the user to specify his symptoms, which are then analyzed by its chatbot. The bot provides possible causes of the symptoms and also a likeliness parameter for the given diagnoses or the option to consult a doctor directly.[1] *OneRemission* is an app designated to cancer patients and survivors. Its chatbot provides diets, exercises and post-cancer activities, empowering the user's independence. The

---

[1] https://ada.com/de/ (accessed: 2023-11-01).

provided information is curated by medical experts, so the user does not always need to rely on a doctor regarding a cancer-specific question.[2] *MediBot* uses an integrated ontology as its knowledge base and provides information on drug medication for Portuguese-speaking users [4]. *DigiCare* combines natural language processing techniques and dynamic Bayesian inference to provide a conversational intelligent tutoring system, aiming to deliver study materials for nursing subjects [25].

In the dementia and care domain, *Elisabot* is a chatbot that supports its users in reminiscence therapy by showing them pictures of past experiences and asking therapy questions about them. The questions regarding the pictures are automatically generated by the chatbot [6]. *AlzBot* offers training for the user to challenge the memory loss of Alzheimer's patients and also provides the opportunity to track the location of the patient to reduce the caregivers' burden [15]. The *Androz Chatbot* and *Companion Chatbot* also provide memory training but also offer features like geo-fencing that offer guidance for PwD that struggle with orientation when wandering around [26, 29].

The *Care* chatbot developed by Müller et al. [17] provided a set of questionnaires, mostly related to biographic contents. In a study they examined the potential use cases and effectiveness of chatbots in the dementia domain. In conclusion, the chatbots were welcomed by the users and provided information, empowering the patients to be more self-reliant, but on the other hand, marked the current limitations and also pointed out the importance of human caregivers that will still remain irreplaceable. Due to the fact that most chatbots are still in their infancy, the use cases remain mostly simple tasks, and more complex user scenarios offer potential for further development.

3   Methods

In chatbot development, several questions have to be addressed. First of all, the exact problem of the caregiver concerning the PwD must be identified to provide suitable knowledge. In addition, depending on the current course of the conversation, a chatbot needs to ask other appropriate questions in order to ensure an optimal diagnosis. In our approach, we addressed this problem through different methods and present a chatbot pipeline that serves as a support for relatives of PwD. Our pipeline is therefore divided into three parts (cf. Fig. 1): interpretation of the user input with the *BERT model (Bidirectional Encoder Representations from Transformers)* [10], prediction of the next diagnosis question with a *Markov logic network (MLN)* and output of relevant knowledge with a given ontology created by domain experts. In the next sections, we will first present the conversation flow with the chatbot and then introduce our ontology-based chatbot pipeline.

---

[2] https://keenethics.com/project-one-remission (accessed: 2023-11-01).

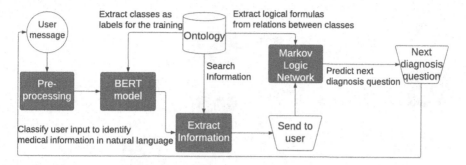

Fig. 1. The figure shows the technical pipeline of the chatbot. First, the user messages are preprocessed, removing umlauts, punctuation (except question marks), double spaces, pronouns and names of reference persons. In addition, only lowercase letters were used. Preprocessed user messages are classified according to medical ontology classes using the BERT model. Based on these identified classes, queries are used to extract information from the ontology that is forwarded to the user as the response. Finally, to ask further diagnostic questions, a Markov logic network is used to predict the most relevant diagnostic question for the current situation.

3.1 Chatbot Conversation Flow

In the course of a chat conversation, the chatbot asks several diagnostic questions until the problem has been sufficiently localized and advice can be given to solve the relative's problem. For this purpose, the chatbot is able to ask open and closed questions, where the closed questions can only be answered with *yes, no* or *maybe*.

This mixture of open as well as closed questions allows the chatbot to effectively recognize medical concepts in the user's chat messages. For each recognized concept, help texts with concrete suggestions for solving the problem (e.g., tips for communication or guidelines to recognize pain in PwD) are provided.

The user can choose for each help text whether to access a long or a short version of the provided content. Furthermore, in certain cases (e.g., more urgent problems), intervention strategies are issued in addition to the help texts to give the relatives concrete recommendations for action. A schematic representation of the conversation flow is shown in Fig. 2.

In addition to interpreting answers to diagnostic questions, the chatbot is also able to recognize other user intents (cf. Table 1) such as asking for regional help or requesting completely different topics.

3.2 Ontology Driven Knowledge Base

In order to provide caregivers helpful knowledge and information such as help texts, advice, intervention strategies as well as contact details of local institutions, it is necessary that the chatbot has a broad domain knowledge in a

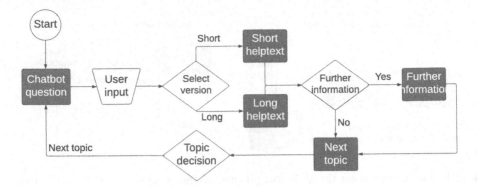

Fig. 2. The figure shows the flow of the conversation with the chatbot. The chatbot first asks a diagnosis question, which the user answers. A help text is then given to the user in order to be able to provide assistance with the user's problem. Since help texts are available in a long and a short version, the user is asked beforehand whether the short or the full long version should be displayed. Afterwards, regardless of the version selected, the user is asked whether further information (e.g., in the form of links) should be delivered. Finally, the user is asked on which topic he would like to have information next in order to be able to ask another diagnosis question.

machine-readable representation. Therefore, our approach uses a topic-specific ontology on the challenging behavior of PwD. An ontology is described as a structured representation of knowledge, encompassing a set of concepts situated in a specific domain, along with the relationship that is linked between these concepts [12].[3]

In our case, different aspects associated with dementia were modeled in the ontology by domain experts (cf. Fig. 3): The *agitation* i.e., the behavior of the PwD, *causes* that can cause the agitation, *consequences* caused by the agitation, characteristics of the *person with dementia* itself (e.g., abilities and medication) and intervention strategies (*interventions*).

In order to narrow down the problem, the approach was limited to only five different types of agitation:

- *Physical aggressive (PA)*: e.g., the PwD is throwing objects or has violent behavior,
- *Physical non-aggressive (PNA)*: e.g., the PwD is wandering around at night or is restless,
- *Verbal aggressive (VA)*: e.g., the PwD offends other people,
- *Verbal non-aggressive (VNA)*: e.g., the PwD keeps repeating the same question,
- *Resisting care (RC)*: e.g., the PwD refuses to be washed or dressed.

---

[3] The *eDEM-CONNECT* ontology was developed in the Web Ontology Language (OWL) using the software *Protégé*: https://protege.stanford.edu/ (accessed: 2023-08-31).

Table 1. Overview of all chatbot intents and representation of corresponding utterances.

Intent	Description	Example user utterances
Answer to diagnosis question	The user answers a question posed by the chatbot	Yes, my husband is in pain
Request for another topic	The user wants information on a completely different topic	I would rather know more about communication
Local help	Provides an overview of aids in the user's local area	Where can I get help near me?
Change helptext version	Changes the available version of the last sent help text	I would prefer to have the long version

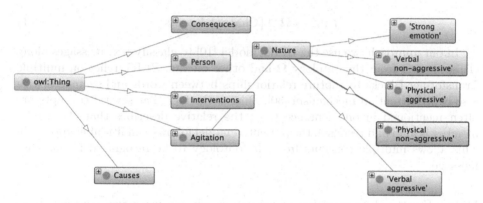

Fig. 3. An excerpt of the classes from the ontology that are relevant for the chatbot. Hierarchical relationships between the concepts are shown. The figure was taken as a screenshot from the software *Protégé*.

Helpful and unknown to the user information is searched in the ontology via $SPARQL^4$ queries, based on the previous conversation history as well as the latest user message. The SPARQL query therefore retrieves all information collected about the situation (e.g., the agitation description of the relative) as input and enables searching the ontology for relevant help texts or other information. The query result is then forwarded to the user as a chat message.

We formally define Γ as the current conversational context that determines which answer or diagnostic question is passed next to the user. Here, the context Γ characterizes the identified problem as a set of nodes ω from the ontology Ω that have been marked as applicable to the situation during the course of the conversation.

Since diagnostic questions can be answered with *yes*, *no* or *maybe*, it is necessary for the chatbot to store the identified ontology nodes with different degrees

---

[4] https://www.w3.org/TR/sparql11-query/ (accessed: 2023-08-31).

of knowledge during the course of the conversation. Due to the different knowledge levels, it is therefore possible to output different help texts for different situations. For example, if the family member is not sure whether the person being cared for is in pain, a help text on the topic of pain recognition can be offered first.

3.3 Interpretation of the User Input

An important step for the communication between chatbot and caregiver is the understanding of the specific problem described in natural language. For the purpose of constraining the problem as well as for further interpretation, we developed a mapping from a chat message $x \in \mathbb{X}$ to a set of medical concepts $c \in \Omega$ and the other defined chatbot intents (e.g., request for local help):

$$f : \mathbb{X} \rightarrow \Omega \cup \{\text{Chatbot Intents}\} \tag{1}$$

In our approach, we use the BERT model [10] to classify text messages along classes $c \in \Omega$ from the ontology Ω and other intents. BERT relies on multiple Transformer-Blocks to capture relationships between words and sentences with a so-called attention mechanism [30]. Due to the fact that several concepts are often mentioned in one sentence (e.g., the relative describes that the family member is loud and restless), the presented model follows a multi-label approach. This allows multiple concepts from the ontology to be recognized in one chat message.

Data. For the demonstration of this approach, we use seven concepts from our ontology as labels for the training: *Physical aggressive (PA)*, *Physical non-aggressive (PNA)*, *Verbal aggressive (VA)*, *Verbal non-aggressive (VNA)* and *Resisting care (RC)*. To answer yes, no and maybe questions, additional concepts for *Yes*, *No* and *Unsure* were added. In order to enable further interactions with the chatbot as described in Sect. 3.1, we added multiple intents to the concept set, such as *Short version*, *Long version* and *Local help*. Furthermore, a rejection class *None* was added to allow the model to select none of the ontology concepts. For this purpose, several sentences about non-medical topics were randomly collected from the English *Wikipedia* and added to the training data set.

The training data set regarding the other concepts was created by experts from the nursing domain by considering possible example sentences users could ask the chatbot. A total of 407 samples were collected and divided into five random folds for the k-fold cross-validation procedure. A similar class distribution was obtained for each fold by stratification. An overview of the total samples per class is shown in Fig. 4.

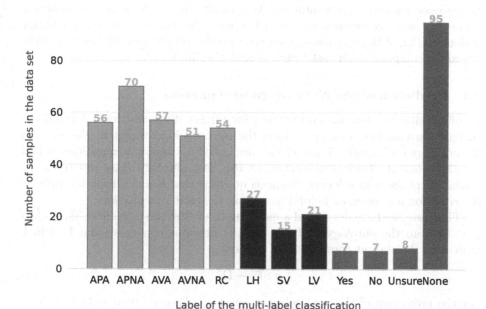

Fig. 4. The graph shows the number of samples used per class. Agitations in green: *Physical aggressive (PA)*, *Physical non-aggressive (PNA)*, *Verbal aggressive (VA)*, *Verbal non-aggressive (VNA)* and *Resisting care (RC)*; intents in blue: *Local help (LH)*, *Short version (SV)* and *Long version (LV)* and *Yes, No* and *Unsure* in light blue. (Color figure online)

Preprocessing and Data Augmentation. Each sample is preprocessed in several steps: Umlauts, punctuations (except for question marks, as these could imply a question) and double spaces were removed. In addition, only lowercase letters were used. To avoid the model learning a gender-specific prediction, all terms such as pronouns and names of reference persons such as husband, mother, etc. were removed and replaced by the token *PwD* (person with dementia).

Due to the small amount of training data, the training data was further augmented using back-translation, which results in a total data set of 1.928 samples. In this method, the sample chatbot queries in German language are first translated into several other languages and then back into the original language [11].

Training. In order to learn the mapping $f : \mathbb{X} \to \Omega \cup \{\text{Chatbot Intents}\}$ (see Eq. 1) from natural language to medical concepts and other intents, the large language model BERT pre-trained on German was fine-tuned within 100 epochs using our generated data set.

The BERT model [10] uses a bidirectional approach, processing input from both left to right and right to left. Therefore, the model is able to understand the context of a phrase considering the previous and subsequent words, resulting in a deeper semantic representation. As a result, the model is able to generate contextual word representations, which allows the model to develop a better understanding of the relationship between words and phrases, making it ideally suited for comprehension tasks such as text classification[5].

3.4   Prediction of the Next Diagnosis Question

To offer suitable questions and content for further diagnosis depending on the current conversation, a mapping from the conversation context to classes from the ontology is necessary. These classes are linked to diagnostic questions as well as other content. Thus, a prediction of the next ontology class describes the prediction of the next relevant diagnosis question that is most likely to apply to the situation and be most helpful in solving the relative's problem.

Therefore, we have developed a mapping to predict the next most likely class $\omega \in \Omega$ from the ontology Ω based on the previous conversational Γ, which represents the current conversational context:

$$g : \Gamma \to \Omega \qquad (2)$$

For the prediction of the next relevant ontology class, we used a *Markov logic network (MLN)*. Markov logic networks combine first-order logic and probabilistic graphical models, enabling the modeling of complex domains with formulas consisting of variables and predicates [21]. Thus, contrary to the direct use of inference in the ontology, the possibility of mapping uncertainties is provided. For this purpose, we have modeled the information about the current situation as well as the domain knowledge as a set of predicates and logical formulas. The objective of the MLN is to determine a probability distribution about which ontology classes might be relevant for the user's problem.

We have modeled an MLN with three observable (knowledge we have gathered so far about the case) and one hidden predicate:

- *Know(X)*: The observable predicate *Know(X)* describes the knowledge gathered in the course of the conversation so far and therefore represents all ontology classes that are reliably applicable to the conversation (verified by asking various diagnostic questions). For example, the predicate *Know(Pain)* indicates that the chatbot knows that the PwD is in pain.
- *Maybe(X)*: The observable predicate *Maybe(X)* describes all the information we have not collected with full certainty about the situation. This is, for example, information that the relative has only indicated with "maybe" or "I don't know".
- *Not(X)*: The observable predicate *Not(X)* was used to make statements that an ontology class is no longer applicable to the situation. For example, a class may no longer be relevant since the relative may have denied questions about that class.

---

[5] Used Python package *Simple Transformers*: https://simpletransformers.ai/ (accessed: 2023-06-29).

- *Question(X)*: The predicate *Question(X)* is the only hidden predicate in the presented MLN. It describes ontology classes that might still apply to the situation and that the chatbot should ask about. For example, the predicate *Question(Communication Problems)* describes that the ontology class *Communication Problems* might be relevant to the relative and the chatbot could ask a related diagnostic question.

In order to include medical knowledge for the calculation of a probability distribution, logical formulas were extracted based on the relations between individual classes defined in the ontology. With the help of the MLN, it is possible to use medical knowledge from the ontology and guide the user through diagnostic questions suitable for the conversational situation.

For this purpose, various relations have been used in the ontology to define the domain knowledge and extract logical formulas in conjunctive normal form that could be used in the MLN:

- Hierarchy relation: The hierarchy of the ontology was used because parent classes often only roughly reflect the subject matter. Therefore, in many cases, it makes sense to generate deeper knowledge and further specify the problem with additional diagnostic questions according to child classes.
- Triggers: Describes from which causes the agitation of the PwD can be triggered.
- Leads to: Describes which agitation leads to which further consequences.
- Exhibits: This is the relation between concepts of the superclasses *Person with Dementia* and *Agitation*. The relation therefore describes which agitation the PwD can exhibit.

The following equations represent the hierarchy (see Eq. 3), triggers (see Eq. 4), leads-to (see Eq. 5) and exhibits (see Eq. 6) relations in the MLN:

$$\forall c, p \in \Omega, p \in parent(c) : \neg Know(p) \lor Question(c) \qquad (3)$$
$$\forall c, p \in \Omega, p \in parent(c) : \neg Maybe(p) \lor Question(c)$$

$$\forall a, b \in \Omega, b \in triggers(a) : \neg Know(a) \lor Question(b) \qquad (4)$$
$$\forall a, b \in \Omega, b \in triggers(a) : \neg Maybe(a) \lor Question(b)$$

$$\forall a, b \in \Omega, b \in leads\ to(a) : \neg Know(a) \lor Question(b) \qquad (5)$$
$$\forall a, b \in \Omega, b \in leads\ to(a) : \neg Maybe(a) \lor Question(b)$$

$$\forall a, b \in \Omega, b \in exhibits(a) : \neg Know(a) \lor Question(b) \qquad (6)$$
$$\forall a, b \in \Omega, b \in exhibits(a) : \neg Maybe(a) \lor Question(b)$$

Assuming the chatbot would recognize a physical-aggressive type of agitation in the relative's chat messages. Since, for example, the relation *physical-aggressive behavior leads to less social contact with other people* is mapped in the ontology, the chatbot would then ask further questions about the social behavior of the person with dementia:

$$\textit{Less social contacts} \in \textit{leads to(Physical aggressive)}: \qquad (7)$$
$$\neg \textit{Know(Physical aggressive)} \vee \textit{Question(Less social contacts)}$$

This enables the chatbot to output help texts on this topic as the conversation progresses. For each extracted relation, a formula with a certain weight $\omega \in \mathbb{R}$ is inserted into the MLN to model the strength of dependencies between predicates. Hierarchical relations were given more weight than other relations because it was assumed that it is more important to generate more information about the current class and thus to explore deeper into the ontology tree.

However, since the predicates are intended to model different degrees of knowledge, the formulas over the *Know* relation were assigned double weight. To model some desired constraints of the real world, we added several hard constraints to our MLN:

- Diagnosis questions may not be asked twice:

$$\forall c \in \Omega : \neg \textit{Know(c)} \vee \neg \textit{Question(c)} \qquad (8)$$
$$\forall c \in \Omega : \neg \textit{Maybe(c)} \vee \neg \textit{Question(c)} \qquad (9)$$

- Classes that are not applicable based on our knowledge may not be asked for:

$$\forall c \in \Omega : \neg \textit{Not(c)} \vee \neg \textit{Question(c)} \qquad (10)$$

- Ask only one thing at a time:

$$\forall a, b \in \Omega : \neg \textit{Question(a)} \vee \neg \textit{Question(b)} \qquad (11)$$

We computed the inference of our defined MLN using the RockIt software[6] from the University of Mannheim. With that, we were able to calculate a probability distribution that delivers a probability for each ontology class of whether the class is applicable to the situation of the relative. In predicting the best diagnostic question, we only consider ontology classes whose probability is above a chosen threshold $\tau \in [0, 1]$. The two ontology classes with the highest probability were then returned to the user so that the user can decide among different options for the next topic.

4   Results

The evaluation was performed on two different data sets. On the one hand, the expert-generated data was divided into five different folds in a k-fold cross-validation. As a result, five different models were trained using four folds respectively as the training set. On the other hand, within a small study, a total of ten relatives of dementia patients were instructed to describe to the chatbot that the PwD refuses to be washed (*Resisting care*). Thus, a total of 20 samples of real chat messages were collected, which were used for the second evaluation. In the process, the model was trained with the entire data set generated by experts.

---

[6] http://executor.informatik.uni-mannheim.de/systems/rockit/ (accessed: 2023-09-08).

4.1   Data Generated by Experts

For each class, the *true positives (TP)*, *true negatives (TN)*, *false positives (FP)*, and *false negatives (FN)* were evaluated. Due to the small number of data for the labels *Yes*, *No* and *Unsure* individual folds could not be evaluated for the corresponding classes. Furthermore, the metrics *Accuracy*, *Precision*, *Recall*, *Specificity* and *F1 Score* were evaluated for each class, with the average calculated across each fold (see Table 2).

Table 2. The table shows the calculated metrics *Accuracy*, *Precision*, *Recall*, *F1 Score* and *Specificity* for all classes: *Physical Aggressive (PA)*, *Physical non-aggressive (PNA)*, *Verbal aggressive (VA)*, *Verbal non-aggressive (VNA)*, *Resisting care (RC)*, *Local help*, *Long version*, *Short version*, *Yes*, *No*, *Unsure* and *None*. The average of all five folds was calculated.

	n	TP	TN	FP	FN	Accuracy	Precision	Recall	F1	Specificity
PA	11.25	8.8	68.6	3.2	2.4	0.93	0.73	0.79	0.76	0.96
PNA	14	9.2	64.6	4.4	4.8	0.89	0.68	0.66	0.67	0.94
VA	11.4	9	68.8	2.8	2.4	0.94	0.76	0.79	0.78	0.96
VNA	10.2	7.3	70.8	2	3	0.94	0.78	0.71	0.74	0.97
Resisting care	10.8	9.8	69.2	3	1	0.94	0.77	0.91	0.83	0.96
Local help	5.4	5	77.6	0	0.4	0.99	1.0	0.93	0.96	1.0
Long version	4.2	3.6	78.6	0.4	0.6	0.99	0.9	0.86	0.88	0.99
Short version	3	2.8	79.2	0.8	0.2	0.99	0.78	0.93	0.85	0.99
Yes	1.75	1.5	80.75	0.25	0.25	0.99	0.86	0.86	0.86	0.99
No	1.75	1.5	80.25	0	0.25	0.99	1.0	0.86	0.92	1.0
Unsure	2	2	81.75	0	0	1.0	1.0	1.0	1.0	1.0
None	19	18.8	64	0	0.2	0.99	1.0	0.99	0.99	1.0

Chat messages for the agitations *Physical aggressive* (F1 value of 0.76), *Verbal aggressive*, *Verbal non-aggressive* and *Resisting care* were recognized similarly well by the trained models. The best values were obtained for the *Resisting care* label (F1 value of 0.82), since with a recall value of 0.92 almost all messages related to this type of agitation were correctly classified. However, the highest precision value (0.83) was achieved for messages concerning the agitation *Verbal aggressive*. Just messages related to the agitation *Physical non-aggressive* were recognized less well than the other labels.

For the evaluation of the entire model, the *macro average*, *micro average* and *weighted average* were calculated for each metric. The macro average calculates the arithmetic mean of the corresponding metric across all classes. With the micro average, on the other hand, the corresponding metric is calculated using the sums of the TP, TN, FP and FN counts. Finally, the weighted average also takes into account the frequency of occurrence of each class when calculating the arithmetic mean. These metrics were evaluated once for all classes, but also evaluated only for these corresponding agitation classes due to the focus on agitation detection. The results of these metrics are shown in Table 3. The evaluation of the model for all classes is about 6–11% better than considering the agitation classes alone. Thereby, the macro, micro and weighted average value for the F1 score is 0.75, 0.76 and 0.76, respectively.

4.2   Data from Relatives of PwD

In the second evaluation with real chat messages from relatives, the model recognized 100% of the descriptions correctly as an agitation of the *Resisting care* type (cf. Table 4). Furthermore, during the evaluation, there were three other messages describing other forms of agitation, which were also recognized without any error.

However, the chatbot also incorrectly recognized some messages of the *Resisting care* class as the agitation *physical non-aggressive* and thus achieved a noticeably worse precision value (0.375) for this class (with only 3 samples). However, because the experiment was designed primarily for the *Resisting care* agitation type and only three samples exist, the metrics for this class offer lower reliability.

5   Discussion

Below, we discuss some advantages of our system compared to the currently popular *ChatGPT*.

The core difference in the developed chatbot lies in the ontology as its main knowledge base for a domain-specific use case. While *ChatGPT*'s main purpose is to provide a conversation partner rather than validated information, its core data set is mostly raw natural language data itself, functioning as its knowledge. With that, *ChatGPT* is very well able to generate a fitting piece of dialogue data that is likely to be a suitable answer to the user's question, but shows limitations in areas where strong concept understanding and association between multiple concepts are required [3,20].

In contrast to that, the *eDEM-CONNECT* pipeline provides a solution in which its knowledge base (the ontology) comes in a form that is on the one hand human-readable and on the other hand provides a conceptional knowledge base for the chatbot. This approach, even though it is more elaborate in its development, allows theoretically faster domain learning for the machine and a result that can be better controlled by the domain experts. Especially in the healthcare domain, where wrong information can potentially cause great harm, it is important to validate such information by domain experts. Currently, our approach has only been tested on a small concept set within the ontology due to the lack of training data for the chatbot. Because of that, a direct comparison between *ChatGPT* and our bot is currently not possible. So any predictions on a larger data set with training data are speculative. Larger data sets provide more complexity and make correct classification of concepts more difficult. The possibility of false classification increases with the growing number of concepts and discrimination between them becomes harder when several concepts are

Table 3. The table shows the metrics for evaluating model performance for all classes using micro, macro and weighted average. The average was calculated over all five folds.

Metric	All classes	Agitation classes only
Macro Average Accuracy	0.97	0.93
Macro Average Precision	0.87	0.76
Macro Average Recall	0.86	0.77
Macro Average F1 Score	0.86	0.75
Macro Average Specificity	0.98	0.96
Micro Average Accuracy	0.97	0.93
Micro Average Precision	0.83	0.74
Micro Average Recall	0.84	0.77
Micro Average F1 Score	0.83	0.76
Micro Average Specificity	0.98	0.96
Weighted Average Accuracy	0.95	0.93
Weighted Average Precision	0.87	0.76
Weighted Average Recall	0.84	0.77
Weighted Average F1 Score	0.83	0.76
Weighted Average Specificity	0.97	0.96

more similar to each other. However, assuming the fact that there is a larger set of training data available in the future, the *eDEM-CONNECT* chatbot might be able to become the initially envisioned intelligent dialog assistant for family caregivers of people with dementia.

Furthermore, the evaluation has shown that the concept of detecting and classifying agitation descriptions in chat messages with a transformer model works fundamentally. The detection of the non-agitation classes (*Yes, No, Unsure, Local help, Long version*, etc.) also works exceptionally well, even with only limited data. The good results of the *Resisting care* class, could be due to the fact that *Resisting care* as a subclass of *Physical non-aggressive* covers a more narrow field than the other classes. However, evaluation of the real data set showed that some samples of the *Resisting care* class were incorrectly classified as *Physical non-aggressive*, too. The reason for this could be the definition of the hierarchy of these classes within the ontology and that the class *Resisting care* was modeled as a subclass of the class *Physical non-aggressive*. A restructuring of the labels could possibly improve this problem.

Responsible for some misclassification of the remaining classes could be the low degree of discrimination between agitations from type *Verbal aggressive* and *Verbal non-aggressive* or from type *Physical aggressive* and *Physical non-aggressive*, because these agitations were often described with very similar words in chat messages. In addition, samples were only labeled by one expert at a time.

Table 4. Confusion matrices of the two agitations from real chat messages of relatives of PwD: *Resisting care* (Left) and *Physical non-aggressive* (Right). The True Positives (TP), False Positives (FP), False Negatives (FN) and True Negatives (TN) were calculated for each class. Furthermore, the table shows the calculated metrics: Accuracy, Precision, Recall, F1 Score and Specificity.

	Actual value				Actual value		
	Positives	Negatives			Positives	Negatives	
Predictions Positives	17	0		Negatives Positives	3	5	
Predictions Negatives	0	3		Negatives Negatives	0	12	
	Resisting care				Physical non-aggressive		

	Accuracy	Precision	Recall	F1 Score	Specificity
Resisting care	1.0	1.0	1.0	1.0	1.0
Physical non-aggressive	0.75	0.375	1.0	0.55	0.71

Due to the fact that humans label samples differently, this might increase the problem of low discriminatory power. An inter-observer reliability analysis could help to solve this problem.

An aspect that will still come up as a challenge in the future will be the transitioning condition between the anamnese step and the phase where the chatbot provides a solution to the user. In contrast to *Ada Health*, where the user is confronted with a large questionnaire, the transition here was intended to be more flexible and faster due to the users needing fast and pithy instructions. A shorter anamnese step will inevitably lead to more faulty instructions in the second phase. Therefore, there has to be some possibility to balance these two steps and maybe even go back to the anamnese status while the intervention phase has been reached.

Several approaches are conceivable here. An approach that has not been tested further would be to train a dialog system by using reinforcement learning and to give the system feedback in the case of good or bad predictions. A bad prediction therefore would be an unsuitable, further topic.

6   Conclusion and Further Work

In the *eDEM-CONNECT* project, we were able to develop a chatbot that uses a domain-specific ontology on challenging behavior of PwD as its main knowledge base. The chatbot is able to identify the concepts of a smaller subset of the ontology when interacting with user inputs and can lead through a dialog in which it provides helpful information regarding a given situation with a PwD.

In the future, a project with a larger set of training data, enabling the chatbot to further deepen its knowledge of the ontology concepts, has very high potential. To realize the initial vision of the chatbot, a scaled-up program with complete ontology coverage and a clearer dialog process would be a suitable option. An alternative to that would be a bot without the ontology, which instead uses a domain-specific GPT, which are currently on the rise [20].

In both cases, a larger-scale user evaluation of the transformer model and the usability of the chatbot in general is also imaginable. Furthermore, the prediction of the next diagnosis question with the Markov logic network has not yet been reliably tested on real user data. The prediction of the next diagnosis question is based on the relationships between the individual ontology classes, which in some cases are difficult to prove medically. Therefore, other methods for predicting the next diagnostic question should be tested for further development to address this problem (e.g., prediction with reinforcement learning would also be conceivable).

Overall, the project provides a proof of concept for a domain-specific chatbot solution that incorporates an integrated ontology as its main knowledge base. This delivers a solid cornerstone for future projects that challenge domain-specific scenarios with the help of smart chatbots. In case of a successful future project that offers broader ontology coverage with good concept recognition, the chatbot will be better able to fulfill its initial project vision. This will improve the stability of the relationships of PwD and their caregiving relatives and professional caregivers will also profit from it. The care domain is continuously challenged by staff shortage and the bot can facilitate the situation by providing individual information to the users. With that, the movement to a retirement home could be prevented or at least delayed, relieving the current care situation in Germany.

References

1. Abdul-Kader, S.A., Woods, D.J.: Survey on chatbot design techniques in speech conversation systems. Int. J. Adv. Comput. Sci. Appl. **6**(7) (2015). https://doi.org/10.14569/IJACSA.2015.060712
2. Al-Zubaide, H., Issa, A.A.: OntBot: ontology based chatbot. In: Fourth IEEE International Symposium on Innovation in Information & Communication Technology, vol. 4, pp. 7–12. IEEE, Piscataway (2011). https://doi.org/10.1109/ISIICT.2011.6149594
3. Azaria, A.: ChatGPT usage and limitations. Preprint (2022). https://doi.org/10.13140/RG.2.2.26616.11526
4. Avila, C., et al.: MediBot: an ontology based chatbot for Portuguese speakers drug's users. In: 21st International Conference on Enterprise Information Systems ICEIS. ICEIS (Setúbal), vol. 21, pp. 25–36. SciTePress, Setúbal (2019). https://doi.org/10.5220/0007656400250036
5. Barros, A., Rajan, R.S., Nili, A.: Scaling up chatbots for corporate service delivery systems. Commun. ACM **64**(8), 88–97 (2021). https://doi.org/10.1145/3446912

6. Caros, M., Garolera, M., Radeva, P., Giro-i Nieto, X.: Automatic reminiscence therapy for dementia. In: Gurrin, C. (ed.) Proceedings of the 2020 International Conference on Multimedia Retrieval, pp. 383–387. ACM Digital Library, Association for Computing Machinery, New York (2020). https://doi.org/10.1145/3372278.3391927

7. Chow, A.R.: How ChatGPT managed to grow faster than TikTok or Instagram (2023). https://time.com/6253615/chatgpt-fastest-growing. Accessed 24 July 2023

8. Clyburn, L.D., Stones, M.J., Hadjistavropoulos, T., Tuokko, H.: Predicting caregiver burden and depression in Alzheimer's disease. J. Gerontol.: Ser. B **55**(1), S2–13 (2000). https://doi.org/10.1093/geronb/55.1.S2

9. Deutsche Alzheimer Gesellschaft e.V.: Zum bundesweiten Tag der pflegenden Angehörigen: Angehörige von Menschen mit Demenz brauchen Entlastung - auch von Bürokratie (2023). https://www.deutsche-alzheimer.de/artikel/zum-bundesweiten-tag-der-pflegenden-angehoerigen-angehoerige-von-menschen-mit-demenz-brauchen-entlastung-auch-von-buerokratie. Accessed 07 Nov 2023

10. Devlin, J., Chang, M., Lee, K., Toutanova, K.: BERT: pre-training of deep bidirectional transformers for language understanding. In: Conference of the North American Chapter of the Association for Computational Linguistics: Human Language Technologies (NAACL-HLT), pp. 4171–4186. Association for Computational Linguistics, Stroudsburg (2019). https://doi.org/10.18653/v1/n19-1423

11. Feng, S.Y., et al.: A survey of data augmentation approaches for NLP. In: Findings of the Association for Computational Linguistics: ACL-IJCNLP 2021, pp. 968–988. Association for Computational Linguistics, Stroudsburg (2021). https://doi.org/10.18653/v1/2021.findings-acl.84, https://aclanthology.org/2021.findings-acl.84

12. Gruber, T.R.: A translation approach to portable ontology specifications. Knowl. Acquisit. **5**(2), 199–220 (1993). https://doi.org/10.1006/knac.1993.1008, https://www.sciencedirect.com/science/article/pii/S1042814383710083

13. Kelle, N., Ehrlich, U.: Situation unterstützender und pflegender Angehöriger von Menschen mit Demenz. dza aktuell - Deutscher Alterssurvey (4) (2022)

14. Kothari, A.N.: ChatGPT, large language models, and generative AI as future augments of surgical cancer care. Ann. Surg. Oncol. **30**(6), 3174–3176 (2023). https://doi.org/10.1245/s10434-023-13442-2

15. Le Xin, T., Arshad, A., Salam, Z.A.B.A.: AlzBot- mobile app chatbot for Alzheimer's patient to be active with their minds. In: 2021 14th International Conference on Developments in eSystems Engineering (DeSE), pp. 124–129. IEEE, Piscataway (2021). https://doi.org/10.1109/DeSE54285.2021.9719410

16. Michalowsky, B., Kaczynski, A., Hoffmann, W.: Ökonomische und gesellschaftliche Herausforderungen der Demenz in Deutschland - Eine Metaanalyse. Bundesgesundheitsblatt Gesundheitsforschung Gesundheitsschutz **62**(8), 981–992 (2019). https://doi.org/10.1007/s00103-019-02985-z

17. Müller, C., Paluch, R., Hasanat, A.A.: Care: a chatbot for dementia care. Mensch und Computer 2022 - Workshopband (2022). https://doi.org/10.18420/MUC2022-MCI-SRC-442

18. Ornstein, K.A., Gaugler, J.E., Devanand, D.P., Scarmeas, N., Zhu, C.W., Stern, Y.: Are there sensitive time periods for dementia caregivers? The occurrence of behavioral and psychological symptoms in the early stages of dementia. Int. Psychogeriatr. **25**(9), 1453–1462 (2013). https://doi.org/10.1017/S1041610213000768

19. Pinkert, C., et al.: Social inclusion of people with dementia - an integrative review of theoretical frameworks, methods and findings in empirical studies. Ageing Soc. **41**(4), 773–793 (2021). https://doi.org/10.1017/S0144686X19001338

20. Ray, P.P.: ChatGPT: a comprehensive review on background, applications, key challenges, bias, ethics, limitations and future scope. Internet Things Cyber-Phys. Syst. **3**, 121–154 (2023). https://doi.org/10.1016/j.iotcps.2023.04.003, https://www.sciencedirect.com/science/article/pii/S266734522300024X

21. Richardson, M., Domingos, P.: Markov logic networks. Mach. Learn. **62**(1–2), 107–136 (2006). https://doi.org/10.1007/s10994-006-5833-1

22. Ruggiano, N., et al.: Chatbots to support people with dementia and their caregivers: systematic review of functions and quality. J. Med. Internet Res. **23**(6), e25006 (2021). https://doi.org/10.2196/25006

23. Schirra-Weirich, L., Wiegelmann, H.: Typenbildung als Beitrag zur Weiterentwicklung von Versorgungsstrukturen für Menschen mit Demenz und ihren versorgenden Angehörigen. Ergebnisse einer Tandem-Studie im Rahmen des Modellprojekts "DemenzNetz StädteRegion Aachen". In: Schäfer-Walkmann, S., Traub, F. (eds) Evolution durch Vernetzung. Edition Centaurus - Perspektiven Sozialer Arbeit in Theorie und Praxis, pp. 59–76. Springer, Wiesbaden (2016). https://doi.org/10.1007/978-3-658-14809-6_4

24. Sosnowski, T., Abuazizeh, M., Kirste, T., Yordanova, K.: Development of a conversational agent for tutoring nursing students to interact with patients. In: Frasson, C., Mylonas, P., Troussas, C. (eds.) ITS 2023. LNCS, vol. 13891, pp. 171–182. Springer, Cham (2023). https://doi.org/10.1007/978-3-031-32883-1_15

25. Sosnowski, T., Yordanova, K.: A probabilistic conversational agent for intelligent tutoring systems. In: Proceedings of the 13th ACM International Conference on Pervasive Technologies Related to Assistive Environments. PETRA 2020. Association for Computing Machinery, New York (2020). https://doi.org/10.1145/3389189.3397978

26. Subhalakshmi, Y., Shivani G.S., Sri Shandhya Devi, T., Sri Raksha Avanthiga, S., Ahila, R.: Androz chatbot for Alzheimer's patients. Int. J. Res. Appl. Sci. Eng. Technol. **11**(5), 3249–3256 (2023). https://doi.org/10.22214/ijraset.2023.52339

27. Thyrian, J.R., et al.: Burden of behavioral and psychiatric symptoms in people screened positive for dementia in primary care: results of the Delphi-study. J. Alzheimer's Dis.: JAD **46** (2015). https://doi.org/10.3233/JAD-143114

28. Valtolina, S., Hu, L.: Charlie: a chatbot to improve the elderly quality of life and to make them more active to fight their sense of loneliness. In: CHItaly 2021: 14th Biannual Conference of the Italian SIGCHI Chapter, pp. 1–5. ACM Digital Library, Association for Computing Machinery, New York (2021). https://doi.org/10.1145/3464385.3464726

29. Varshini, M.P., Surabhi, S., Keerthan Kumar, T.G.: The companion chatbot for dementia patients. Int. J. Adv. Sci. Technol. **29**, 6582–6592 (2020)

30. Vaswani, A., et al.: Attention is all you need. In: Advances in Neural Information Processing Systems, vol. 30, pp. 5998–6008. Curran Associates, Inc., Red Hook (2017)

Digital Imaging and Communications in Medicine (DICOM). Biomedical, and Health Informatics

A Cascade Approach for Automatic Segmentation of Coronary Arteries Calcification in Computed Tomography Images Using Deep Learning

Alan de C. Araújo[1]([✉])[iD], Aristófanes C. Silva[1][iD], João M. Pedrosa[2],
Italo F. S. Silva[1][iD], and João O. B. Diniz[3][iD]

[1] Applied Computing Group - Federal University of Maranhão (NCA/UFMA),
São Luís, MA 65080040, Brazil
alan.araujo@nca.ufma.br, {ac.silva,italo.francyles}@ufma.br
[2] Institute for Systems and Computer Engineering, Technology and Science
(INESC TEC), 4200-465 Porto, Portugal
joao.m.pedrosa@inesctec.pt
[3] Federal Institute of Education, Science and Technology (IFMA),
Grajaú, MA 65940-000, Brazil
joao.bandeira@ifma.edu.br

Abstract. One of the indicators of possible occurrences of cardiovascular diseases is the amount of coronary artery calcium. Recently,
approaches using new technologies such as deep learning have been used
to help identify these indicators. This work proposes a segmentation
method for calcification of the coronary arteries that has three steps:
(1) extraction of the ROI using U-Net with batch normalization after
convolution layers, (2) segmentation of the calcifications and (3) removal
of false positives using Modified U-Net with EfficientNet. The method
uses histogram matching as preprocessing in order to increase the contrast between tissue and calcification and normalize the different types of
exams. Multiple architectures were tested and the best achieved 96.9%
F1-Score, 97.1% recall and 98.3% in the OrcaScore Dataset.

Keywords: Coronary artery calcium · Segmentation · U-Net ·
EfficientNetB0 · OrcaScore Dataset

1 Introduction

Cardiovascular diseases are the leading causes of global mortality [4]. One indicator of the potential occurrence of cardiovascular disease is the amount of coronary artery calcification (CAC) [2]. CAC is commonly computed through computed tomography scans, which can be performed with or without contrast. The
contrast-enhanced scan, known as coronary CT angiography (CCTA), involves
the injection of an ionizing substance that highlights soft tissues, aiding in the

A. Cunha et al. (Eds.): MobiHealth 2023, LNICST 578, pp. 95–109, 2024.
https://doi.org/10.1007/978-3-031-60665-6_7

visualization of both soft tissues (heart, arteries, and veins) and hard tissues (bone structures). However, due to the use of a radioactive substance, this examination is contraindicated for certain patients. In such cases, a non-contrast CT scan (CSCT) is performed, which, in turn, exhibits a lower contrast between soft and hard tissues, making their visualization more challenging [3].

In the past, human interaction was required to differentiate calcium in the arteries from other calcifications, such as the aorta and bones [5]. Due to technological advancements, new methods of working with images and large amounts of data have emerged, and artificial intelligence has brought new approaches to problems involving imaging. Consequently, methods have been developed to automatically identify CAC, including deep learning-based approaches [7]. These approaches have been successfully applied to medical images, aiding in monitoring, particularly in detecting subtle findings that a physician might overlook and small details invisible to the naked eye [1].

Despite significant efforts to support the development of automatic CAC identification methods primarily based on deep learning, there is still room for new experiments and improvements. Therefore, the paper's main objective is to propose a cascaded method for segmenting calcifications in the coronary arteries. The proposed method utilizes histogram matching to enhance the contrast between calcification and tissue, simulating the contrast-enhanced scan, thus eliminating the need for the patient to undergo the contrast-enhanced examination. The method involves using a U-Net with batch normalization after the convolutional layers to extract the region of interest (ROI) and a U-Net with the encoder replaced by EfficientNetB0 for calcification segmentation. Additionally, a specific step is included to remove false positives, which are prevalent in this segmentation problem.

This paper is organized as follows: In Sect. 2, we discuss related works on calcifications in coronary arteries segmentation, exploring advancements in previously published methods. Section 3 provides detailed information about the proposed method for calcification segmentation. The results are presented in Sect. 4.3, and finally, Sect. 5 concludes the paper by summarizing the findings and discussing future work.

2   Related Works

In this section, we present works from the literature that are related to the proposed problem. The criteria for selecting related works were studies that employed fully convolutional networks (FCNs) for cardiac calcification segmentation and did not utilize contrast-enhanced examinations.

In [7], a DenseRAUnet is employed, which combines a Dense U-Net, ResNet, and dilated convolution. The images are preprocessed by resizing them to 512 × 512 pixels. The loss function is a combination of Bootstrap and IoU to effectively balance the background class and the calcification class. The model is trained on non-contrast thoracic CT scans in a 2.5D approach and evaluated on cardiac CT scans. The results show a remarkable F1-Score of 95.4% and a precision of

99.1%. However, it does not perform preprocessing to minimize the issues caused by the low contrast between tissues and calcifications in non-contrast CT scans.

In contrast, [2] introduces a multi-task model for simultaneous segmentation of both the coronary artery region and calcifications. The model was trained and evaluated on three datasets, namely DISCHARGE, OrcaScore, and CADMAN. During training, the authors utilized the weighted uncertainty loss [9]. The proposed method achieved an F1-Score of 92.8% for the calcification segmentation task. However, this method does not have a way to mitigate the differences in scans performed on different CT scanners, which hinders the learning process of the network.

In [3], the authors employ five 3D U-Net models trained from zero using the ADAM optimizer and Dice as the loss function. Each of them was trained with a different distribution os the dataset. The final result is obtained by majority voting among the five models. As a preprocessing step, the resolution of the scans is reduced to either 2.5 or 3 mm. To recover lost information, all voxels above 130 HU in the original image are intensified in the reduced-resolution image. A total of 783 patients are used for training the five 3D U-Net models. The method achieves an F1-Score of 97.4% on the OrcaScore Dataset. However, this model does not have a mechanism to prevent or remove false positives, which are common in this problem due to calcifications in regions such as the aorta and mitral valve.

Despite the numerous proposed methods, achieving accurate segmentation of calcifications remains challenging due to the low contrast between tissues and calcifications in contrast-free examinations, as well as the variations between scans acquired from different tomography machines. Consequently, developing a segmentation method that uses preprocessing to enhance the contrast between tissue and calcification in non-contrast CT scans, as well as normalize the various scans performed on different CT scanners, can facilitate their identification. Additionally, incorporating a specific step for false positive removal, which is common in this problem of coronary arteries calcification segmentation, would be beneficial.

3   Material and Methods

This section presents information regarding the dataset used, the proposed method, and the applied techniques.

3.1   Datasets

A separate image database was utilized for each step of the method. For the ROI extraction step, the CT Heart database, consisting of 1000 computed tomography scans with heart annotations, was employed. This database contains a total of 2532 slices. The dataset was divided into 60% for training, 20% for validation, and 20% for testing. Three data augmentation techniques were applied during training, including horizontal flipping, vertical flipping, and 45° rotation. Ultimately, the distribution consisted of 6076 images for training, 506 images for validation, and 506 images for testing.

For the calcification segmentation step, the OrcaScore database was used, which consists of computed tomography scans from 32 patients, totaling 1540 slices. This database includes scans acquired from four different tomography machines in four distinct hospitals, providing a greater diversity of examinations. The dataset was divided into 20 patients for training, 4 patients for validation, and 8 patients for testing. Data augmentation techniques were applied to the training set, including horizontal flipping, vertical flipping, and 45° rotation. Ultimately, the distribution consisted of 4248 images for training, 150 images for validation, and 301 images for testing.

The image database for the false positive removal step was formed through preprocessing, which involved extracting a 96 × 96 pixel ROI from the predictions made in the calcification segmentation step, as well as ROIs from the masks in the OrcaScore database. Thus, the database consists of 198 true-positive images and 32 false positive images. The distribution of true-positive images is 80% for training, 10% for validation, and 10% for testing. As for the false positive images, they are divided as follows: 60% for training, 20% for validation, and 20% for testing. Due to the limited amount of data, data augmentation techniques are applied to generate new images. For the true-positive training set, horizontal flipping, vertical flipping, and 45° rotation techniques are performed, resulting in a total of 540 true-positive images. For the false positive set, a larger number of images is generated to balance the database. The augmentation techniques applied include horizontal flipping, vertical flipping, and rotation from 10 to 70° in 5° increments, resulting in a total of 240 false positive images.

3.2   Proposed Method

The proposed method follows a cascaded approach, whereby the output of each step serves as the input for the subsequent step. It is divided into three steps, namely ROI extraction, calcification segmentation, and false positive removal. Each step is designed to address a specific aspect of the task, as illustrated in Fig. 1.

3.2.1   ROI Extraction

Computed tomography scans can vary significantly depending on the tomography machine, vendor, hospital, and other factors. Therefore, histogram matching [12] was applied to make the diverse scans more similar to each other and enhance the contrast between the ROI and other regions. Additionally, this preprocessing step also increases the contrast between calcifications and surrounding tissue, which aids in subsequent stages. To determine the reference image, we performed an initial ROI segmentation. The patient slice with the highest F1-Score in this initial segmentation was selected as the reference image. An example of the application of histogram matching can be seen in Fig. 2.

The architecture of the network used in the first stage was the modified U-Net proposed by [6]. The structure consists of down-sampling and up-sampling

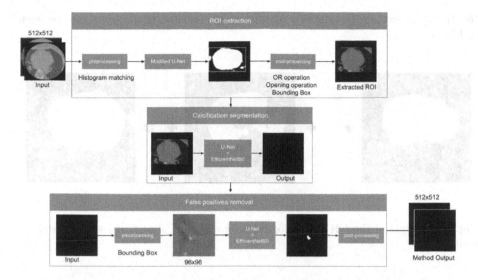

Fig. 1. Overview of the proposed method.

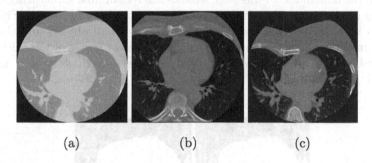

  (a)   (b)   (c)

Fig. 2. Histogram matching application: (a) original image (b) reference image e (c) modified histogram image.

layers, giving it a U-shaped format. The down-sampling blocks consist of successive 3 × 3 convolution layers and batch normalization layers, followed by rectified linear unit (ReLU) activation functions and 2 × 2 max-pooling operations. The number of filters is doubled in each block, starting with 64 filters and reaching a total of 1024. On the other hand, the up-sampling blocks consist of 2 × 2 convolution layers, with each respective block from the down-sampling section having a corresponding 3 × 3 convolution layer. The last layer includes a transposed convolution that outputs an image with the same dimensions as the input image.

After the initial segmentation of the ROI, a final mask is formed by performing an OR morphological operation [12] on all the segmentations of the patient's slices. This means that for each pixel in the final mask, if at least one segmentation predicts it as part of the ROI, it will be marked as belonging to the ROI. An example of the OR operation applied to the problem can be seen in Fig. 3.

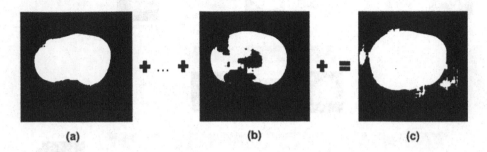

(a)   (b)   (c)

Fig. 3. Example of the OR morthological operation: (a) slice 1, (b) slice N, and (c) final mask.

In addition, an opening operation [12] is applied to eliminate possible artifacts present in the final mask. In this step, a fixed-size rectangular structuring element of 7×7 is used. An example of the opening operation can be seen in Fig. 4.

It can be observed that the operation removes small objects and thin lines from the image while preserving the shape and size of larger objects. Finally, a bounding box is created around the final mask to ensure that the ROI has been extracted, as shown in Fig. 5.

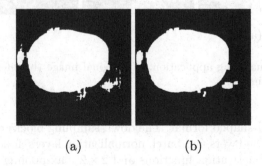

(a)   (b)

Fig. 4. Example of opening operation: (a) original image and (b) resulting image.

3.2.2   Calcification Segmentation

In the calcification segmentation stage, the initial segmentation of calcifications in the coronary arteries is performed using the chosen architecture. Due to the fact that the input image in this stage is only the ROI extracted in the previous stage, some false positives are avoided in regions such as the sternum and spine. However, there are still false positives within the ROI, mainly calcifications in the aorta.

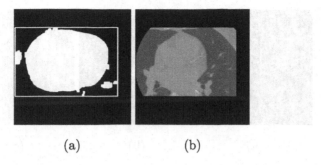

(a)   (b)

Fig. 5. Example of: (a) bounding box after postprocessing and (b) extracted ROI from first step

The neural network architecture used in the second and third stages was the modified U-Net with the encoder path based on EfficientNetB0. The standard U-Net structure is present in the up-sampling layers, while the down-sampling part features the EfficienteNetB0 model, which includes a 3×3 convolutional layer with 64 filters. Following that, there are 5 blocks of deep convolution, each consisting of a 3×3 convolutional layer and a 1×1 convolutional layer. Each decoding block contains a transposed convolutional layer of size 2×2 obtained from the previous layer with a stride of 2, concatenated with a 1×1 convolution for each respective block in the down-sampling section. In the last layer, a transposed convolution takes place, returning an output image with the same dimensions as the input image.

3.2.3 False Positive Removal

In the false positive removal step, preprocessing and post-processing techniques are applied to remove false positives caused mainly by calcifications in other regions of the ROI that are not part of the coronary arteries, such as the aorta.

During the preprocessing sub-step, a bounding box is created around the predictions made in the calcification segmentation step. These bounding boxes are expanded to 96×96 pixels size and then an ROI is formed from the 512×512 image as shown in Fig. 6. In this way, the ROI provides contextual information about the location of the calcification segmentation, aiding in its identification.

During the post-processing sub-step, the output images of this step are 96×96 pixels. Then, these images are placed in the same location in the original image from which they were extracted (512×512 image), resulting in an output image of the method that is 512×512 pixels, the same size as the input image (Fig. 7).

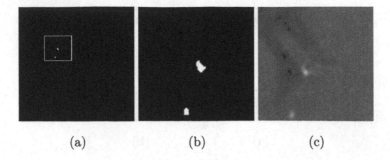

(a)   (b)   (c)

Fig. 6. Example of: (a) 512×512 image with bounding box represented by red square (b) bounding box 96×96 and (c) 96×96 ROI extracted from original image

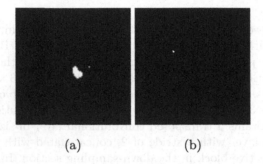

(a)   (b)

Fig. 7. Example of: (a) output image 96×96 and (b) method output image 512×512

4   Experiment Setup

This section presents information regarding the configurations of the experiments such as dataset division, the metrics used to evaluate the method and the results of differents architectures and between other methods.

4.1   Experiments Setup

For the training of the ROI extraction step, the Dice loss [11] was chosen as the loss function due to its superior performance compared to the Focal loss and cross-entropy. The CT Heart dataset was used, consisting of 6076 images for training, 506 images for validation, and 506 images for testing. Training was conducted for 70 epochs, with a batch size of 2 and a learning rate of 1e−4. Additionally, the Early Stopping technique was employed with a patience of 7 epochs. These experiments, along with all others, were conducted on hardware with the following configuration: an NVIDIA GTX 1660 Super graphics card with 6 GB of VRAM.

For the second step training, the focal loss [10] was used as the loss function because it provides better results when there is class imbalance. The OrcaScore dataset was used, consisting of 4248 images for training, 150 images for validation, and 300 images for testing. Training was conducted for 70 epochs, with a batch size of 4 and a learning rate of 1e−4. Was also used the Early Stopping technique employed with a patience of 5 epochs.

For the training of the third step, Focal Loss was used. The dataset was divided into 1266 images for training, 36 images for validation, and 36 images for testing. Training was conducted for 50 epochs, with a batch size of 24 and a learning rate of 1e−4. Additionally, the Early Stopping technique was employed with a tolerance of 7 epochs.

4.2   Results Evaluation

For the results evaluation, the metrics of F1-Score, precision, and recall were used [8]. Precision measures the proportion of correct positive class predictions compared to the total number of samples classified as positive (Eq. 1). Recall measures the proportion of true positive samples that were correctly classified by the model compared to the total number of positive samples (Eq. 2). F1-Score is the harmonic mean between precision and recall (Eq. 3).

$$Precision = \frac{TP}{TP + FP} \tag{1}$$

$$Recall = \frac{TP}{VP + FN} \tag{2}$$

$$F1 - Score = 2 \times \frac{Precision \times Recall}{Precision + Recall} \tag{3}$$

where TP stands for true positives, FP, in turn, stands for false positives, and FN represents false negatives.

4.3   Results and Discussion

In Table 1, an improvement can be observed in the modified U-Net compared to the original U-Net for the ROI extraction task. It is important to note that these metrics were obtained by testing only on the CT Heart dataset, as it contains heart annotations. The ROI extraction was performed on the OrcaScore dataset, and it can be visualized in Fig. 8.

Table 1. Comparison between architectures for ROI extraction

Image	F1-Score (%)	Precision (%)	Recall (%)
Original U-Net	63,0	83,2	93,3
Modified U-Net	**85,0**	**85,4**	**96,8**

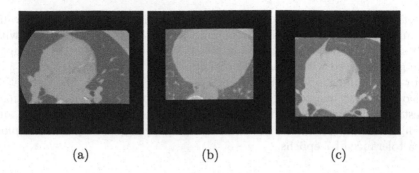

(a)   (b)   (c)

Fig. 8. ROI extraction examples in OrcaScore dataset: (a) patient 1 (b) patient 2 and (c) patient 3

Tests were conducted with images with and without histogram matching in order to validate the improvement of metrics when different types of images are more similar to each other, as well as to enhance the contrast between calcifications and tissues. The comparison between these tests can be visualized in Table 2.

Table 2. Comparison between images with and without histogram matching

Image	F1-Score (%)	Precision (%)	Recall (%)
Without histogram matching	12,3	11,3	13,7
With histogram matching	**81,7**	**84,2**	**95,0**

After comparing the preprocessing, experiments were conducted using other architectures, specifically the U-Net with other modifications in the encoder path, such as ResNet-50 and EfficientNetB3. This allowed us to evaluate architectures with more parameters and deeper structures. Table 3 shows the metrics obtained by each network in the task of segmenting coronary arteries calcifications.

Table 3. Comparison between architectures for calcification segmentation

Architecture	F1-Score (%)	Precision (%)	Recall (%)
U-Net + Resnet-34	95,8	97,9	96,6
U-Net + Resnet-50	95,6	**98,2**	95,4
U-Net + Resnet-101	94,6	97,5	96,1
U-Net + EfficientNetB0	**96,6**	98,0	97,2
U-Net + EfficientNetB3	96,0	97,5	**97,5**
U-Net + EfficientNetB5	90,7	93,4	90,5

The modified U-Net with EfficientNetB0 was chosen because it yielded a higher F1-Score, thus achieving a higher harmonic mean between Precision and Recall. After confirming the effectiveness of the architecture for segmenting calcifications in coronary arteries, the method was validated using cross-validation. Table 4 displays the metric values, mean, and standard deviation for each validation fold. Since the train-test split was 75%/25%, cross-validation was performed with 4 folds.

Table 4. Cross validation results

Fold number	F1-Score (%)	Precision (%)	Recall (%)
1	94,8	95,6	97,2
2	93,1	96,2	95,7
3	**96,6**	**98,0**	**97,2**
4	90,8	94,4	93,3
Mean	93,8	95,9	96,2
Standard Deviation	2,4	1,2	2,1

The model analyzed so far had some false positive predictions, mainly in the central area of the heart, where there were calcifications in the aorta, as observed by the red arrows in Fig. 9. These calcifications are not part of the coronary arteries, so even though they are calcifications, they are false positives that should be avoided. In this context, the third step of the model (false positive removal) is necessary.

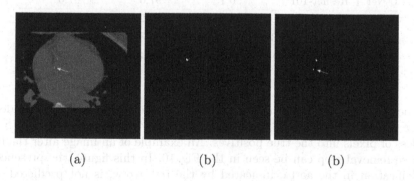

(a)   (b)   (b)

Fig. 9. Calcification segmentation example: (a) original image (b) ground-truth and (c) prediction

A comparison between the model with and without the false positive removal step can be observed in the Table 5.

Table 5. Comparison between model with and without false positive removal step

Model	F1-Score (%)	Precision (%)	Recall (%)
Without false positive removal step	96,6	98,0	**97,2**
With false positive removal step	**96,9**	**98,3**	97,1

As can be seen, there was an improvement in F1-Score and Precision due to the fact that some false positives were removed. However, Recall decreased due to the loss of some true positive pixels. Despite the loss of some pixels, the calcifications continue to be identified, thus maintaining the objective of segmenting them.

Similarly as made in the second step, experiments with the multiple architectures were conducted, such as U-Net with modifications in the encoder path (ResNet-34 and EfficientNetB5). Table 6 shows the metrics obtained by each network in the task of false positive removal.

Table 6. Comparison between architectures for false positive removal step

Architecture	F1-Score (%)	Precision (%)	Recall (%)
U-Net + Resnet-34	95,9	97,5	96,8
U-Net + Resnet-50	95,8	97,2	96,4
U-Net + Resnet-101	96,1	97,6	97,0
U-Net + EfficientNetB0	96,8	98,2	97,0
U-Net + EfficientNetB3	96,2	97,3	96,9
U-Net + EfficientNetB5	**96,9**	**98,3**	**97,1**

The modified U-Net with EfficientNetB5 was chosen because it yielded a higher F1-Score, Recall and Precision, thus removing false positives with the less loss of pixels into the true positives. An example of an image after the false positive removal step can be seen in the Fig. 10. In this figure, the presence of a calcification in the aorta, indicated by the red arrow, is not predicted as a calcification by the model, demonstrating the effectiveness of the false positive removal step.

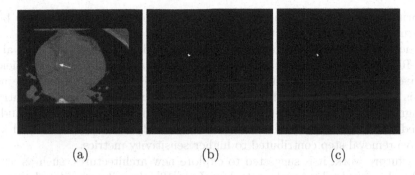

(a)   (b)   (c)

Fig. 10. Calcification segmentation example: (a) original image (b) ground-truth and (c) prediction

4.4 Related Works Comparison

In the calcifications segmentation, the proposed method achieves positive results close to other previous works that were tested in the same dataset (OrcaScore), as can be seen in the Table 7.

Table 7. Methods on the segmentation of coronary arteries calcifications

Method	F1-Score (%)	Precision (%)	Recall (%)
[2]	92,8	98,4	96,1
[3]	**97,5**	**99,5**	96,8
[7]	95,4	99,1	91,1
Proposed method	96,9	98,3	**97,1**

The proposed method exhibited metrics close to those of [3]. His method employs 5 3D U-Nets for segmentation voting, which requires high computational cost and powerful hardware configuration, as well as utilizing a more complex architecture compared to the proposed method. Based on this, the proposed method outperformed [3] recall metric, which is used to evaluate true positives. This is due to the use of histogram matching and the proposed architecture, and the specific step for false positive removal made the precision increased. It is worth noting that the proposed method also surpassed the F1-Score of [2] and [7].

5 Conclusion

The study aimed to develop a method for segmenting coronary artery calcifications in the OrcaScore Dataset. Several experiments were conducted to improve the results, including preprocessing, data augmentation, post-processing, and exploring different architectures. The results presented are based on the best-performing metrics obtained thus far.

The experiments using the U-Net and modified U-Net architectures, along with ROI extraction, histogram matching, and false positive removal, yielded positive outcomes. It is worth noting that only CSCT exam images were used in this work, excluding the less common CCTA exams that involve contrast. Histogram matching, a preprocessing step not employed in previous studies, showed noticeable improvements in the results. Additionally, a dedicated false positive removal step contributed to higher sensitivity metrics.

As future work, it is suggested to explore new architectures, such as attention blocks or hybrid networks with DeepLab [13], since it uses dilated convolutions and captures information from broader contexts without increasing computational complexity, in addition to showing promising results in segmentation tasks.

Acknowledgements. The authors acknowledge the Coordenação de Aperfeiçoamento de Pessoal de Nível Superior (CAPES), Brazil - Finance Code 001, Conselho Nacional de Desenvolvimento Científico e Tecnológico (CNPq), Brazil, and Fundação de Amparo à Pesquisa Desenvolvimento Científico e Tecnológico do Maranhão (FAPEMA) (Brazil), Empresa Brasileira de Serviços Hospitalares (Ebserh) Brazil (Grant number 409593/2021-4) for the financial support.

References

1. de Vos, B.D., Wolterink, J.M., Leiner, T., de Jong, P.A., Lessmann, N., Išgum, I.: Direct automatic coronary calcium scoring in cardiac and chest CT. IEEE Trans. Med. Imaging **38**(9), 2127–2138 (2019)
2. Follmer, B., et al.: Active multitask learning with uncertainty-weighted loss for coronary calcium scoring. Med. Phys. **49**(11), 7262–7277 (2022)
3. Gogin, N., et al.: Automatic coronary artery calcium scoring from unenhanced-ECG-gated CT using deep learning. Diagn. Intervent. Imaging **102**(11), 683–690 (2021)
4. Wang, H., et al.: systematic analysis for the global burden of disease study 2015. Lancet **388**(10053), 2127–2138 (2019)
5. Wang, W., et al.: Coronary artery calcium score quantification using a deep-learning algorithm. Clin. Radiol. **75**(3), 237-e11 (2020)
6. Yoshida, A., Lee, Y., Yoshimura, N., Kuramoto, T., Hasegawa, A., Kanazawa, T.: Automated heart segmentation using U-net in pediatric cardiac CT. Sensors **18**(3), 100127 (2021)
7. Zhang, W., Zhang, J., Du, X., Zhang, Y., Li, S.: An end-to-end joint learning framework of artery-specific coronary calcium scoring in non-contrast cardiac CT. Computing **101**(3), 667–678 (2020)
8. Chinchor, N., Sundheim, B.M.: MUC-5 evaluation metrics. In: Fifth Message Understanding Conference (MUC-5): Proceedings of a Conference Held in Baltimore, Maryland, pp. 25–27 (2020)
9. Kendall, A., Gal, Y., Cipolla, R.: Multi-task learning using uncertainty to weigh losses for scene geometry and semantics. In: Proceedings of the IEEE Conference on Computer Vision and Pattern Recognition, pp. 7482–7491 (2018)

10. Lin, T.-Y., Goyal, P., Girshick, R., He, K., Dollar, P.: Focal loss for dense object detection. In: Proceedings of the IEEE International Conference on Computer Vision, pp. 2980–2988 (2017)
11. Sudre, C.H., Li, W., Vercauteren, T., Ourselin, S., Jorge Cardoso, M.: Generalised dice overlap as a deep learning loss function for highly unbalanced segmentations. In: Cardoso, M.J., et al. (eds.) DLMIA/ML-CDS -2017. LNCS, vol. 10553, pp. 240–248. Springer, Cham (2017). https://doi.org/10.1007/978-3-319-67558-9_28
12. Gonzalez, R.C.: Digital Image Processing, 2nd edn. Pearson Education, India (2009)
13. Wang, C., et al.: A three-stage self supervised deep learning network for automatic calcium scoring of cardiac computed tomography images. In: 2022 International Conference on Digital Image Computing: Techniques and Applications (DICTA). IEEE (2022)

Evaluation of Transfer Learning with a U-Net Architectures for Kidney Segmentation

Caio Eduardo Falcão Matos[1]($\boxtimes$) (iD), João Guilherme Araújo do Vale[3] (iD),
Marcos Melo Ferreira[1] (iD), Geraldo Braz Júnior[2] (iD),
and João Dallyson Sousa de Almeida[2] (iD)

[1] Federal Institute of Education, Science and Technology of Maranhão,
São Luís, Brazil
caio.matos@ifma.edu.br, marcos.ferreira@discente.ufma.br

[2] Applied Computer Group, Federal University of Maranhão, São Luís, Brazil
{geraldo,jdallyson}@nca.ufma.br

[3] Federal University of Maranhão, São Luís, Brazil
jga.vale@discente.ufma.br

Abstract. Kidney cancer emerges as one of the primary causes of mortality due to neoplasms on a global scale. Early detection and diagnosis of this disease often allow for more treatment options, contributing to the reduction of death rates. In this way, a correct delimitation of kidneys and renal tumor areas provides better analysis and diagnosis of suspicious lesions, contributing to treatment planning. This task is usually performed manually, making the process susceptible to fatigue (physical and visual) and distraction. Therefore, computational techniques, such as deep neural networks, are presented with great prominence as alternatives to improve segmentation precision and contribute to the early diagnosis of kidney cancer. In this work, we propose a methodology for kidney segmentation in computed tomography images by transfer learning to the U-Net network architecture. The KiTS19 dataset was used to evaluate the proposed methodology and obtained the best result for kidney segmentation of 96.0% of average Dice coefficient and average Jaccard index of 94.4%, using a pre-trained EfficentNet as an encoder for a U-Net.

Keywords: Kidney Segmentation · EfficentNet · U-Net · Transfer Learning

The authors thank the Higher Education Personnel Improvement Coordination (CAPES) - Finance Code 001, National Council for Scientific and Technological Development (CNPq) and the Foundation for Research and Scientific and Technological Development of the State of Maranhão (FAPEMA) for the financial support for the development of this work.

A. Cunha et al. (Eds.): MobiHealth 2023, LNICST 578, pp. 110–121, 2024.
https://doi.org/10.1007/978-3-031-60665-6_8

1   Introduction

Cancer is an ailment characterized by the uncontrolled growth and spread of certain cells within the body. It has the potential to initiate in nearly any part of the human body, comprised of trillions of cells [25,26]. According to the World Health Organization (WHO) report, cancer is the second leading cause of death worldwide, accounting for about 9.6 million deaths in 2018 alone [22].

Kidney cancer is also called renal cancer, is among the 14 most common types of cancer in the world, with over 400,000 diagnoses and over 170,000 deaths in 2020 alone [14]. An estimated 79,000 new cases of kidney cancer will be diagnosed this year 2022 in the United States, where 13 thousand of these will result in deaths [1].

Individuals identified in the early stages of the disease, where there is no spread, exhibit approximately a 93% relative survival rate of around 93% over a five-year span. Conversely, if the diagnosis occurs at an advanced stage with disease metastasis, the rate drops to 12%, underscoring the significance of early detection [2]. In this context, the early diagnosis assumes a pivotal role as an indispensable tool for prognosis and treatment, significantly augmenting the prospects of curative outcomes for the patient.

In recent years, medicine in general has made great strides in prevention, detection and treatment. Imaging tests, such as computed tomography (CT), represent a non-invasive alternative to obtain additional information to assist the physician. In this way, advances in computer-aided detection and diagnosis (CAD) methodologies have contributed to the early detection of kidney cancer, indicating suspicious areas and accurately diagnosing abnormalities. Renal area segmentation is an essential step for computer-assisted diagnosis or urological treatment. Therefore, several approaches based on deep learning have been widely applied in this task. Convolutional neural networks, especially the U-Net [24] networks and their various variations, have achieved excellent results in the semantic segmentation task focused on medical images [16,21,27,33].

This work aims to explore the transfer learning approach using a pre-trained EfficientNet to improve the coding step of a U-Net architecture and segment the kidney regions in a CT image. Furthermore, the contributions of this work include (1) the adaptation and integration of architectural models based on CNNs (Inception, ResNet, VGG, MobileNet, and EfficientNet) as the encoders for the U-Net architecture, (2) the evaluation of previous models with transfer learning for renal segmentation in computed tomography images.

2   Related Work

The task of segmenting kidneys and kidney tumors on computed tomography images aims to assist specialists in diagnosing kidney cancer. For both tasks, computational techniques can be applied to reduce the risks of radiation exposure (radiological examinations) and invasive procedures such as renal biopsy. Thus, the application and development of techniques aimed at image processing and deep learning are investigated by several works to analyze and segment kidneys and suspicious tumor regions.

Mu et al. [19] introduced a multi-resolution strategy combined with V-Net networks to automatic segment kidneys and renal tumors in CT images, training two V-Nets using images with different resolutions to determine the region of interest (kidneys and tumors).

Approaches that apply successive semantic segmentation networks to locate objects in images are called cascade architecture. The works of Zhang et al. [32] and Hou et al. [10] develop this approach for targeting kidneys and renal tumors. In the first one presents a two-stage approach utilizing a 3D UNet model. In the first stage, a rudimentary model is employed to identify the kidney's location and crop sub-volume patches encompassing the entire organ. Subsequently, the second stage involves a multitask 3D UNet model, which concurrently segments both the kidney and tumors based on the patches obtained from the initial stage. Conversely, the second work proposes a three-stage semantic segmentation pipeline based on 3D U-Nets, where the first two projects are based on nnUNet and are responsible for segmenting kidneys and the third stage for segmenting kidney tumors.

Isensee and Maier-Hein [15] propose an approach that integrates three networks, namely Plain 3D U-Net, Residual 3D U-Net, and Pre-activation Residual 3D U-Net, based on the U-Net architecture for the segmentation of kidneys and tumors. Türk, Lüy and Barışçı [30] demonstrate a hybrid model using the superior features of existing V-Nets models is presented. This model presents modifications in the encoding and decoding phases in the standard architecture.

Cruz et al. [6] presents um método baseado em três estágios, Scope Reduction, Segmentação dos rins e redução de falsos positivos. A primeira utiliza a rede AlexNet para efetuar slices classification. The second utiliza a rede U-Net para segmentação dos rins. At last, reduction of false positives by removing small segmented fragments.

Adaptations aimed at the U-Net network were applied using the methods proposed by [28] and [5] for kidney segmentation in the Kits19 dataset. The first method proposes the 2.5D MFFAU-Net (Multi-level Feature Fusion Attention U-Net), which uses a 2.5D model to learn to combine representations of 2D slices applied in a ResConv architecture in MFFAU-Net for kidney segmentation. The other method applies a deep learning model, which is an ensemble of U-Net models developed after testing various model variations.

A modification of the convolution blocks of the U-Net network architecture is proposed by Hou et al. [11]. According to this work, dilated convolution blocks (DCB) are applied to replace the traditional pooling operations of the U-Net network. Such changes aim to retain semantic information better. This approach additionally employs three networks (reduced resolution, complete resolution, and refinement) for the segmentation of renal structures and tumors.

When reviewing the relevant literature, it becomes evident that variations in the architecture of the convolutional neural network U-Net [24] have been consistently employed across all proposed methodologies. This underscores the inherent potential of encoder-decoder-based convolutional neural networks. Consequently, the approach proposed in this study aims to harness the full capabilities of the U-Net convolutional network by leveraging a diverse set of pretrained architectures as encoders for the task of segmenting kidneys in computed tomography images.

3   Materials and Methods

This section presents the proposed methodology for segmenting the kidneys in computed tomography images. For the development of the experiments, CT images were used from the KiTS19 database [9]. Then, we applied a preprocessing step for each volume to improve the contrast of the organs. In the next step, we applied pre-trained CNN architectures as an encoder of the U-Net to evaluate how the transfer of learning can positively influence the segmentation of the kidneys in CT images. We use a U-Net network because it could be easily customizable, changing the encode (and adapting the decode) and improving the skip connections. We hypothesize that transfer learning techniques could generate more reliable and precise results. Figure 1 illustrates the steps of the proposed methodology. In the following subsections, each of these steps is detailed.

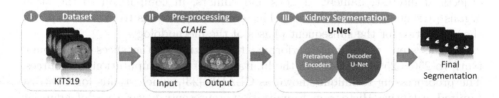

Fig. 1. Steps of the proposed method.

3.1   Dataset

In this work, we used a database with CT images aimed at the challenge of segmenting kidney tumors called KiTS19.

This dataset comes from patients undergoing nephrectomy for renal tumors at the University of Minnesota Medical Center (USA) between 2010 and 2018. A total of 300 exams were collected in this survey. Of which, 210 were made available for training and validation and 90 to test according to the challenge. In addition to imaging exams, a manual segmentation, performed by medical students under the supervision of Dr. Christopher Weight, is made available representing the kidneys and tumors for each patient [9]. CT images and masks (Ground Truth), available in NIFTI format for each volume, are converted into slices, each image being grayscale with a resolution of 512×512, where the number of slices varies between patients (Fig. 2).

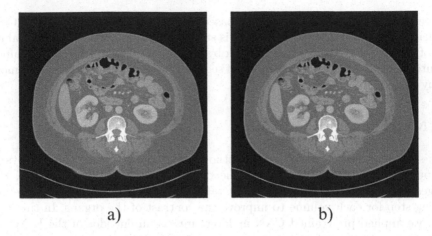

a)   b)

Fig. 2. Example from the KiTS19 dataset. (a) CT scan slice and (b) provided kidney and tumor annotations.

3.2 Image Pre-processing

The objective of this preprocessing stage is to augment the contrast of the objects of interest, namely, kidneys and tumors, in comparison to the other organs present in the examination. This enhancement aims to provide superior characteristics for the subsequent phases of the methodology.

In this step, we initially performed the resizing of the slices and ground truth to 256×256 pixels due to the limitations of the computational resources. The preprocessing technique known as CLAHE [23], which stands for Contrast Limited Adaptive Histogram Equalization, represents a variation of adaptive histogram equalization (AHE) aimed at mitigating excessive contrast amplification. This method functions within localized image regions referred to as "blocks" rather than operating on the entire image. In this approach, each pixel of the original image resides at the center of its respective contextual region. The process entails clipping the histogram of the original image and redistributing the pixels across the various gray levels. Then, the CLAHE was applied to the KiTS19 base images using a grid size of 8×8 and a clip contrast limit 2.0. The application of this technique aims to increase the contrast of the object of interest, the kidneys, in relation to the other organs present in the abdominal region. Figure 3 depicts the technique's application on the KiTS19 dataset.

3.3 Kidney Segmentation

CNN architectures focused on semantic segmentation typically incorporate encoding and decoding networks such as the U-Net network. This property aims to reduce and restore the image resolution to capture the most relevant details in their respective encoding and decoding phases. Therefore, we apply the

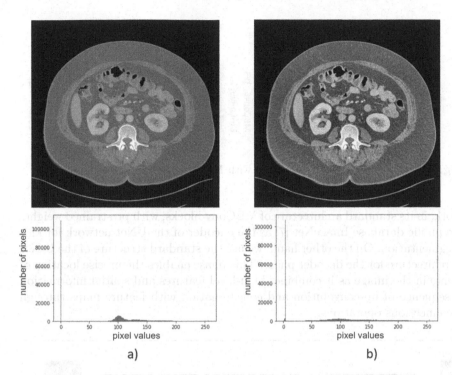

Fig. 3. Result of applying CLAHE with the respective histograms. (a) original image and (b) preprocessed image.

CNN-based architecture of the EfficientNet network as an alternative to replace the U-Net network's encoder for segmentation of the kidneys.

EfficientUNet Architecture. EfficientNet's architecture is based on convolutional neural networks and has a method called Compound Scaling that uniformly scales all dimensions of depth/width/resolution using a composite coefficient. The architecture of this network has 8 variations from B0 to B7, where each model number refers to variants with a more significant number of [29] parameters. The inverted residual block called MBConv developed in the MobileNetV2 [12] architecture became the basis for constructing EfficientNet networks, where each of the 8 models (B0–B7) share standard blocks with subtle complexities in their architectures. Thus, in this work, we use the EfficientNet-B3 architecture composed of 7 MBConv blocks, where each of the blocks presents the size of the applied filter (3×3 or 5×5) and the default activation function used, which can be, respectively, ReLU [20] and ReLU6 [13] for blocks MBConv1 and MBConv6. An overview of the architecture can be seen in Fig. 4.

Figure 5 presents the architecture evaluated in this work. This approach modifies the standard U-Net network by replacing the encoder phase with a CNN-based architecture with pre-trained weights. We adopted an EfficientNet-B3

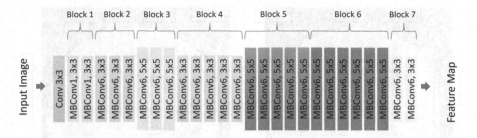

Fig. 4. Architecture of EfficientNet-B3 with MBConv as basic building blocks.

network, in its standard architecture of MBConv blocks, with pre-trained weights in the public database ImageNet [7] as the encoder of the UNet network for kidney segmentation. On the other hand, we use the standard structure of the U-Net [24] architecture for the decoder phase. This phase enables the precise location of elements in the image as it combines high-level features and spatial information by a sequence of up-convolution and concatenation with feature maps through skip connections operations.

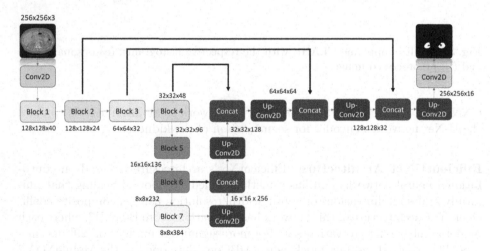

Fig. 5. Proposed architecture of EfficientNet-B3 as encoder in U-Net.

4   Results

In this section, we present the results of the experiments carried out in evaluating the proposed methodology. The utilized metrics encompassed the Sørensen-Dice index, commonly referred to as the Dice coefficient (DSC) [8] and Jaccard index (JCD) [17].

We divided the 210 exams provided by the KiTS19 dataset into three datasets respecting the proportions 70% (147 exams) for training, 20% (42 exams) for validation, and 10% (21 exams) for the test. A random separation of the data sets was conducted based on patients (exams) to ensure the integrity of the slices in the training, testing, and validation sets.

To study the effect of different encoders, beyond EfficientNet, we perform experiments with VGG16, ResNet50, InceptionV3, SE-Resnet-152, MobileNetv2 and EfficientNetB3. The architecture formed by each of the encoders combined with the UNet decoder was trained for 50 epochs, using a *batch* size equal to 16, Adam optimizer with a learning rate of 0.0001 and DiceLoss + BinaryFocalLoss as a loss function. This set of parameters was defined after several experiments, and this set produced the best results. Table 1 shows that the EfficientNet-B3, when used as an encoder for a U-Net obtained the best results among other tested encoders.

Table 1. Results of the combination of pre-trained models with U-Net for kidney segmentation.

Method	DSC	JCD	Error
U-Net + InceptionV3	89.19%	85.82%	0.1209
U-Net + Resnet-50	91.32%	89.15%	0.0965
U-Net + SE-Resnet-152	91.33%	88.95%	0.0954
U-Net + VGG-16	91.76%	89.59%	0.0906
U-Net + MobileNetV2	93.93%	92.20%	0.0658
U-Net + EfficientNetB3	**96.04%**	**94.47%**	**0.0445**

Table 1 shows that the MobileNet and EfficientNet networks outperformed the other applied networks. The results of 89.1% Dice and 85.8% Jaccard obtained by the Inception network demonstrate limitations in kidney identification and segmentation, as it performed the worst among the networks. The ResNet, SE-ResNet, and VGG networks achieved relatively close results in terms of Dice, Jaccard, and error rates. Among these three networks, VGG achieved the highest scores with Dice, Jaccard, and Error rates of 91.7%, 89.5%, and 0.09, respectively.

However, EfficientNet and MobileNet networks focus on the foreground and produce better results for kidney segmentation, as reflected in their Dice, Jaccard, and Error values. When comparing these two networks, it is observed that EfficientNet outperformed MobileNet in all metrics. Considering only the Dice coefficient, the EfficientNet network scored 2% points higher than MobileNet, reaching 93.9%.

Figure 6 provide examples of kidney segmentation carried out by the MobileNet and EfficientNet networks, respectively. It is observed that both networks exhibit good performance in distinguishing the kidneys from other abdominal organs and structures.

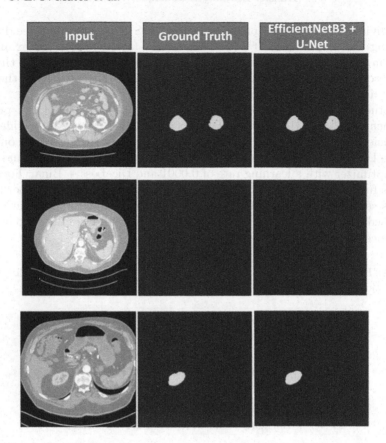

Fig. 6. Examples of kidney segmentation using the EfficientNetB3 + U-Net network. From left to right: input slice, expert annotation (ground truth), and segmentation performed by the network.

In Table 2, we compare the performance of the proposed methodology with the works that represent the state of the art in the KiTS19 database. It is important to note that the methods cited do not provide information about the exact procedures for splitting the training, testing, and validation datasets, nor do they specify how slices are divided within the datasets. As a result, it is not possible to make an exact comparison of the results.

The EfficientNet-B3 has proven to be the best encoder when used in conjunction with the U-Net network. This combination yields results comparable to the ensemble methods employed by most of the studies, as well as the hybrid approach of the V-Net network, which is considered the benchmark for the best-performing method in kidney segmentation. The proposed methodology achieved Dice and Jaccard scores of 96% and 94.4%, respectively, with only a 1.7% point difference from the method proposed by [30]. Furthermore, it offers significantly fewer hyperparameter choices and a customizable architecture for supplementary tasks.

Table 2. Comparison of the proposed method with works aimed at kidney segmentation using the KiTS19 dataset.

Work	Technique	DSC	JCD
Ma (2019) [18]	Ensemble Networks	97.3%	-
Zhang et al. (2019) [32]	Cascade	97.4%	-
Mu et al. (2019) [19]	MR-VB-Net	97.4%	-
Hou et al. (2019) [10]	Cascade	96.7%	-
Isensee et al. (2019) [15]	Ensemble Deep Net	97.4%	-
Trk et al. (2020) [30]	Hybrid V-Net	**97.7%**	-
Cruz et al. (2020) [6]	U-Net 2D	96.3%	93.0%
Hou et al. (2020) [11]	U-Net Modified	96.7%	-
Xie et al. (2020) [31]	SE-ResNeXT	96.7%	-
Jason et al. (2021) [5]	Ensemble of U-Net	94.9%	-
Peng et al. (2023) [28]	2.5D MFFAU-Net	92.4%	-
Proposed Method	**EfficientNetB3 + U-Net**	**96.0%**	**94.4%**

5 Conclusion

The development of methodologies and architectures for semantic segmentation aimed at identifying organs and tumor lesions in computed tomography scans presents itself as a challenging task, especially in abdominal CT scans, which encompass a wide variety of organs such as kidneys, spleen, bladder, among others. The methodology proposed in this study sought to evaluate the application of some of the leading fully convolutional networks (FCNs), particularly the EfficientNet network, as an encoder and feature extractor for the U-Net network, applied to the segmentation of kidneys and renal tumors in CT scans.

The methodology proposed in this work sought to explore and evaluate the learning transfer of CNN-based architectures using the EfficientNet network as an encoder and feature extractor of the U-Net network for segmenting kidneys in CT scans.

The results obtained for the kidney segmentation task demonstrate that the EfficientNet network applied as an encoder of the U-Net network produces an efficient approach for identifying kidneys in CT images. In addition, the proposed methodology obtained results comparable to the literature for kidney segmentation. Thus, the results for this task indicate that architectures with different encoders and decoders emerge as a research area where they allow the construction of methods with the integration of different networks aimed at kidney segmentation. We also observe that the application of the standard U-Net decoder can reconstruct features at each stage of both backbones, thus obtaining information oriented towards both local context and global information.

Despite promising results, the proposed method could be improved in some ways. As future works, the adaptation of the pre-trained EfficientNet-B3 model applied to variations of the U-Net network such as Attention U-Net [21], U-Net++ [33], BCDU-Net [4], LSTM-UNet [3] could contribute to a better identification of the kidneys in CT scans.

References

1. ACS: American cancer society - key statistics about kidney cancer (2022). https://www.cancer.org/cancer/kidney-cancer/about/key-statistics.html
2. ACS: American cancer society - survival rates for kidney cancer (2022). https://www.cancer.org/cancer/kidney-cancer/detection-diagnosis-staging/survival-rates.html
3. Arbelle, A., Raviv, T.R.: Microscopy cell segmentation via convolutional LSTM networks. In: 2019 IEEE 16th International Symposium on Biomedical Imaging (ISBI 2019), pp. 1008–1012. IEEE, Hilton Molino Stucky, Venice (2019)
4. Azad, R., Asadi-Aghbolaghi, M., Fathy, M., Escalera, S.: Bi-directional ConvLSTM U-net with densley connected convolutions. In: Proceedings of the IEEE/CVF International Conference on Computer Vision Workshops. IEEE, Seoul (2019)
5. Causey, J., et al.: An ensemble of U-net models for kidney tumor segmentation with CT images. IEEE/ACM Trans. Comput. Biol. Bioinf. **19**(3), 1387–1392 (2021)
6. da Cruz, L.B., et al.: Kidney segmentation from computed tomography images using deep neural network. Comput. Biol. Med. **123**, 103906 (2020)
7. Deng, J., Dong, W., Socher, R., Li, L.J., Li, K., Fei-Fei, L.: ImageNet: a large-scale hierarchical image database. In: 2009 IEEE Conference on Computer Vision and Pattern Recognition, pp. 248–255. IEEE, Miami (2009)
8. Fleiss, J.L., Levin, B., Paik, M.C., et al.: The measurement of interrater agreement. Stat. Methods Rates Proport. **2**(212–236), 22–23 (1981)
9. Heller, N., et al.: The KiTS19 challenge data: 300 kidney tumor cases with clinical context, CT semantic segmentations, and surgical outcomes. arXiv preprint arXiv:1904.00445 (2019)
10. Hou, X., Xie, C., Li, F., Nan, Y.: Cascaded semantic segmentation for kidney and tumor. Submissions to the (2019)
11. Hou, X., et al.: A triple-stage self-guided network for kidney tumor segmentation. In: 2020 IEEE 17th International Symposium on Biomedical Imaging (ISBI), pp. 341–344. IEEE, Iowa City (2020)
12. Howard, A., Zhmoginov, A., Chen, L.C., Sandler, M., Zhu, M.: Inverted residuals and linear bottlenecks: mobile networks for classification, detection and segmentation (2018)
13. Howard, A.G., et al.: MobileNets: efficient convolutional neural networks for mobile vision applications. arXiv preprint arXiv:1704.04861 (2017)
14. Internacional, W.: World cancer research fund international - kidney cancer statistics (2022). https://www.wcrf.org/cancer-trends/kidney-cancer-statistics/
15. Isensee, F., Maier-Hein, K.H.: An attempt at beating the 3D U-net. arXiv preprint arXiv:1908.02182 (2019)
16. Isensee, F., et al.: nnU-Net: self-adapting framework for U-net-based medical image segmentation. arXiv preprint arXiv:1809.10486 (2018)
17. Jaccard, P.: The distribution of the flora in the alpine zone. 1. New Phytol. **11**(2), 37–50 (1912)
18. Ma, J.: Solution to the kidney tumor segmentation challenge 2019 (2019)

19. Mu, G., Lin, Z., Han, M., Yao, G., Gao, Y.: Segmentation of kidney tumor by multi-resolution VB-nets (2019)
20. Nair, V., Hinton, G.E.: Rectified linear units improve restricted Boltzmann machines. In: ICML. Omnipress, Madison (2010)
21. Oktay, O., et al.: Attention U-net: Learning where to look for the pancreas. arXiv preprint arXiv:1804.03999 (2018)
22. OPAS/OMS: Pan-American health organization - cancer. 2022 (2022). https://www.paho.org/pt/topicos/cancer
23. Pizer, S.M., et al.: Adaptive histogram equalization and its variations. Comput. Vision Graph. Image Process. **39**(3), 355–368 (1987)
24. Ronneberger, O., Fischer, P., Brox, T.: U-net: convolutional networks for biomedical image segmentation. In: Navab, N., Hornegger, J., Wells, W.M., Frangi, A.F. (eds.) MICCAI 2015. LNCS, vol. 9351, pp. 234–241. Springer, Cham (2015). https://doi.org/10.1007/978-3-319-24574-4_28
25. Roy, N.K., Bordoloi, D., Monisha, J., Anip, A., Padmavathi, G., Kunnumakkara, A.B.: Cancer-an overview and molecular alterations in cancer. Fusion Genes Cancer 1–15 (2017)
26. Sprouffske, K., Athena Aktipis, C., Radich, J.P., Carroll, M., Nedelcu, A.M., Maley, C.C.: An evolutionary explanation for the presence of cancer nonstem cells in neoplasms. Evol. Appl. **6**(1), 92–101 (2013)
27. Sun, J., Darbehani, F., Zaidi, M., Wang, B.: SAUNet: shape attentive U-net for interpretable medical image segmentation. In: Martel, A.L., et al. (eds.) MICCAI 2020. LNCS, vol. 12264, pp. 797–806. Springer, Cham (2020). https://doi.org/10.1007/978-3-030-59719-1_77
28. Sun, P., et al.: 2.5 d MFFAU-Net: a convolutional neural network for kidney segmentation. BMC Med. Inform. Decis. Making **23**(1), 1–11 (2023)
29. Tan, M., Le, Q.: EfficientNet: rethinking model scaling for convolutional neural networks. In: International conference on machine learning. pp. 6105–6114. PMLR, Long Beach (2019)
30. Türk, F., Lüy, M., Barışçı, N.: Kidney and renal tumor segmentation using a hybrid V-Net-based model. Mathematics **8**(10), 1772 (2020)
31. Xie, X., Li, L., Lian, S., Chen, S., Luo, Z.: SERU: a cascaded se-ResNeXT U-Net for kidney and tumor segmentation. Concurr. Comput.: Pract. Exp. **32**(14), e5738 (2020)
32. Zhang, Y., et al.: Cascaded volumetric convolutional network for kidney tumor segmentation from CT volumes. arXiv preprint arXiv:1910.02235 (2019)
33. Zhou, Zongwei, Rahman Siddiquee, Md Mahfuzur, Tajbakhsh, Nima, Liang, Jianming: UNet++: a nested U-Net architecture for medical image segmentation. In: Stoyanov, D., et al. (eds.) DLMIA/ML-CDS -2018. LNCS, vol. 11045, pp. 3–11. Springer, Cham (2018). https://doi.org/10.1007/978-3-030-00889-5_1

Training U-Net with Proportional Image Division for Retinal Structure Segmentation

Pedro Victor de Abreu Fonseca[1], Alexandre Carvalho Araújo[1], João Dallyson S. de Almeida[1(✉)], Geraldo Braz Júnior[1], Aristófanes Correa Silva[1], and Rodrigo de Melo Souza Veras[2]

[1] Federal University of Maranhão - UFMA, Applied Computing Group - NCA/UFMA, São Luís, Brazil
jdallyson@nca.ufma.br
[2] Federal University of Piauí - UFPI, Teresina, Brazil

Abstract. Cup and optic disc segmentation has become one of the main objects of study in the field of creating and improving machine learning-oriented models due to the importance of vision for human beings and the ability to assist physicians in diagnosing ocular problems. Within this context, this study presents a new method based on the proportional division of images concerning features extracted from the sample set. These samples go through a pre-processing step involving image resizing before going to deep feature extraction and K-means clustering, thus dividing the set for validation and training. Soon after, the amount of samples is increased through data augmentation before going on to the U-Net training. The proposed method has been evaluated on the public RIM-ONE and DRISHTI-GS datasets, and presented promising results in the segmentation of both structures, with emphasis on obtaining the value of 92.2% of Dice for the segmentation of the optic cup in the DRISHTI-GS test dataset and 95.9% of Dice for the optic disc in the RIM-ONE.

Keywords: Segmentation · Retinal fundus · Proportional Image Division · U-Net

1 Introduction

Vision is one of the most important senses for human beings because we can understand the world around us. However, the organ connected to this sense, the human eye, is susceptible to pathologies leading to partial or total loss of this sense. Part of these problems include Glaucoma and Cataracts, which represent a large part of the cases related to the loss of sight [6,25]. Moreover, according to [31], Glaucoma is a pathology that, due to its silent way of acting, may soon become the leading cause of blindness, estimating a total of 118.8 million people worldwide will be affected.

© ICST Institute for Computer Sciences, Social Informatics and Telecommunications Engineering 2024
Published by Springer Nature Switzerland AG 2024. All Rights Reserved
A. Cunha et al. (Eds.): MobiHealth 2023, LNICST 578, pp. 122–138, 2024.
https://doi.org/10.1007/978-3-031-60665-6_9

These eye diseases can be detected early with examinations that physicians can perform, such as the use of structural tests for a clinical analysis of the optic disc on OCT images. Functional tests are based on standard automated perimetry, which is an analysis of the individual's field of vision [28]. Early treatment can be initiated by analyzing and checking retinal structures such as the cup and the optic disc. Due to the human effort required for these tasks and the growing number of cases linked to these diseases, algorithms that use Deep Learning for the segmentation and classification of the structures of the human eye have been developed and improved to provide concise and robust results, facilitating the work done by professionals in the area [2,5,8,14].

The optic disc and cup are the structures most targeted in the retinal segmentation task. However, such a task proves to be challenging for even the most refined neural networks, with emphasis on the optic cup due to its size, tonality, and the presence of other surrounding structures such as blood vessels [32]. Such structures are arranged in Fig. 1. To deal with the difficulty of this task, image processing techniques have been used, such as extraction of a region of interest (ROI) that aims to highlight only the part of the original image that contains the structures [21,32] and the extraction of the green channel from the image [15]. Important highlighted is the use of architectures using Deep Learning that has created near state-of-the-art learning models.

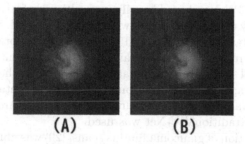

(A)   **(B)**

Fig. 1. (A) represents the disc and optic cup area, while (B) delimits these areas. The larger circle is the disc, and the smaller one is the optic cup. Adapted from [24]

We propose an approach that works directly with the optic cup and disc segmentation region to have a balanced set of samples. Differing from related work that has been heavily concerned with preprocessing the images laid out for training [12,16,21], using as architecture the U-Net neural network with encoder from ResNet-34 presented by [32]. The proposed method includes an initial step of proportional separation of the images used in the training/validation of the model, according to features extracted concerning the disc and the optic cup, seeking a balancing in the number of samples arranged in each set of images aiming to improve the generalization of the segmentation model produced.

Our study contributes to segmenting fundus images, precisely the optic cup and optic disc, by sampling the results and obtaining an approach heavily based on sample separation by balancing the sets used for training using feature extraction previously extracted from the samples available for training.

This paper is organized as follows: Sect. 2 presents the related works to the fundus retinal structures segmentation in images. Section 3 details the materials and method of this work, including datasets, the proposed method with proportional division approaches, and the experiment set-up. In Sect. 4, we present the results of the proposed method. Section 5 discusses the results. Finally, Sect. 6 presents the conclusions and suggestions for future work.

2   Related Works

Segmentation of retinal structures is one of the most addressed tasks in the literature, in which several approaches are used to obtain good results. [34] used entropy techniques in union with a uniform set of fundus examination samples used by a convolutional neural network based on boosting filters. As much as modifications to the architectures have been widely applied, [12] preferred to use the standard U-Net architecture without modifications to it by applying image processing techniques working with eye fundus scans in an even smaller proportion when compared to the works cited here. [21] using image processing techniques, extracted a region of interest from the set of fundus exams for segmentation of the optical cup, which soon after is passed to U-Net architecture for segmentation. [26] proposed for the segmentation of retinal structures an architecture named ResFPN-Net, based heavily on multi-scale feature extraction that combined previously extracted features with new ones found. Such methodology allowed the segmentation of the disc and the optic cup to obtain positive results when compared to related works. [16] aimed at the segmentation of the optic cup and the optical disk through operations directly on the masks contained in the training set, applying modifications to the pixels contained in the edges, which were binary values of 0 or 1, to numbers generated through probabilities, as architecture the traditional U-Net was used.

For the classification of glaucoma fundus scans, [29] was able to achieve better results than related works on a sample set using as architecture implementation of U-Net, named U-Net++. In addition, hyperparameter optimization was used with a loss function that combined the binary entropy with the Dice coefficient function, performing a subtraction between the two equations.

Using only the DRISHTI-GS dataset, [30] construed a framework to aid the classification of Glaucoma in fundus examination samples. To accomplish such a task, two custom CNNs were implemented, each used for disk and optic cup segmentation. In addition, image processing techniques, such as edge detection, image dilation, and erosion application, were used to ensure that good results were obtained in segmenting the targeted structures.

As much as our study performs the segmentation of retinal structures separately, works regarding the simultaneous segmentation of the optic cup and the optic disc have been developed as [1]. The authors used a more diversified training concerning the number of samples available for training with the accession of a new set of fundus exams, the ORIGA dataset, in addition to the use of the DenseNet architecture for the simultaneous segmentation of the optic disc and the optic cup, obtaining results superior to the methods used as a reference in large datasets. As a result of the advance in segmentation-oriented neural networks, hybrid architectures have emerged, increasing the potential of convolutional networks already known by the scientific community. An example is the integration of residual backbones that provide robust and dynamic learning due to the number of parameters and *shortcuts* that the final model presents [32]. Due to these advantages, good results were obtained by [32] integrating the pre-trained residual backbone of ResNet-34, thus avoiding training from the beginning, together with the U-Net, for the segmentation of retinal structures.

3 Materials and Method

3.1 Image Datasets

The public retinal image datasets DRISHTI-GS [23] and RIM-ONE [10] were selected for the experiments. These datasets were chosen because both are widely used for training architectures focused on the segmentation/classification of retinal fundus images. The DRISHTI-GS dataset contains 101 images in its entirety with a resolution of 2896 × 1944 pixels and with a field-of-view of 30°. In comparison, the RIM-ONE presents 159 images with a resolution of 2144 × 1424 pixels. Each image was used without cropping, without ROI extraction, thus differentiating from the works used as references [21,32]. The bases were used together for the training process. The Fig. 2 and Fig. 3 shows a sample of the Drishti-GS and RIM-ONE dataset respectively.

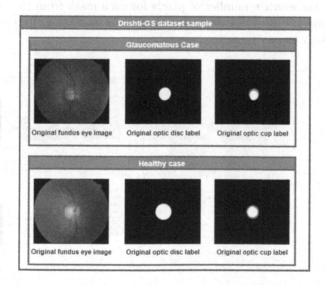

Fig. 2. Original sample of the Drishti-GS dataset. Originally, each mask contained in the dataset is composed of several markings for the optical cup and optical disk.

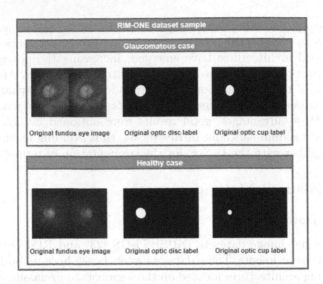

Fig. 3. Original sample of the RIM-ONE dataset. Each sample is composed of a pair of the same fundus eye exam.

3.2 Proposed Method

The proposed method is organized in the following steps: (1) preprocessing, (2) proportional split of samples, which can be done by extracting deep features or working with the average number of pixels for each mask from the training set, (3) data augmentation, (4) U-net with ResNet-34 backbone. Figure 4 presents the methodology steps.

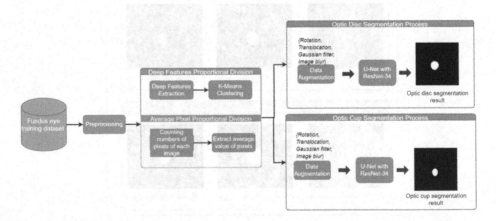

Fig. 4. Proposed Method. The proposed method uses mostly the same operations for both optical cup and optical disk segmentation.

Preprocessing. In the preprocessing step, the images were resized to 256×256 pixels, aiming to test the performance of the proposed method in an even smaller image than [32], which used the dimensions 512×512 pixels, thereby using fewer computational resources for model generation. Due to the change in the dimensions of the samples to a smaller value than the original shape, one can expect more difficulty from the architecture used for training in segmenting the structures, particularly that of the optic cup.

Proportional Division. Both datasets present for each image the disc delimitation and optic cup to be used in training, emphasizing the DRISHTI-GS masks with several labelings performed by experts. Thus, for each image in the DRISHTI-GS dataset, the demarcation with the smallest segmentation region was selected because, as previously mentioned, regions with small segmentation areas are challenging to segment, so to test the proposed methodology, such a choice was made. The RIM-ONE dataset has, for each image, only one label.

The proportional splitting approach was inspired by the work of [9], in which they proposed proportional splitting based on tumor size and pixel intensity to better distribute images from CT scans of the kidneys into the training, validation, and test sets. To define the division based on texture, the authors have defined a threshold (pixel intensity) that separates the reference cases into cases with light and dark tumors. Their goal of segmenting kidney tumors was improved with proportional splitting. In our study, we evaluate proportional splitting based on the area and texture of the regions of interest. In the latter approach, we set the split automatically using deep features and clustering using k-means.

Area Based Proportional Division. The mask annotations area of the training samples was initially used as the separation parameter to divide the training set evenly. The optic cup and the optic disc are represented by a set of white pixels in the masks in both datasets used. The area was obtained considering the number of pixels in each segmentation region. Next, the entire set of images for training is traversed to obtain the average area that references the region of interest contained in the masks. Thereafter, images are categorized as "large region of interest" or "small region of interest" according to their area compared to the average area. The perfect distribution would be 50% of images with the large area and 50% with the small area. However, this task is challenging due to the original arrangement of the DRISHTI-GS and RIM-ONE datasets that are originally unbalanced. Thus, the dataset's proportional splitting shows a variation of 20% concerning the perfect balancing in the worst-case distribution for this approach. The representation of this approach can be seen in Fig. 5.

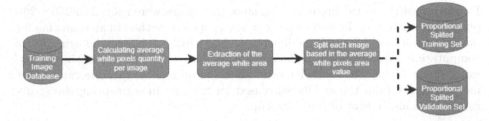

Fig. 5. Flow of operations for the proportional division based on the segmentation area.

Splitting Based on Deep Features + K-Means. This approach differs from the previous one because a network was used for feature extraction on the training set. The purpose of this new method was to verify the effectiveness of the texture features in the activity of the image's proportional division. After several experiments, the ResNet-34 model was used to perform feature extraction, which proved to be more efficient than other architectures previously used for the same task, such as VGG19, ResNet-50, and VGG16. Figure 6 shows steps for this approach.

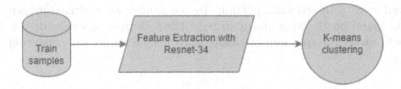

Fig. 6. Feature Extraction Approach using the ResNet-34 model.

After extraction, samples with similar characteristics are clustered using the K-means algorithm [11]. The silhouette coefficient was used to define the value for the number of clusters. This coefficient is calculated using Eq. 1.

$$S(x) = \frac{b(x) - a(x)}{\max(b(x), a(x))} \tag{1}$$

In which x represents an element in the π cluster, a(x) is the average distance of x to all elements in the π cluster, and b(x) represents the average distance of x from all points in another γ cluster. The interval of values for Eq. 1 is $[-1, 1]$, where the closer to 1 the better defined the clusters are [22]. An interval [2–5] of k values was evaluated. At the end of the process, the selected number with the best silhouette coefficient was K = 2.

Data Augmentation. To increase the number of dataset images, new images were generated performing operations of rotation, contrast change, and blur through the transformations of the Albumentation framework [7]. This generator moves the images at 45° angles in a scaling limit of 0.5, rotates the images vertically and horizontally with a probability of 50%, and also, in this same probability, applies filters and lighting effects such as Gaussian noise. It is important to note that due to the 50% value, previously established, each image may or may not be modified with all the operations determined.

To define a test set for the RIM-ONE dataset, of the 159 images initially contained in the same dataset, a percentage of 20% of these images were destined for the creation of a test set, totaling 30 images from the RIM-ONE for post-training evaluation and 129 images from the same dataset for training. Overall, 129 samples from the RIM-ONE combined with 50 images from the DRISHTI-GS, totaling 179 images, proceeded to be distributed into ten folds used during the k-folding technique to ensure a more reliable and robust validation process [19]. After repartitioning, each fold went through a data augmentation step, resulting in a total of 4,180 images summing all the samples in each fold. The test datasets remained unchanged without data augmentation.

Network Architecture. The neural network architecture used was U-Net [20] modified with the path encoder based on ResNet-34, as proposed in [32]. The standard U-net structure is present in the up-sampling decoding layers, while the down-sampling layer features the ResNet-34 model, containing a 7×7 convolutional layer and 64 filters. After that, there are 4 residual blocks, containing each block two 3×3 convolutional layers presenting *shortcuts* between each connection [32].

Each residual block has, respectively, 3 connections in the first block, 4 in the second, 6 in the third and 3 in the last, with each block of 3 connections having batch normalization, and an exponential increase in the number of filters by a factor of 2, thus starting with 64 filters and ending at 512 in the last block. Each decoding block contains a 2×2 convolution transposed layer obtained from the previous layer with a stride of 2, concatenated with a 1×1 convolution for each respective block contained in the down-sampling section. The already concatenated tensor goes through the batch normalization process before proceeding to the next decoding layer. Finally, in the last layer, the last transposed convolution occurs, which returns an image with the same dimensions as the input image. Figure 7 illustrates the complete architecture of the neural network used.

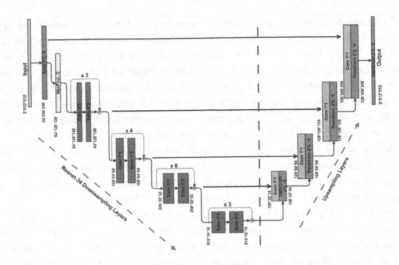

Fig. 7. Hybrid U-Net architecture with the ResNet-34 backbone. Adapted from [32]

3.3   Evaluation Metrics

We used as evaluation metrics the Dice coefficient (DiceScore) (Eq. 2), which aims to measure the similarity between two samples. In this work, the similarity between the generated mask prediction and the reference mask and the Jaccard index (JaccardScore) (Eq. 3) is calculated by dividing the pixels of the prediction concerning the reference mask of the image.

$$DiceScore = \frac{2 \times TP}{2 \times TP + FP + FN} \tag{2}$$

$$JaccardScore = \frac{TP}{TP + FP + FN} \tag{3}$$

In which TP represents pixels correctly labeled as being from the optic cup or optic disc, FP represents pixels misclassified as the optic cup or optic disc, and FN pixels misclassified as not being optic disc or optic cup.

3.4   Experimental Set-Up

In the network training, binary entropy weighted cross entropy was chosen as the loss function [18]. Its purpose is to act with a better proportion of the weights contained in each image and its respective mask, assigning for each class (0 and 1) a corresponding weight. This function is described in Eq. 4. The choice of such a function made it possible to avoid class unbalances.

$$Loss = (\alpha \times \mathbf{t} \times \mathbf{p} + \alpha \times ((\mathbf{t} - 1) \times (\mathbf{p} - 1))) - (\alpha - 1) \tag{4}$$

where α remains at the negative value of -1, t represents the target value, the mask of the image according to experts, and p is a prediction image that was generated by the network.

Each *fold* was trained for 30 epochs with a batch size of value 4 with a learning rate set at 1e-4 with a decay of 0.5 every 10000 steps. In addition, the Early Stopping technique was used with the patience set to 3 epochs [13]. These parameters were set after performing training in addition to using the HyperOpt library [4]. All experiments were performed on hardware configured with NVIDIA GeForce GTX 1660 TI video card with 6 GB of RAM.

4   Results

Using the DRISHTI-GS and RIM-ONE test datasets, this section aims to demonstrate the values obtained to measure the accuracy of the model generated by the proposed method. The DRISHTI-GS dataset initially presented 50 images for training and 51 for testing, while the RIM-ONE had 159 images without division. After the augmentation, the number of images in the DRISHTI-GS and RIM-ONE datasets composing the training samples was 1,150 and 3,030, respectively.

Initially, experiments were performed to evaluate the performance of the chosen architecture, comparing the metrics obtained with a set of distinct architectures. It is important to note that the IOU metric in the following tables represents the JaccardScore equation seen in Sect. 3.3. Results for these experiments are shown in Table 1, for the DRISHTI-GS test dataset, and in Table 2, for the RIM-ONE test dataset. Importantly, these results were obtained without extracting Deep Features but using only the proportional division based on the image area. These architectures were chosen to measure the methodology's effectiveness on a deeper residual architecture with more layers (ResNet-50) and one with fewer training parameters (MobileNetV2).

Table 1. Optic disc and optic cup segmentation results. DRISHTI-GS test dataset. (*) means using proportional division based on area.

Architecture	Optic Disc		Optic Cup	
	Dice Score	IOU Score	Dice Score	IOU Score
U-Net with Resnet-50	95.4	92.2	89.0	78.9
U-Net with Resnet-50 (*)	96.0	**93.1**	90.2	80.4
U-Net with MobileNetV2	94.3	91.1	88.0	77.3
U-Net with MobileNetV2 (*)	95.0	91.0	89.2	79.1
U-Net with Resnet-34	96.0	92.2	89.5	79.9
U-Net with Resnet-34 (*)	**96.1**	92.4	**90.4**	**81.6**

After analyzing the values in both tables, it is possible to notice that the proposed U-Net model with ResNet-34 using proportional division is the most effective in segmenting the optic cup and the optic disc in the test sets of both datasets used in the experiments. Notably, the values obtained in the optic cup

Table 2. Optic disc and optic cup segmentation results. RIM-ONE test dataset. (*) means using proportional division based on area.

Architecture	Optic Disc		Optic Cup	
	Dice score	IOU score	Dice score	IOU score
U-Net with Resnet-50	96.0	92.0	84.6	72.5
U-Net with Resnet-50 (*)	96.0	**92.4**	85.0	73.3
U-Net with MobileNetV2	95.4	91.0	81.9	67.5
U-Net with MobileNetV2 (*)	96.0	91.1	83.4	68.7
U-Net with Resnet-34	95.2	91.3	85.1	73.4
U-Net with Resnet-34 (*)	**96.3**	91.8	**85.4**	**73.6**

segmentation stand out in both test samples, thus demonstrating that the application of proportional division proves beneficial regarding the results obtained in the tested networks.

For both optic cup and optic disc segmentation, the pre-trained U-Net model with the Resnet-34 backbone was used by modifying only the images for training and validation. Table 3 and Table 4 show the results obtained on the DRISHTI-GS and RIM-ONE test dataset, respectively, compared to the results of the works used as reference. It is important to point out that our work differs from the related works in a large number of parameters, from the number of folds used in the cross-validation, to the architecture and image base itself, so it is very difficult to make a direct comparison with each of the authors cited in the results tables. This time, there is the inclusion of the proposed methodology that couples proportional splitting with feature extraction and K-means clustering.

Table 3. Optic disc and optic cup segmentation results. DRISHTI-GS test dataset. (*) means using proportional division.

Method	Optic Disc		Optic Cup	
	Dice score	IOU score	Dice score	IOU score
[34]	97.3	91.4	87.1	85.0
[21]	–	–	85	75
[1]	94.9	90.4	82.8	71.1
[32]	96.4	94.2	88.7	78.0
[12]	–	–	95.0	79.0
[26]	91.6	–	73.3	–
[16]	93.0	**95.7**	93.3	**94.4**
[29]	97.0	94.7	95.0	93.2
[30]	**98.7**	93.2	**97.1**	92.1
Area based (*)	96.1	92.4	91.6	83.4
Deep Feature Extraction (*)	96.3	93.2	92.2	84.3

Table 4. Optic disc and optic cup segmentation results. RIM-ONE test dataset. (*) means using proportional division.

Method	Optic Disc		Optic Cup	
	Dice score	IOU score	Dice score	IOU score
[34]	94.2	89.0	82.4	80.2
[21]	95.0	89.0	82.0	69.0
[1]	90.3	82.8	69.0	55.6
[32]	96.1	**92.5**	84.4	74.2
[12]	96.1	88.3	**89.0**	76.2
[26]	87.3	–	75.9	–
[16]	93.2	88.4	78.6	65.9
[29]	-	92.0	–	**89.0**
Area based (*)	**96.4**	91.8	87.2	76.7
Deep Feature Extraction (*)	95.9	91.1	87.8	77.1

Analyzing the results shown in Table 3, the proposed method presents favorable and promising results, approaching the highest values of related works. It is important to note that in most cases, the proportional splitting with deep feature extraction and K-means clustering presented higher metrics when compared to the area method based, highlighting the gain in Dice and Jaccard results in the segmentation of the optic cup. Examples of the predictions generated by the proposed method on the DRISHTI-GS test dataset of both the optic cup and the optic disc can be seen in Fig. 8 and Fig. 9, respectively, while Fig. 10 presents the optic cup segmentation with the lowest Dice value obtained on the DRISHTI-GS test dataset, which was 83%.

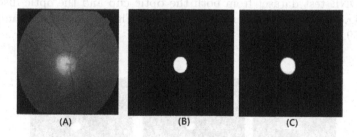

Fig. 8. Segmentation of the optic cup. With (A) meaning the original image, (B) the ground truth and (C) the prediction. Sample of the DRISHTI-GS test dataset.

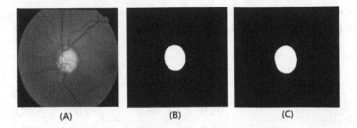

Fig. 9. Optic Disc Segmentation. With (A) meaning the original image, (B) the ground truth and (C) the prediction. Sample of the DRISHTI-GS test dataset.

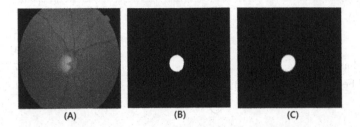

Fig. 10. Optic cup segmentation result with the smallest Dice value of 83%. With (A) meaning the original image, (B) the ground truth and (C) the prediction. Sample of the DRISHTI-GS test dataset.

For the RIM-ONE test dataset, the proposed model follows the same pattern seen in the DRISHTI-GS test samples, with results close to the highest values found in reference works and an increase in the metrics with the use of feature extraction for the segmentation of the optic cup. There was a decrease concerning the metrics obtained of 0.5% points for the Dice metric and 0.7% points for the Jaccard metric. Examples of predictions generated by the proposed method on the RIM-ONE test dataset from both the optic cup and the optic disc can be seen in Fig. 11 and Fig. 12, respectively, while Fig. 13 presents a sample that obtained 69.7% Dice value.

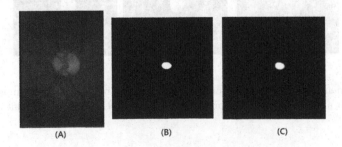

Fig. 11. Segmentation of the optic cup. With (A) meaning the original image, (B) the ground truth and (C) the prediction. Sample of the RIM-ONE test dataset.

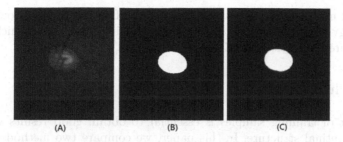

Fig. 12. Segmentation of the optic disc. With (A) meaning the original image, (B) the ground truth and (C) the prediction. Sample of the RIM-ONE test dataset.

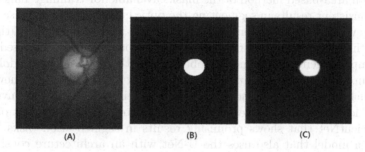

Fig. 13. Optic cup segmentation result with the smallest Dice value of 69.7%. With (A) meaning the original image, (B) the ground truth and (C) the prediction. Sample of the RIM-ONE test dataset.

5   Discussion

After analyzing the set of values obtained through the experiments performed, the application of proportional division showed promising results in the segmentation tasks, both of the disc and the optic cup, with emphasis on the latter, in which the values surpassed those of [32] that used the same architecture for the segmentation of the same structures. Notably, the results were achieved according to the best parameters that made it possible to find the set of best metrics until now.

Furthermore, integrating feature extraction and sample clustering using the K-means technique improved the optic cup and the optic disc segmentation. Overall, the experiments conducted with the U-Net model modified with ResNet-34, with proportional splitting, demonstrated through the results, show that a robust learning procedure using a distributed training set of samples assists in obtaining better results in the segmentation of the optic cup and the optic disc.

The effectiveness of using a balanced training set through a balanced division of the samples was shown. Even if there is room for improvement, our study presents robust results approaching the best values in the tables shown in the results section. However, our method cannot perform an utterly proportional division of the training samples when using the area method-based due to the unbalanced nature of the RIM-ONE and DRISHTI-GS datasets. However, this methodology comes very close to the balanced division approach, which involves Deep Feature Extraction and K-Means clustering.

6   Conclusion

A good set of training samples is essential to obtain good results when segmenting a retinal structure. In this paper, we compare two methods that aim to work directly on the division of samples from the training set so that we have the most balanced training set at the end of the process. First, we used the division area-based method of the masks available for training. This method showed consistent results in segmenting the optic cup and the optic disc in both datasets, even though it presented an unbalanced sample rate. Next, the separation with Deep Feature Extraction and K-means clustering was used, which showed improvements in the metrics obtained by the previous methodology.

In future works, we intend to expand the set of images by adding new image dataset such as ORIGA [33] and REFUGE [17]. It is also intended to investigate new deep learning architectures, such as the use of a hybrid network of U-Net with EfficientNet that shows promising results in segmentation tasks [3] and, together, a model that also uses the U-Net with an architecture consisting of hierarchical bottlenecks that prove to be useful for multi-segmentation tasks [27].

Acknowledgement(s). The authors acknowledge the Coordenação de Aperfeiçoamento de Pessoal de Nível Superior (CAPES) - Finance Code 001, Brazil, Conselho Nacional de Desenvolvimento Científico e Tecnológico (CNPq), Brazil, and Fundação de Amparo à Pesquisa e ao Desenvolvimento Científico e Tecnológico do Maranhão (FAPEMA), Brazil, for the financial support.

Disclosure Statement. No potential conflict of interest was reported by the author(s).

References

1. Al-Bander, B., Williams, B.M., Al-Nuaimy, W., Al-Taee, M.A., Pratt, H., Zheng, Y.: Dense fully convolutional segmentation of the optic disc and cup in colour fundus for glaucoma diagnosis. Symmetry **10**(4), 87 (2018)
2. Araújo, J.D.L., et al.: Glaucoma diagnosis in fundus eye images using diversity indexes. Multimed. Tools Appl. **78**(10), 12987–13004 (2019)
3. Baheti, B., Innani, S., Gajre, S.S., Talbar, S.N.: Eff-UNet: a novel architecture for semantic segmentation in unstructured environment. In: 2020 IEEE/CVF Conference on Computer Vision and Pattern Recognition Workshops (CVPRW), pp. 1473–1481 (2020)
4. Bergstra, J., Yamins, D., Cox, D.D., et al.: Hyperopt: a python library for optimizing the hyperparameters of machine learning algorithms. In: Proceedings of the 12th Python in Science Conference, vol. 13, p. 20. Citeseer (2013)

5. Bilal, A., Sun, G., Mazhar, S., Imran, A., Latif, J.: A transfer learning and U-net-based automatic detection of diabetic retinopathy from fundus images. In: Computer Methods in Biomechanics and Biomedical Engineering: Imaging & Visualization, pp. 1–12 (2022)

6. Bourne, R., et al.: Trends in prevalence of blindness and distance and near vision impairment over 30 years: an analysis for the global burden of disease study. Lancet Glob. Health 9(2), e130–e143 (2021)

7. Buslaev, A., Iglovikov, V.I., Khvedchenya, E., Parinov, A., Druzhinin, M., Kalinin, A.A.: Albumentations: fast and flexible image augmentations. Information 11(2), 125 (2020)

8. Claro, M., et al.: An hybrid feature space from texture information and transfer learning for glaucoma classification. J. Vis. Commun. Image Represent. 64, 102597 (2019)

9. da Cruz, L.B., et al.: Kidney tumor segmentation from computed tomography images using DeepLabv3+ 2.5 D model. Expert Syst. Appl. 192, 116270 (2022)

10. Fumero, F., Sigut, J., Alayón, S., González-Hernández, M., González de la Rosa, M.: Interactive tool and database for optic disc and cup segmentation of stereo and monocular retinal fundus images. In: 23rd International Conference in Central Europe on Computer Graphics, Visualization and Computer Vision (WSCG 2015), pp. 91–97. Václav Skala-UNION Agency (2015)

11. Hartigan, J.A., Wong, M.A.: Algorithm as 136: a k-means clustering algorithm. J. Roy. Stat. Soc. Ser. C (Appl. Stat.) 28(1), 100–108 (1979)

12. Joshua, A.O., Nelwamondo, F.V., Mabuza-Hocquet, G.: Segmentation of optic cup and disc for diagnosis of glaucoma on retinal fundus images. In: 2019 Southern African Universities Power Engineering Conference/Robotics and Mechatronics/Pattern Recognition Association of South Africa (SAUPEC/RobMech/PRASA), pp. 183–187. IEEE (2019)

13. Li, M., Soltanolkotabi, M., Oymak, S.: Gradient descent with early stopping is provably robust to label noise for overparameterized neural networks. In: International Conference on Artificial Intelligence and Statistics, pp. 4313–4324. PMLR (2020)

14. Lima, A., Júnior, G.B., de Almeida, J.D., de Paiva, A.C., Veras, R.: An automated CNN architecture search for glaucoma diagnosis based on neat. Multimed. Tools Appl. 81(10), 13441–13465 (2022)

15. Lima, A., Maia, L.B., dos Santos, P.T.C., Junior, G.B., de Almeida, J.D., de Paiva, A.C.: Evolving convolutional neural networks for glaucoma diagnosis. In: Anais do XVIII Simpósio Brasileiro de Computação Aplicada à Saúde. SBC (2018)

16. Mangipudi, P.S., Pandey, H.M., Choudhary, A.: Improved optic disc and cup segmentation in glaucomatic images using deep learning architecture. Multimed. Tools Appl. 80(20), 30143–30163 (2021)

17. Orlando, J.I., et al.: Refuge challenge: a unified framework for evaluating automated methods for glaucoma assessment from fundus photographs. Med. Image Anal. 59, 101570 (2020)

18. Pedregosa, F., et al.: Scikit-learn: machine learning in python. J. Mach. Learn. Res. 12, 2825–2830 (2011)

19. Rodriguez, J.D., Perez, A., Lozano, J.A.: Sensitivity analysis of k-fold cross validation in prediction error estimation. IEEE Trans. Pattern Anal. Mach. Intell. 32(3), 569–575 (2009)

20. Ronneberger, O., Fischer, P., Brox, T.: U-net: convolutional networks for biomedical image segmentation. In: Navab, N., Hornegger, J., Wells, W.M., Frangi, A.F. (eds.) MICCAI 2015. LNCS, vol. 9351, pp. 234–241. Springer, Cham (2015). https://doi.org/10.1007/978-3-319-24574-4_28

21. Sevastopolsky, A.: Optic disc and cup segmentation methods for glaucoma detection with modification of u-net convolutional neural network. Pattern Recognit Image Anal. **27**(3), 618–624 (2017)

22. Shutaywi, M., Kachouie, N.N.: Silhouette analysis for performance evaluation in machine learning with applications to clustering. Entropy **23**(6), 759 (2021)

23. Sivaswamy, J., Krishnadas, S., Chakravarty, A., Joshi, G., Tabish, A.S., et al.: A comprehensive retinal image dataset for the assessment of glaucoma from the optic nerve head analysis. JSM Biomed. Imaging Data Pap. **2**(1), 1004 (2015)

24. Sivaswamy, J., et al.: Drishti-GS: Retinal image dataset for optic nerve head (ONH) segmentation. In: 2014 IEEE 11th International Symposium on Biomedical Imaging (ISBI), pp. 53–56 (2014). https://api.semanticscholar.org/CorpusID:18432155

25. Steinmetz, J.D., et al.: Causes of blindness and vision impairment in 2020 and trends over 30 years, and prevalence of avoidable blindness in relation to vision 2020: the right to sight: an analysis for the global burden of disease study. Lancet Glob. Health **9**(2), e144–e160 (2021)

26. Sun, G., et al.: Joint optic disc and cup segmentation based on multi-scale feature analysis and attention pyramid architecture for glaucoma screening. Neural Comput. Appl. 1–14 (2021)

27. Tang, S., Qi, Z., Granley, J., Beyeler, M.: U-net with hierarchical bottleneck attention for landmark detection in fundus images of the degenerated retina. In: Fu, H., Garvin, M.K., MacGillivray, T., Xu, Y., Zheng, Y. (eds.) OMIA 2021. LNCS, vol. 12970, pp. 62–71. Springer, Cham (2021). https://doi.org/10.1007/978-3-030-87000-3_7

28. Tatham, A.J., Weinreb, R.N., Medeiros, F.A.: Strategies for improving early detection of glaucoma: the combined structure-function index. Clin. Ophthalmol. **8**, 611–621 (2014)

29. Tulsani, A., Kumar, P., Pathan, S.: Automated segmentation of optic disc and optic cup for glaucoma assessment using improved UNet++ architecture. Biocybern. Biomed. Eng. **41**(2), 819–832 (2021)

30. Veena, H., Muruganandham, A., Kumaran, T.S.: A novel optic disc and optic cup segmentation technique to diagnose glaucoma using deep learning convolutional neural network over retinal fundus images. J. King Saud Univ.-Comput. Inf. Sci. **34**(8), 6187–6198 (2022)

31. Wu, Y., et al.: Measures of disease activity in glaucoma. Biosens. Bioelectron. **196**, 113700 (2022)

32. Yu, S., Xiao, D., Frost, S., Kanagasingam, Y.: Robust optic disc and cup segmentation with deep learning for glaucoma detection. Comput. Med. Imaging Graph. **74**, 61–71 (2019)

33. Zhang, Z., et al.: ORIGA-light: an online retinal fundus image database for glaucoma analysis and research. In: 2010 Annual International Conference of the IEEE Engineering in Medicine and Biology, pp. 3065–3068. IEEE (2010)

34. Zilly, J., Buhmann, J.M., Mahapatra, D.: Glaucoma detection using entropy sampling and ensemble learning for automatic optic cup and disc segmentation. Comput. Med. Imaging Graph. **55**, 28–41 (2017)

Eff-Unet for Trachea Segmentation on CT Scans

Arthur Guilherme Santos Fernandes$^{(\boxtimes)}$ ⓘ, Geraldo Braz Junior,
João Otávio Bandeira Diniz, Marcos Melo Ferreira ⓘ,
José Ribamar Durand Rodrigues Junior ⓘ,
Mackele Lourrane Jurema Da Silva ⓘ, and Lucas Araújo Gonçalves

Applied Computing Group, Federal University of Maranhão,
Av. Portugueses 1996, São Luís, MA, Brazil
{arthurgsf,geraldo,joao.bandeira}@nca.ufma.br,
{marcos.ferreira,durand.jose,mackele.ljs,araujo.lucas}@discente.ufma.br

Abstract. Organ at Risk segmentation has an important role in the meticulous planning of radiotherapy for cancer treatment. Its primary objective is to safeguard the surrounding healthy tissues while precisely directing radiation to target cancer cells. Currently, this task needs manual intervention by physicians, a process that can be time-consuming and susceptible to errors. Consequently, the integration of automatic segmentation methods offers the potential to accelerate the delineation of organs during radiotherapy planning. In this study, we applied Eff-Unet, a fully convolutional neural network model, and trained it to perform the semantic segmentation of trachea in computed tomography images. This approach yielded a noteworthy 78.9% dice score, underscoring its capability to enhance the efficiency and precision of organ segmentation during the radiotherapy planning process.

Keywords: Deep Learning · Semantic Segmentation · Radiotherapy · Fully Convolutional Neural Networks · Organs at Risk

1 Introduction

Radiation therapy represents a form of cancer treatment wherein substantial doses of intense radiation are directed towards malignant cells, destroying it or reducing the tumor's size [5]. The initial phase of radiation therapy planning revolves around pinpointing the precise location of the tumor and the adjacent organs. This crucial step is instrumental in mitigating the counter effects of

---

This work received the support of the Coordination for the Improvement of Higher Education Personnel - Brazil (CAPES) - Financing Code 001, National Council for Scientific and Technological Development (CNPq), Maranhão Research Support Foundation (FAPEMA) and Brazilian Company of Hospital Services (Ebserh) (Proc. 409593/2021-4).

© ICST Institute for Computer Sciences, Social Informatics and Telecommunications Engineering 2024
Published by Springer Nature Switzerland AG 2024. All Rights Reserved
A. Cunha et al. (Eds.): MobiHealth 2023, LNICST 578, pp. 139–150, 2024.
https://doi.org/10.1007/978-3-031-60665-6_10

ionizing radiation over healthy cells. The healthy organs that encircle the tumor are commonly referred to as "Organs at Risk" (OaR) [7,14]. The task of manually delineating these OaRs from images acquired through Computed Tomography (CT) falls under the purview of a medical practitioner.

CT is a diagnostic imaging technique that helps physicians to assess the condition of soft and hard tissues within the body. This method involves an X-ray machine that circumnavigates the patient while radiation detectors on the opposing end register radiation levels as the X-rays pass through the biological tissue and ultimately convert them into a digitized image [2,11]. The outcome is a three-dimensional image that is further dissected into two-dimensional slices for enhanced visualization [9]. For illustrative purposes, Fig. 1 showcases instances of CT cross-sections.

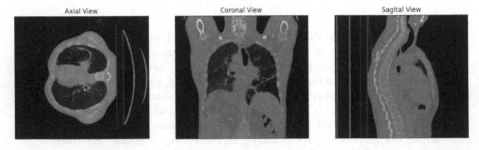

Fig. 1. Examples of 2D images obtained from a CT scan.

Accurate manual segmentation of Organs at Risk (OaR) holds significant importance, as it provides precise information regarding the proximity of healthy tissue to the tumor. This information allows specialists to precisely target the radiation beam exclusively at the cancerous tissue, effectively minimizing unwarranted X-ray exposure and decreasing the likelihood of adverse side effects from radiation therapy, which may encompass issues such as inflammation, fibrosis, ulceration, and in severe cases, organ failure [18]. However, this process relies on the physician's clinical experience and can be time-consuming and susceptible to errors. Small organs, such as the trachea, present unique challenges for segmentation due to their size, textural similarities with surrounding tissues, and limited detail. Consequently, recent research endeavors concentrated on developing automated methods for segmenting organs at risk (OaR).

Given the significance of Organ-at-Risk (OaR) segmentation in cancer treatment and the papers available on automated medical image processing, this research tackles the challenge of automating the segmentation of the trachea from CT exams by applying image preprocessing techniques alongside a convolutional neural network architecture known as Eff-Unet [4]. The primary contributions of this are: **(a)** A methodology for automated trachea segmentation utilizing Eff-Unet, **(b)** evaluating the performance of the Eff-Unet [4] neural network for the trachea segmentation task, **(c)** minimizing neural network resource usage by applying the eff-Unet [4] architecture. The EfficientNet [17] is used as a feature extractor backbone, leading to a leaner model suitable for embedded or mobile systems.

2 Related Work

Automated segmentation facilitates the data processing time and guides clinicians by providing task-specific visualizations and measurements [3]. Semantic segmentation of Organs at Risk serves as an initial phase in radiotherapy planning, aiding the identification of task-relevant specific regions. Specifically about trachea region segmentation, certain studies have devised techniques for trachea segmentation by employing encoder/decoder fully convolutional networks or by integrating transformers within these network architectures.

In response to recent advancements in transformer architecture applied to image segmentation, [21] demonstrated that these techniques paired with U-Net [15] achieved relative success segmenting various Organs at Risk (OaR), including the trachea.

Other approaches harness the 3D characteristics of tomography to extract contextual information from CT scans, as seen in [19] and [20].

Alternately, some methods combined U-Net [15] with other convolutional network architectures for OaR segmentation. For instance, [8] employs a contextual pyramid fusion module that extracts features from various scales and merges them, while [22] utilizes Generative Adversarial Networks in conjunction with U-Net [15] to perform semantic segmentation of various organs in CT scans.

Efforts have been made to curate publicly available datasets for OaR segmentation. In the case of [13], the authors prepared a CT scan collection containing 60 volumes from different patients that were diagnosed with lung cancer. With this data, they trained a simplified U-NET [15] model. Out of these 60, 40 CT scans have been made publicly accessible, forming the SEGTHOR dataset.

Within the existing literature, many methodologies have sprung from the U-NET [15] architecture, frequently without placing a central emphasis on network efficiency concerning the number of trainable parameters. In pursuit of a leaner model, this study assesses the adoption of the Eff-Unet [4] fully convolutional network design. It incorporates the robust yet compact EfficientNet [17] as an encoder within the U-Net [15] encoder/decoder framework, aiming to achieve semantic segmentation of tracheal regions in computed tomography images with lower resource consumption, enabling the model to be embedded into larger medical systems.

3 Materials and Methods

This section introduces the adopted methodology, outlining its stages. Figure 2 provides an overview of the overall workflow in this study, commencing with image acquisition, progressing through preprocessing, Eff-Unet [4] model training, and concluding with the generation of predicted segmentation masks.

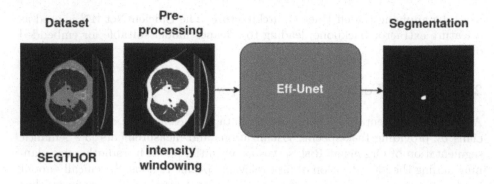

Fig. 2. Methodology Overview

3.1 Dataset

The images were obtained from the SEGTHOR [13] dataset, which contains 60 CT volumes obtained from lung cancer patients. From those 60 patients, only 40 were made public by the dataset owners. This yields 7420 2D cross-section images, where 1987 images depict the trachea, while the remaining 5433 do not, resulting in an imbalanced dataset. Slices without trachea do not participate during the training phase. The training, test and validation were separated patient-wise as follows: 30% (12) of the 40 patients were used for testing, while 62,5% (25) were separated for training, and the remaining 7,5% (3) patients were used for validation (Fig. 3).

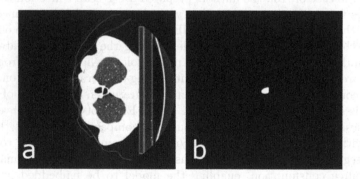

Fig. 3. a) Example of a slice that contains trachea; b) Physician-made delineation of the trachea.

Pre-processing: We implemented an intensity windowing technique to enhance contrast, restricting pixel values within a specific range and eliminating irrelevant information. Following this step, we conducted image normalization and resizing.

Intensity Windowing: In radiology, intensity windowing is a valuable tool to enhance CT imaging. It involves clipping the pixel values outside a given interval, say $[\alpha, \beta]$, to the closest boundary value while letting pixels within the interval remain unaffected. These intervals are known as "windows", and each one enhances different tissues. Figure 4 depicts the application of various windows to the same image.

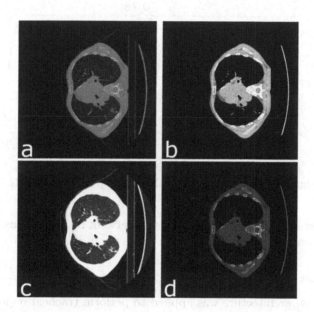

Fig. 4. Example of various windows clipping the same image intensities.

According to [6], an intensity interval of $[-1000, 60]$ is commonly used to visualize the trachea, as it effectively raises contrast between muscle and air. These boundaries are appropriate for human visualization but might not be optimal for convolutional network training, so a hyper-parameter optimization of the interval $[\alpha, \beta]$ is applied to find the best window for trachea segmentation.

We performed the hyper-parameter optimization using Bayesian optimization [1]. The optimization was executed for 100 trials, estimating the α and β boundaries for the intensity windowing preprocessing step. The best parameters were found in trial 48, obtaining **78.35%** dice score for the test with $\alpha = -890$ and $\beta = 66$. The learning rate for the ADAM was also optimized. The best parameter found was 0.0008. Figure 5 demonstrates the dice score behavior along the 100 trials.

Normalization: Following the application of intensity windowing, a subsequent step involves normalization. It entails subtracting the image mean from pixel values and dividing by the image's standard deviation. This process aims to create more uniform data, facilitating the model's learning process.

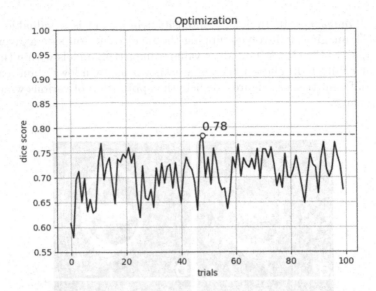

Fig. 5. The dice score curve along the optimization trials.

Resizing: After normalization, the images underwent resizing, transitioning from 512×512 dimensions to 256×256.

3.2   Eff-Unet

The Eff-Unet [4] architecture was applied to perform tracheal region segmentation. It is composed of an EfficientNet [17] feature extraction backbone acting as the encoder in the U-Net [15] framework, merging feature maps from different layers, and restoring them to the input size via transposed convolution, the result is a segmentation mask. Figure 6 depicts the model architectural overview.

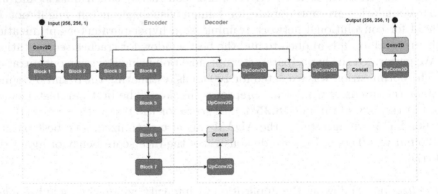

Fig. 6. Architectural overview of Eff-Unet.

EfficientNet: Engineered with efficiency resource usage as a main consideration, this network family comprises variants derived from a base model obtained
via Neural Architecture Search (NAS) [23]. The foundational network is denoted
as "b0", while additional models span from "b1" to "b7". These models vary in
terms of input resolution, channel count, and layer configurations within each
stage. Consequently, the numerical designation in the network's name corresponds to its size, with larger numbers indicating more extensive models in
terms of parameters. In this work, the **EfficientNetB0** was chosen as the feature extractor for the U-Net. A concise overview of the core structure of the
"b0" model is provided in Table 1.

Table 1. EfficientNet B0 architecture [17].

Stage	Operator	Resolution	#Channels	#Layers
1	Conv 3×3	224×224	32	1
2	MBConv1 3×3	112×112	16	1
3	MBConv6 3×3	112×112	24	2
4	MBConv6 5×5	56×56	40	2
5	MBConv6 3×3	28×28	80	3
6	MBConv6 5×5	14×14	112	3
7	MBConv6 5×5	14×14	192	4
8	MBConv6 3×3	7×7	320	1
9	Conv 1×1 & Pooling & FC	7×7	1280	1

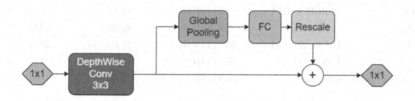

Fig. 7. Schematic diagram of MBConv.

The fundamental building blocks at the core of EfficientNet are the MBConv
blocks, initially introduced in MobileNetV2 [16]. These blocks represent an
inverted residual bottleneck architecture characterized by an expansion of the
channel count in intermediate layers, followed by a subsequent reduction to their
original size. Figure 7 provides a visual representation of the MBConv block. The
numeric value following the name, such as in "MBConv1" and "MBConv6", indicates the number of filters in the initial 1×1 convolutional layer on the left. For
instance, if the input channels number 4, then the MBConv1 block will have 4
filters, while the MBConv6 block will have 24 (4 * 6).

3.3 Results

A series of experiments were conducted to assess the viability of our proposed method. The training ran on an Intel Core™ i5-10400F CPU@2.90 GHz computer, complemented by an Nvidia® GPU RTX-3060 with 12GB of memory. The model is implemented in Python, with libraries such as TensorFlow, Keras, and Segmentation Models [10].

The patient-wise division for training, testing, and validation occurs as follows: Out of the 40 patients in the dataset, 30% (12) were designated for the testing set, while 62.5% (25) stands for the training set. The remaining 7.5% (3) of patients were separated for validation. It's crucial to underscore that our results derive from a dataset that incorporates 30% less data than previous studies on the same dataset. This discrepancy originated because 20 CT scans were hidden in a challenge platform and were used only to perform model evaluation, but the challenge ended, and the 20 volumes are still not public.

The train lasted for 100 epochs and employed the ADAM [12] (Adaptive Moment Estimation) to update weights. The chosen loss function was Dice Loss. The best-performing model reached 78.35% test dice score. This result was found with EfficientNetB0, the most compact model of the EfficientNet family, which has only *10 million* trainable parameters, as opposed to the literature's best performer [19], which has *120 million*. Table 2 summarizes the dice score for the main methods of the literature for trachea segmentation in comparison to this paper's method.

Table 2. Contrast with Relevant Studies.

Paper	Method	Dataset	Dice Score (%)	#Params
[19]	MultiRes 3D U-Net	SEGTHOR	92.17	120M
[20]	U-Net 2.5D	SEGTHOR	92.56	23M
[8]	U-Net/SPP Module	SEGTHOR	89.00	26M
[22]	U-Net/ GAN	SEGTHOR	88.30	~
Current Work	Eff-Unet	SEGTHOR (-30%)	78.35	10M

3.4 Discussion

To visually evaluate what the achieved 78.35% dice score represents for a segmentation model, some case studies are illustrated below. The network demonstrates robust performance in accurately segmenting the central regions of the trachea, as exemplified in Fig. 8. In this example, the Eff-Unet [4] model correctly identified the trachea's shape and precise location. The prediction is indicated in the left image, in gray contour, while the ground truth is on the right image, marked in orange.

Some other regions of the organ poses a more intricate challenge, primarily due to the organ's shape variations depending on its depth within the body. In certain depths, the trachea may bifurcate into two separate tubes. Figure 9

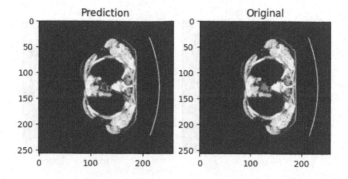

Fig. 8. Case Study: Forecasting the Central Segment of the Trachea. The leftmost image is overlapped with model's prediction, tinted in green. Right image represents the ground truth, provided by a physician, and is marked with orange (Color figure online)

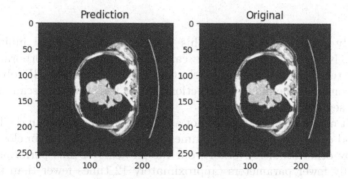

Fig. 9. Case Study: 2D slice featuring trachea division into two tubes. The leftmost image displays the model's prediction, highlighted in green and overlapped with the original. On the right, the ground truth, validated by a physician, is presented in orange. (Color figure online)

contains a 2D slice where the trachea splits into two. Despite the adversity and varying shape, it is clear that the model found no issue labeling the tracheal region pixels in the image.

For peripheral tracheal slices (those near the organ's ends) or images lacking tracheal presence, the model encounters difficulties in providing accurate outputs. This occurs due to specific image regions displaying textural features and shapes closely resembling the trachea. Consequently, the network generates false positives, as illustrated in Fig. 10. It's worth noting that while this CT slice does not contain the trachea, another body structure shares a similar shape and texture, leading the model to misclassify this region as the trachea. This false positive area is highlighted in green.

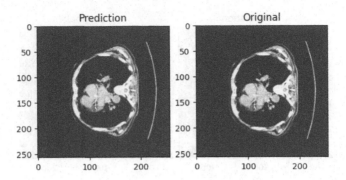

Fig. 10. Case Study: The primary limitations of the method are evident in slices devoid of trachea presence. In the leftmost image, the model's prediction is highlighted in green and overlapped. On the right, the ground truth, supplied by a physician, corresponds to an image without trachea presence, hence no markings are present. (Color figure online)

Precisely delineating slices of this nature poses a central limitation for the model. Nevertheless, this hurdle can be mitigated by incorporating post-processing techniques, specifically selecting solely the largest 3D object. This approach considers the model's predictions across the entire CT scan, ultimately enhancing segmentation accuracy.

While it may not claim the top spot as the highest dice score in the literature, this method consistently delivers commendable results that are in close to those achieved by other studies. Notably, our model achieves this performance with substantially fewer parameters (approximately 12 times fewer than the model presented in [19]). This reduced parameter count signifies a compact fully convolutional neural network, that operates with significantly reduced computational resource demands compared to its counterparts.

This efficiency is achieved by leveraging the EfficientNet [17] architecture, which is renowned for its compact and scalable design philosophy. It has been purposefully engineered to address resource constraints while maintaining robust performance, making it an ideal choice for applications where computational efficiency is a priority.

4   Conclusion

In this study, we introduced an automated approach for trachea segmentation in CT images, employing the Eff-Unet [4] neural network architecture. The obtained results exhibit relative competitiveness within the field. The utilization of Eff-Unet architecture led to a **compact model** for trachea segmentation that can be embedded into broader healthcare systems, being a valuable tool in the realm of medical image analysis, particularly in Organ at Risk segmentation and Radiotherapy planning.

There is ample room for future enhancements in this methodology, with the potential to elevate its effectiveness further. Some promising avenues for improvement are: **(a):** adding neighboring slices information to the network input, enabling a richer understanding of the 3D context and potentially improving segmentation performance, **(b):** implementing post-processing methods to refine the model's output, such as false positive reduction and segmentation refinement.

Ultimately, these improvements can potentially improve the quality of life for individuals dealing with cancer through the optimization of treatment planning processes.

References

1. Akiba, T., Sano, S., Yanase, T., Ohta, T., Koyama, M.: Optuna: a next-generation hyperparameter optimization framework. In: Proceedings of the 25th ACM SIGKDD International Conference on Knowledge Discovery and Data Mining (2019)
2. Amaro, E.J., Yamashita, H.: Aspectos básicos de tomografia computadorizada e ressonância magnética. Braz. J. Psychiatry **23** (2001)
3. Azad, R., et al.: Medical image segmentation review: the success of U-net (2022)
4. Baheti, B., Innani, S., Gajre, S., Talbar, S.: Eff-UNet: a novel architecture for semantic segmentation in unstructured environment. In: 2020 IEEE/CVF Conference on Computer Vision and Pattern Recognition Workshops (CVPRW), pp. 1473–1481 (2020). https://doi.org/10.1109/CVPRW50498.2020.00187
5. Baskar, R., Lee, K.A., Yeo, R., Yeoh, K.W.: Cancer and radiation therapy: current advances and future directions. Int. J. Med. Sci. **9**(3), 193 (2012)
6. Consídera, D.P., et al.: A tomografia computadorizada de alta resolução na avaliação da toxicidade pulmonar por amiodarona. Radiol. Bras. **39**, 113–118 (2006)
7. Diniz, J., Ferreira, J., Silva, G., Quintanilha, D., Silva, A., Paiva, A.: Segmentação de coração em tomografias computadorizadas utilizando atlas probabilístico e redes neurais convolucionais. In: Anais do XXI Simpósio Brasileiro de Computação Aplicada à Saúde, pp. 83–94. SBC, Porto Alegre (2021). https://doi.org/10.5753/sbcas.2021.16055, https://sol.sbc.org.br/index.php/sbcas/article/view/16055
8. Feng, S., et al.: CPFNet: context pyramid fusion network for medical image segmentation. IEEE Trans. Med. Imaging **39**(10), 3008–3018 (2020). https://doi.org/10.1109/TMI.2020.2983721
9. Gupta, T., Narayan, C.A.: Image-guided radiation therapy: physician's perspectives. J. Med. Phys./Assoc. Med. Phys. India **37**(4), 174 (2012)
10. Iakubovskii, P.: Segmentation models (2019)
11. Kalender, W.A.: X-ray computed tomography. Phys. Med. Biol. **51**(13), R29 (2006)
12. Kingma, D.P., Ba, J.: Adam: a method for stochastic optimization (2017)
13. Lambert, Z., Petitjean, C., Dubray, B., Ruan, S.: SegTHOR: segmentation of thoracic organs at risk in CT images (2019). https://doi.org/10.48550/ARXIV.1912.05950, https://arxiv.org/abs/1912.05950
14. Noël, G., Antoni, D., Barillot, I., Chauvet, B.: Délinéation des organes à risque et contraintes dosimétriques. Cancer/Radiothérapie **20**, S36–S60 (2016). https://doi.org/10.1016/j.canrad.2016.07.032, https://www.sciencedirect.com/science/article/pii/S1278321816301676. Recorad: Recommandations pour la pratique de la radiothérapie externe et de la curiethérapie

15. Ronneberger, O., Fischer, P., Brox, T.: U-net: convolutional networks for biomedical image segmentation. In: Navab, N., Hornegger, J., Wells, W.M., Frangi, A.F. (eds.) MICCAI 2015. LNCS, vol. 9351, pp. 234–241. Springer, Cham (2015). https://doi.org/10.1007/978-3-319-24574-4_28

16. Sandler, M., Howard, A., Zhu, M., Zhmoginov, A., Chen, L.C.: MobileNetv2: inverted residuals and linear bottlenecks (2019)

17. Tan, M., Le, Q.: EfficientNet: rethinking model scaling for convolutional neural networks. In: Chaudhuri, K., Salakhutdinov, R. (eds.) Proceedings of the 36th International Conference on Machine Learning. Proceedings of Machine Learning Research, vol. 97, pp. 6105–6114. PMLR (2019). https://proceedings.mlr.press/v97/tan19a.html

18. Tekatli, H., et al.: Normal tissue complication probability modeling of pulmonary toxicity after stereotactic and hypofractionated radiation therapy for central lung tumors. Int. J. Radiat. Oncol.* Biol.* Phys. 100(3), 738–747 (2018)

19. Wang, Q., et al.: 3D enhanced multi-scale network for thoracic organs segmentation. SegTHOR@ ISBI 3(1), 1–5 (2019)

20. Wang, S., et al.: Conquering data variations in resolution: a slice-aware multi-branch decoder network. IEEE Trans. Med. Imaging 39(12), 4174–4185 (2020). https://doi.org/10.1109/TMI.2020.3014433

21. Yan, X., Tang, H., Sun, S., Ma, H., Kong, D., Xie, X.: After-UNet: axial fusion transformer UNet for medical image segmentation. In: 2022 IEEE/CVF Winter Conference on Applications of Computer Vision (WACV), pp. 3270–3280. IEEE Computer Society, Los Alamitos (2022). https://doi.org/10.1109/WACV51458.2022.00333, https://doi.ieeecomputersociety.org/10.1109/WACV51458.2022.00333

22. Zhao, W., Chen, H., Lu, Y.: W-net: a network structure for automatic segmentation of organs at risk in thorax computed tomography. In: Proceedings of the 2020 2nd International Conference on Intelligent Medicine and Image Processing, IMIP 2020, pp. 66-69. Association for Computing Machinery, New York (2020). https://doi.org/10.1145/3399637.3399642

23. Zoph, B., Le, Q.: Neural architecture search with reinforcement learning. In: International Conference on Learning Representations (2017). https://openreview.net/forum?id=r1Ue8Hcxg

A Vision Transformer Approach to Fundus Image Classification

Danilo Leite[1], José Camara[1], João Rodrigues[3], and António Cunha[1,2(✉)]

[1] University of Trás-os-Montes and Alto Douro, Vila Real, Portugal
{danilol,acunha}@utad.pt
[2] INESC TEC—Institute for Systems and Computer Engineering, Technology and Science,
4200-465 Porto, Portugal
[3] LARSyS & ISE, Universidade do Algarve, 8005-226 Faro, Portugal
jrodrig@ualg.pt

Abstract. Glaucoma is a condition that affects the optic nerve, with loss of retinal nerve fibers, increased excavation of the optic nerve, and a progressive decrease in the visual field. It is the leading cause of irreversible blindness in the world. Manual classification of glaucoma is a complex and time-consuming process that requires assessing a variety of ocular features by experienced clinicians. Automated detection can assist the specialist in early diagnosis and effective treatment of glaucoma and prevent vision loss. This study developed a deep learning model based on vision transformers, called ViT-BRSET, to detect patients with increased excavation of the optic nerve automatically. ViT-BRSET is a neural network architecture that is particularly effective for computer vision tasks. The results of this study were promising, with an accuracy of 0.94, an F1-score of 0.91, and a recall of 0.94. The model was trained on a new dataset called BRSET, which consists of 16,112 fundus images of patients with increased excavation of the optic nerve. The results of this study suggest that ViT-BRSET has the potential to improve early diagnosis through early detection of optic nerve excavation, one of the main signs of glaucomatous disease. ViT-BRSET can be used to mass-screen patients, identifying those who need further examination by a doctor.

Keywords: Fundus Image · Vision transformers · BRSET

1 Introduction

Glaucoma is one of the leading causes of irreversible or disabling blindness worldwide. The World Health Organization (WHO) estimates that in 2040 there will be 112 million disease cases [1]. The earlier glaucoma is diagnosed and treated, the greater the chances of preserving vision. Manual classification of glaucoma is a complex and time-consuming process that requires assessing several ocular features [2]. Screening is essential for early diagnosis and treatment of glaucoma, as early intervention can help prevent vision loss. The cup-to-disc ratio (CDR), a widely used measure by experts to detect glaucoma, calculates the proportion between the size of the cup and the size of the disc, as well as the area of the cup and the location of the disc [3].

A. Cunha et al. (Eds.): MobiHealth 2023, LNICST 578, pp. 151–162, 2024.
https://doi.org/10.1007/978-3-031-60665-6_11

Computerized diagnostic systems (CAD) based on modern deep learning models, such as Vision Transformers (ViT), can help classify glaucoma with greater accuracy and speed than manual classification. Recent work [4–7] explores the efficacy of modern transformer architectures based on ViT in the diagnosis of retinal diseases, showing promising results. As these CADs are developed and improved, they can revolutionize the diagnosis of glaucoma, making it more accurate, faster, and accessible. However, a large amount of data is required to train Deep Learning (DL) models. Several datasets are available to help train these models and make them more efficient. Recently, a new sizeable Brazilian dataset of fundus images was published, called the Brazilian Multilabel Ophthalmological Dataset (BRSET) [8]. In addition to the pictures, BRSET includes several clinical parameters, including increased optic nerve excavations, an essential factor in diagnosing glaucoma. In Fig. 1, we see a normal eye (A) and one eye with increased excavation (B). Images A1 and B1 show the optic nerve head. Visually, we can see that the cup in B2 is enlarged compared to A1.

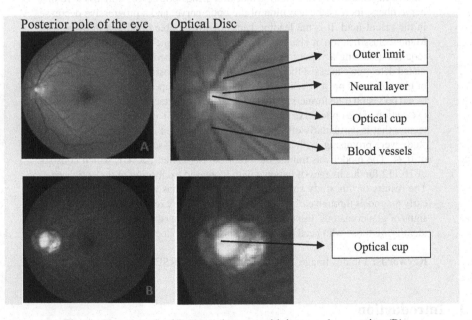

Fig. 1. Shows eye health (A) and an eye with increased excavation (B)

The optic nerve head, optic disc, or optic papilla is an oval-shaped structure, orange in color, located approximately 3 to 4 mm nasal to the center of the retina through which nerve cell fibers pass, called ganglion cell fibers, which form the nervous layer (more orange layer) and carry electrical stimuli created in the retina from visible light to the cerebral cortex, where they will be interpreted. In the central part of the optic nerve head is the emergence of retinal vessels, and the cup or excavation or optic cup is represented by a more yellowish color in the center of the optical disc due to the absence of ganglionic fibers. In the progression of the glaucomatous disease, we observe irregularities on the inner edge of the neural layer and increased excavation represented by the death of ganglion fibers. In Fig. 1, we see a normal eye (A) with increased excavation (B). Images A1 and B1 show the optic nerve head. Visually, we can see that the cup in B2 is enlarged compared to A1.

Increased excavation in the optic nerve head is one of the main signs of the glaucomatous papilla; however, in diagnosing glaucoma, the change in the neural layer of the papilla must correspond to the difference in the visual field.

A diagnosis of glaucoma can only be made by a doctor. Therefore, this work built a model based on a promising DL approach called ViT [7]. It compared its preliminary results with other DL models in the literature for glaucoma detection. The model built was trained with the BRSET dataset. The results obtained in this study are promising and suggest that the ViT model can be a valuable tool for glaucoma detection. This study also seeks to contribute to the constant evolution of this critical ophthalmological condition's early and effective detection.

2 Literature Review

In the early stages of the disease, it can be difficult for experts to identify early changes in the optic nerve head. Recently, there have been significant advances in machine learning (ML) to diagnose glaucoma. A recent study [9] developed a convolutional neural network (CNN) for glaucoma detection. The proposed model achieved an accuracy of 0.96 with the LAG dataset and 0.82 with the RIM-ONE dataset. The algorithm uses an attention prediction subnetwork to create focused and cropped maps of fundus images, which are then used for glaucoma detection and measurement using statistical methods.

In another study [3], the authors evaluated models trained on significant public datasets to detect glaucoma in retinal images acquired by retinography and mobile devices classification methods produced model activation maps to support predictions. Segmentation methods evaluated the cup-to-disc ratio (CDR), a frequently used indicator in practice by experts to screen the optic nerve. The segmentation of the disc and cup achieved DICE 0.8 and IoU 0.7.

Another study [4] compared the DeiT (Data-efficient image Transformer) and ResNet-50 models trained on fundus photographs from the Ocular Hypertension Treatment Study (OHTS). The DeiT demonstrated performance similar to ResNet-50 on the OHTS test sets. The DeiT and ResNet-50 achieved AUROC 0.91 and 0.82, respectively. The authors highlight that image transformers can improve generalization and interpretability in ML models, detecting eye diseases and possibly other medical conditions that rely on images for clinical diagnosis and treatment.

Finally, a study [10] proposed a 13-layer CNN architecture. SoftMax and Support Vector Machine (SVM) classifiers were used to classify the images. The CNN accuracy with the SoftMax classifier was 0.93, while the CNN with an SVM classifier achieved an accuracy of 0.95. The dataset used for this investigation consisted of images collected from various public datasets and a private research centre.

The literature review in glaucoma diagnosis using ML has demonstrated significant advances, with ML being capable of detecting the disease with accuracy comparable to that of experts. However, there are still challenges to be overcome, such as the need for more robust datasets and the need to improve the interpretability of the models.

3 Datasets

3.1 Brazilian Multilabel Ophthalmological Dataset (BRSET)

The Brazilian Multilabel Ophthalmological Dataset (BRSET) [8] is a high-quality ophthalmological dataset of 16.266 images from 8.524 Brazilian patients. The images are in color and include photographs of the retinas of both eyes, along with demographic, anatomical, and clinical data. BRSET was designed to enhance the development of the scientific community and validate machine learning models. The demographic data includes age, gender, nationality, diabetes, duration of diabetes, and insulin usage. Anatomical parameters include data on the optic disc, vessels, and macula. Clinical parameters encompass diabetic retinopathy, macular edema, scars, nevi, vascular occlusion, hypertensive retinopathy, drusen, hemorrhages, retinal detachment, myopic fundus, and increased excavation.

BRSET is a valuable resource for researchers studying eye diseases. It allows machine learning models to predict demographic characteristics and classify multilabel diseases using fundus retina images.

In addition to BRSET, other publicly available datasets can be used to train machine learning models for glaucoma detection. These datasets are HRF, Drishti-GS1, RIM-ONE, sjchoi86-HRF, and ACRIMA. Table 1 provides an overview of the characteristics of these datasets [2].

Table 1. Public databases for glaucoma.

Data base	Glaucoma	Normal	Total
HRF	27	18	45
Drishti-GS1	70	31	101
RIM-UM	194	261	455
sjchoi86-HRF	101	300	401
ACRIMA	396	309	705

It is important to note that these datasets exhibit heterogeneity in their characteristics, such as lighting, field of view, and resolution. These variations can affect the performance of models trained on different datasets.

4 Fundamentals of Deep Learning

Deep learning (DL) is a subfield of machine learning that relies on the analysis of data through the representation of successive layers, inspired by the functioning of the human brain. Each layer can filter specific properties and highlight relevant features, with significant applications in medical diagnostic problems. This enables the learning of complex representations and the decomposition of these representations into intermediate spaces represented by the intermediate layers.

Deep learning has exhibited significant potential for application in the medical field, enhancing the precision of image processing and the detection pertinent diagnostic features in various examinations, including X-rays, computed tomography, ultrasounds, histological analyses of organs and tissues, as well as the scrutiny of photographic images. This methodology enables the discernment of intricate elements within extensive datasets by employing multiple intermediary layers between the input and output. Each layer is adept at refining the input signal to suit the subsequent layer, thereby unveiling progressively abstract insights.

For these methods to be successful, it is essential to have sufficient data for training and evaluation of the system. In addition, the validation of these methods requires a reference standard that can be used for comparison, which emphasizes the importance of public retinal databases that meet well-defined requirements [6, 11]. Within deep learning, convolutional neural networks (CNNs) are the most widely used architecture for image classification in computer vision.

5 Transformers

Convolutional neural networks (CNNs) have demonstrated remarkable superiority in various visual tasks over the past decade. They are particularly effective at capturing spatial features in images and are invariant to translations. CNNs have consistently proven their performance on a variety of benchmark metrics. However, they have some limitations related to how the models operate and learn from images due to the restriction on the receptive field, which results in a localized understanding of images [4, 7]. To address these limitations in visual tasks, so-called vision transformers have emerged. These architectures were developed to overcome the shortcomings of CNNs, particularly the need for a global understanding of images. After demonstrating their effectiveness in natural language processing tasks, vision transformers have also gained prominence in computer vision applications [12, 13].

In the study of[12], Dosovitskiy et al. adopt an approach of dividing the image into patches and applying self-attention calculations on each patch. When trained with sufficient data, the results achieved surpassed those obtained by CNNs regarding accuracy and computational efficiency. In addition, vision transformers can outperform CNNs in various tasks by applying multiple training techniques. Transfer learning or modifying the transformer architecture can further improve the performance of vision transformers. A notable limitation of CNNs is their restriction to the receptive field, which represents the area of the image processed by a single convolutional layer. This can make it difficult to understand complex images that contain information from different parts of the image.

6 Methodology

The dataset used was BRSET, which contains 16,112 retinal images from 8,524 Brazilian patients. The images were classified as positive for glaucoma (3,181) or negative (12,931), with an average age of 57.09 ± 18.1 years. The workflow developed is presented in Fig. 2, detailing the three main stages executed throughout this study: data collection and processing, model training and construction, and performance evaluation.

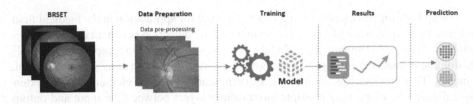

Fig. 2. The model pipeline for glaucoma screening

6.1 Data Preparation and Augmentation

Data preprocessing and data augmentation are essential steps in developing machine learning models. These processes help ensure that the data is in the correct format and that the model is trained on a representative dataset.

Data Preprocessing

This work used preprocessing to prepare images for training an object classification model. Each image were preprocessed as follows [14]:

- The region of interest (ROI) was extracted from the image to ensure that the model is trained only on the parts of the idea that are relevant to the classification task (Fig. 3).
- The image pixels were normalized to have a mean of 0 and a standard deviation of 1. This helps to ensure that the data are on the same scale and that the model is not biased towards any particular color channel.
- The color channels in the image were standardized to have the same range of values, which helps to ensure that the data are on the same scale and that the model is not biased towards any color channel.
- The noise in the image was reduced using a Gaussian filter, which helped to improve the image quality and increase the model's accuracy.
- The image was resized to a resolution of 224 × 224 pixels due to hardware limitations, which helps to ensure that the model can be run on hardware with memory or processing constraints.

To extract the ROI, we apply image thresholding to the grayscale image. This converts the image to a binary image, where bright areas are white and dark regions are black. The optic disc appears as a white area in the binary image. Finally, we extract a sub image from the original colored image that contains the optic disc. This sub image is input to a machine learning model to classify the image as glaucomatous or non-glaucomatous. Figure 2 shows a summary of this step.

Data Augmentation

After preprocessing, the data were divided into 3 folders: training, validation, and test.

- The model was trained on a set of images, and its performance was evaluated on a separate set of images. This helps to ensure that the model is balanced with the training data and that it can generalize to new data.

Data augmentation was used on the training dataset to mitigate overfitting and address potential data imbalances. Data augmentation is a powerful technique used to expand

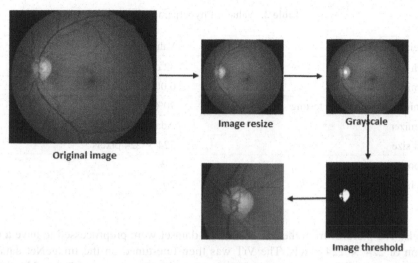

Fig. 3. Preprocessing steps

the training dataset's size and diversity, thereby enhancing the model's accuracy and its ability to generalize effectively.

6.2 Training

The dataset was randomly divided into three subsets in the following proportions: 70% for training, 15% for validation, and 15% for testing. This division of the data is essential to ensure that the model is trained on a representative dataset and evaluated on an independent dataset [15]. This division of the data into three subsets helps to ensure that the model is trained and assessed relatively. The training subset is used to train the model, and the validation and test subsets are used to evaluate the model's performance. To ensure that the class distribution was representative of the real-world data, stratified cross-validation with 10 folds was used. Stratified cross-validation is a cross-validation method that ensures that each class in the dataset is represented in each training and validation subset. After some trial and error, the best hyperparameters for the model were found, as summarized in Table 2.

6.3 Model

The Vision Transformer (ViT) is a deep learning model that uses transformers, a neural network efficient at processing sequences. The ViT can capture spatial and temporal features of images by dividing them into patches, which are then processed individually by the transformers. The transformers can then learn the relationships between the patches, allowing them to capture spatial and temporal features. The ViT was trained on the ImageNet-21k dataset, which consists of 21,841,116 images and 21.841 classes. The ImageNet-21k dataset is a large and diverse dataset created to train computer vision

Table 2. Values of hyperparameters

Hyperparameters	Values
Batch Size	32 data
Learning rate	0,001
Training, validation and testing	70%, 15%, 15%
Optimizer	Adam
Input size	224 × 224 pixels
Dropout	0.3
Epoch	20

models. The pictures from the ImageNet-21k dataset were preprocessed to have a resolution of 224 × 224 pixels. The ViT was then fine-tuned on the ImageNet dataset, consisting of 1 million images and 1.000 classes, with a resolution of 224 × 224 pixels.

This work aims to classify images into two classes including increased optic nerve excavations, an essential factor in diagnosing glaucoma. To do this, the pre-trained classification heads of each ViT model were removed. Then, a new classification head or (softmax) was added to the model with the two class labels: normal or increased optic nerve excavations. Pulling the pre-trained classification heads allowed the ViT models to be fine-tuned for classifying glaucoma images [12]. Figure 4 illustrates the architecture of the ViT.

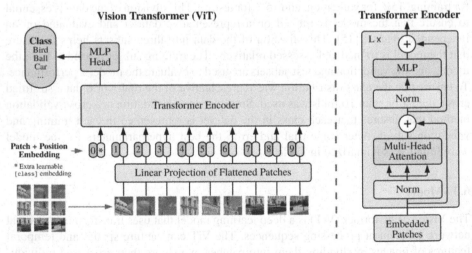

Fig. 4. Visualisation for ViT architecture

6.4 Evolution

Accuracy is one of the most critical factors in evaluating machine learning models, and it encompasses two crucial dimensions: discrimination and reliability. Discrimination measures the model's ability to distinguish between data classes, while reliability assesses its capacity to yield consistent predictions. Several techniques are available to evaluate the performance of machine learning models. However, for this study, we chose to use the accuracy (1), precision (2), recall (3), and F1-score (4) metrics. These metrics comprehensively overview the model's performance [14].

$$ACC = \frac{TP + FN}{TP + TN + FP + FN} \tag{1}$$

$$P = \frac{TP}{TP + FP} \tag{2}$$

$$R = \frac{TP}{TP + FN} \tag{3}$$

$$F1 = 2 * \frac{P*R}{P + R} \tag{4}$$

6.5 Results

Therefore, accuracy and sensitivity in glaucoma detection are of great importance. In this study, we used the following classification for the accuracy, f1-score, and recall metrics in the model evaluation [15]: Excellent: > 0.90; Good: 0.80–0.90; Acceptable: 0.70–0.80; Poor: 0.60–0.70; No acceptable discrimination ability: < 0.60. The results obtained in this study are presented in Table 3.

Table 3. Results

Models	Accuracy	F1-score	Recall
VIT-BRSET	**0.94**	**0.91**	**0.94**
Xception	0.91	0.89	0.90
VGG16	0.90	0.90	0.91
VGG19	0.89	0.88	0.90
MobileNetV2	0.90	**0.91**	0.91
InceptionV3	0.93	**0.91**	0.92
NASNetMobile	0.89	0.90	0.90

Table 3 presents the results of the performance of different DL models for eye disease detection trained on the BRSET. The results show that the ViT model achieved the best results in all metrics. The accuracy of 0.94 indicates that the model correctly classified 94% of the images. Additionally, the F1-score of 0.91 and the recall of 0.94 suggest that the VIT can accurately identify most cases of glaucoma (high sensitivity) while maintaining a good balance between accuracy and sensitivity. This combination is crucial in medical applications, where accurate glaucoma identification is essential for referring patients for appropriate treatment.

The Xception model achieved the second-best performance, followed by the VGG16, VGG19, MobileNetV2, InceptionV3, and NASNetMobile models. These results suggest that the ViT is an effective neural network architecture for eye disease detection [6].

7   Discussion

Manual classification of glaucoma is a complex and time-consuming process that requires assessing a range of ocular features by experienced clinicians. Automated detection plays a crucial role in early diagnosis and effective management of glaucoma, as early intervention can prevent vision loss. DL models have been developed and deployed to identify glaucoma early, improving patient quality of life and slowing disease progression. CNNs are the most widely used DL models in developing solutions for detecting and classifying glaucoma early. They have achieved promising results in automated glaucoma detection, and their popularity is growing steadily. In addition, recent research [4–7] has explored the efficiency of other DL architecture's vision transformers. This approach is highly efficient, achieving good results in computer vision tasks. This study used a new Brazilian dataset, the Brazilian Multilabel Ophthalmological Dataset (BRSET), to train a vision transformer model to detect normal or increased optic nerve excavations, an essential factor in diagnosing glaucoma. BRSET is a high-quality dataset with well-segmented and labeled fundus images.

The results obtained in this work showed that the ViT could detect increased optic nerve excavations with high accuracy, surpassing the results of other DL models used in the literature. The model achieved an accuracy of 0.94, beating the results of the DeiT (0.91) and ResNet-50 (0.88) models of Fan et al. [4] and Souza et al. [6]. The model also achieved an accuracy of 0.916, AUROC of 0.968, and F1-score of 0.915, although it still falls below the 0.99 result obtained by He et al. [5].

In the work of Fan et al. [4], they compared the Data-efficient image Transformer (DeiT) and ResNet-50 models trained on fundus images. DeiT performed similarly to ResNet-50 on the OHTS test sets. The accuracy of DeiT and ResNet-50 were 0.91 and 0.88, respectively. However, the authors note that vision transformers can improve generalization and interpretability in machine learning models, detecting eye diseases and possibly other medical conditions that rely on images for clinical diagnosis and treatment. He et al. [5] present an interpretable transformer network for classifying retinal diseases using optical coherence tomography (OCT). The network is based on the Swin Transformer model, which is a transformer architecture that has been modified to be more interpretable. The network was trained on a dataset of OCT images from patients with various retinal diseases. The results showed that the network achieved an accuracy of 0.99 in the classification of retinal diseases. In this work, the authors obtained a better result.

The AlterNet-K model was presented in the study conducted by Souza et al. [6], a computer vision model that combines ResNets and MSAs to improve generalization.

The researchers conducted a comprehensive comparison, evaluating the performance of AlterNet-K against transformer-based models, such as ViT, DeiT-S, and the Swin Transformer, as well as against conventional deep convolutional neural network (DCNN) models, including ResNet, EfficientNet, MobileNet, and VGG. The results obtained by the authors were an accuracy of 0.916, an AUROC of 0.968, and an F1-score of 0.915. However, the results presented by Souza et al. were similar to those of the present study.

The results presented in the table indicate that Vision Transformers have a promising potential in the early increased optic nerve excavations, an essential factor in diagnosing glaucoma. The VIT-BRSET model, trained on data from fundus images of Brazilian patients, achieved an impressive accuracy of 0.94, surpassing the DL models tested in this study. Finally, we emphasize that further studies are needed to assess the efficacy of CNNs and Vision Transformers in detecting glaucoma in broader contexts. Additionally, it is crucial to develop more interpretable models, as they allow physicians to understand the decisions made by the models, increasing the confidence of healthcare professionals in using these tools to improve patient care.

8 Conclusion

This study investigated the potential of the ViT base-patch16-224 model for increased optic nerve excavations, an essential factor in diagnosing glaucoma. The ViT base patch 16-224 was trained on a dataset of fundus eye images and evaluated on an independent test dataset. The model achieved an accuracy of 0.94, an F1-score of 0.91, and a recall of 0.94, which is a promising result. The results indicate that ViT base-patch16-224 could be an effective tool to detect increased optic nerve excavations.

However, further studies are needed to assess the effectiveness of other transformers on more extensive and diverse datasets and under different clinical conditions. An important future task is to use technology to make ViT's decision-making more transparent to increase user confidence in the results. Additionally, it is essential to test the model's generalization with other datasets to ensure it can be applied to various populations and conditions.

Acknowledgements. This work was supported by the Portuguese Foundation for Science and Technology (FCT), project LARSyS - FCT Project UIDB/50009/2020 and National Funds finance this work through the Portuguese funding agency, FCT - Fundação para a Ciência e a Tecnologia, within project LA/P/0063/2020.

References

1. Tham, Y.C., Li, X., Wong, T.Y., Quigley, H.A., Aung, T., Cheng, C.Y.: Global prevalence of glaucoma and projections of glaucoma burden through 2040: a systematic review and meta-analysis. Ophthalmology **121**(11), 2081–2090 (2014). https://doi.org/10.1016/j.ophtha.2014.05.013
2. Camara, J., Rezende, R., Pires, I.M., Cunha, A.: Retinal glaucoma public datasets: what do we have and what is missing? J. Clin. Med. **11**(13), 3850 (2022). https://doi.org/10.3390/JCM11133850

3. Neto, A., Camera, J., Oliveira, S., Cláudia, A., Cunha, A.: Optic disc and cup segmentations for glaucoma assessment using cup-to-disc ratio. Proc. Comput. Sci. **196**(2021), 485–492 (2021). https://doi.org/10.1016/j.procs.2021.12.040

4. Fan, R., et al.: Detecting glaucoma from fundus photographs using deep learning without convolutions transformer for improved generalization. Ophthalmol. Sci. **3**, 100233 (2023). https://doi.org/10.1016/j.xops.2022.100233

5. He, J., Wang, J., Han, Z., Ma, J., Wang, C., Qi, M.: An interpretable transformer network for the retinal disease classification using optical coherence tomography. Sci. Rep. **13**, 3637. https://doi.org/10.1038/s41598-023-30853-z. 123AD

6. D'Souza, G., Siddalingaswamy, P.C., Pandya, M.A.: AlterNet-K: a small and compact model for the detection of glaucoma **1**, 3. https://doi.org/10.1007/s13534-023-00307-6

7. Karrothu, A., Chunduru, A.: Glaucoma detection using computer vision and vision transformers (2023). https://journal.uob.edu.bh/handle/123456789/5206. Accessed 13 Sept 2023

8. Nakayama, L.F., et al.: A Brazilian multilabel ophthalmological dataset (BRSET) v1.0.0 (2023). https://physionet.org/content/brazilian-ophthalmological/1.0.0/. Accessed 13 Sept 2023

9. Li, L., et al.: A large-scale database and a CNN model for attention-based glaucoma detection. IEEE Trans. Med. Imaging **39**(2), 413–424 (2020). https://doi.org/10.1109/TMI.2019.2927226

10. Ajitha, S., Akkara, J.D., Judy, M.V.: Identification of glaucoma from fundus images using deep learning techniques. Indian J. Ophthalmol. **69**(10), 2702–2709 (2021). https://doi.org/10.4103/IJO.IJO_92_21

11. Teixeira, I., Morais, R., Sousa, J.J., Cunha, A.: Deep learning models for the classification of crops in aerial imagery: a review. Agriculture **13**(5) (2023). https://doi.org/10.3390/AGRICULTURE13050965

12. Dosovitskiy, A., et al.: An image is worth 16×16 words: transformers for image recognition at scale. In: ICLR 2021 - 9th International Conference on Learning Representations, October 2020. Accessed 14 Sept 2023. https://arxiv.org/abs/2010.11929v2

13. Wassel, M., Hamdi, A.M., Adly, N., Torki, M.: Vision transformers based classification for glaucomatous eye condition. In: Proceedings - International Conference on Pattern Recognition, vol. 2022-August, pp. 5082–5088 (2022). https://doi.org/10.1109/ICPR56361.2022.9956086

14. Leite, D., et al.: Machine Learning automatic assessment for glaucoma and myopia based on Corvis ST data. Proc. Comput. Sci. **196**(2021), 454–460 (2021). https://doi.org/10.1016/j.procs.2021.12.036

15. Leite, D.R.A., de Moraes, R.M., Lopes, L.W.: Different performances of machine learning models to classify dysphonic and non-dysphonic voices (2022). https://doi.org/10.1016/j.jvoice.2022.11.001

Glaucoma Grading Using Fundus Images

Mackele Lourrane Jurema da Silva[1]([✉])(iD), Marcos Melo Ferreira[1,2](iD),
Geraldo Braz Junior[1](iD), João Dallyson Sousa de Almeida[1](iD),
and Arthur Guilherme Santos Fernandes[1](iD)

[1] Federal University of Maranhao, Sao Luis, MA, Brazil
{mackele.ljs,marcos.ferreira}@discente.ufma.br,
{geraldo,jdalyson,arthurgsf}@nca.ufma.br
[2] Federal Institute of Maranhao, Sao Luis, MA, Brazil

Abstract. Glaucoma is a chronic, progressive eye disease caused by gradual damage to the optic nerve and is considered the major cause of irreversible visual damage. Because it is impossible to reverse the loss of vision caused by the disease, early detection is essential that interventions can be carried out in the early stages of the disease to stop its progression. Fundus imaging is one of the main methods used to diagnose the disease, making it possible to assess the cup-to-disc ratio by a specialist. In this work, we propose a method based on deep learning, which uses fundus images to help detect the disease in its early stages. In this way, the proposed method can have clinical use and be used to develop tools for classifying more serious disease cases. As a best result, the proposed method achieved a kappa value of 0.83.

Keywords: Glaucoma · Diagnosis · Deep Learning

1 Introduction

Glaucoma is an ophthalmological disease identified as the second leading cause of blindness and the main cause of irreversible visual damage, [8,28]. It is estimated that the total number of people with glaucoma worldwide is approximately 80 million [24], with 1.5 million cases registered in Brazil, according to the Brazilian Council of Ophthalmology (CBO) [7]. However, the number of registered cases does not reflect the total number of people with the disease due to the difficulty of early diagnosis since there are no symptoms in the early stages [20]. According to a survey [21] carried out by the Brazilian Society of Glaucoma (SBG), 41% of the people interviewed do not know what glaucoma is, and 39% are unaware of the probability of blindness. These data suggest that there is little concern with

This work was carried out with the support of the Coordination for the Improvement of Higher Education Personnel - Brazil (CAPES) - Financing Code 001, Maranhão Research Support Foundation (FAPEMA), National Council for Scientific and Technological Development (CNPq) and Brazilian Company of Hospital Services (Ebserh) Brazil (Proc. 409593/2021-4).

A. Cunha et al. (Eds.): MobiHealth 2023, LNICST 578, pp. 163–172, 2024.
https://doi.org/10.1007/978-3-031-60665-6_12

disease prevention and that most cases will only be detected when symptoms are present. This indicates an advanced stage of the disease in which visual damage and blindness cannot be avoided.

The disease is a disorder in which excessive intraocular pressure (IOP) causes damage to the optic nerve. This damage leads to a progressive loss of peripheral vision, which can progress to total vision loss [29]. CBO estimates point out that in Brazil, there are 1.6 million blind people, with glaucoma being one of the three main causes of blindness [6]. Although irreversible, the loss can be avoided if medical procedures are performed in the early stages of the disease. According to the World Health Organization (WHO) [28], only 11% of people who received timely diagnosis and treatment reported having acquired moderate or severe damage resulting from the most severe forms of the disease.

The necessary interventions to avoid visual damage caused by increased intraocular pressure must be carried out in the early stages of the disease. Glaucoma can be detected using medical images such as fundus images and Optical Coherence Tomography (OCTs) [1]. Analyzing fundus images makes it possible to detect changes in clinical parameters that indicate the disease, such as increased excavation of the optic nerve [22]. However, the analysis of a large number of exams takes a lot of time, being exhausting for the specialist [13]. In this context, automatic methods that can help specialists detect glaucoma using medical images may have great potential for clinical use. Approaches based on deep learning have shown promising results in image classification tasks [14, 27].

This study presents a method based on deep learning for automatically classifying the glaucoma stage using fundus images from different datasets. The main objective of this work is to present a method that can be used to develop tools that can facilitate the early diagnosis of the disease. In this work, the performance of an optimized Convolutional Neural Network with an architecture that combines convolutional blocks from two SOTA models [16, 23], which received fundus images as input, was investigated.

The main contributions of this work are a) a CNN architecture optimized for grading the glaucoma stage based on medical images (fundus images); b) an easily configurable method and expandable convolutional neural network architecture that combines Dense and Inception blocks for glaucoma grading.

The remaining sections are organized as follows. Section 2 presents some related works. Section 3 presents the proposed method. Section 4 presents the results and evaluation of our method. Section 5 concludes this paper.

2   Related Work

Several methods have been proposed for the detection of glaucoma using fundus images. Most methods are based on deep learning, and more recently, *Vision Transformers* [9]. Another characteristic present in most of the proposed methods is the capture of the optic disc region for classification since the main biological marker for the detection of glaucoma is the excavation of the optic disc [5].

An architecture that combines features extracted from fundus images and images containing only the optic disc region was presented in [12]. The work aims to classify the images from the GAMMA dataset into early, progressive, and non-glaucoma. Feature extraction was performed using a network with two extraction levels, with the Resnet34 CNN as the backbone.

The work developed in [17] aims to segment and classify fundus images. The model was named EffUnet-SpaGen and contains two stages, a U-shaped convolutional neural network where the method segments the optical disc and the cup, EffUNet. The model also presents a spatial generative algorithm, SpaGen. The model outputs 99.7% AUROC in the Origa dataset.

In [10], a method was proposed that performs the decomposition of the optic disc region present in fundus images, the BEMD, (*Bi-dimensional Empirical Mode Decomposition*). The research presents a VGG 19 with multiple inputs, thus being a multilevel network. The original image will feed the network, and from the image, the BEMD will be made, and the decompositions will serve as input for the other network inputs; after the convolution stage, they have concatenated all the outputs. Finally, the SVM classifier classifies in glaucoma or not glaucoma. The proposed method, trained on the Refuge dataset, presents 99.0% and 96.9% accuracy when tested on the Refuge and Origa-light datasets, respectively.

Li et al. [18] evaluates the performance of four CNN Resnet models (Resnet34/50/101/152) for glaucoma stage classification on the GAMMA test set. The best result was a kappa value of 0.699, using the ResNet34 model. In [4], supervised contrastive learning was used to train a ResNet model to perform feature extraction from fundus images. As the best result, a kappa value of 0.728 and an accuracy of 0.830 were achieved.

Tian et al. [25] present a GC-Net to classify images from the GAMMA dataset into non-glaucoma, early-stage glaucoma, and progressive glaucoma, using as input optic disc regions. A pre-trained CNN forms the proposed architecture used as a feature extractor and an attention module formed by a global attention block and a class attention block, achieving as best result a kappa value of 0.894.

In [11], a comparison was made to evaluate the classification capacity between a CNN (ResNet50 model) and a DeiT network (*Distilling Vision Transformers*) [26]. The two networks were trained on a private dataset and were tested on five public datasets, with the Deit network achieving superior results compared to CNN ResNEt50.

3 Materials and Method

The proposed method uses a convolutional network based on the DenseNet [16] and Inception [23] models for predicting stages in early or progressive glaucoma (intermediate and advanced glaucoma). The proposed method uses fundus images for model training and evaluation. In this work, we optimized the model's hyperparameters, evaluating the number of dense blocks and the number of layers per block and searching for the best architecture for prediction. The method used for developing this research comprises five main steps: Image acquisition, image preprocessing, model construction, model tuning, and model evaluation.

The steps of the proposed method, along with some keywords that summarize each step, are shown in Fig. 1.

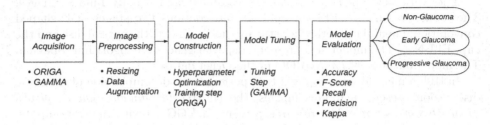

Fig. 1. Steps of the proposed method.

3.1   Image Acquisition

Origa [30] and Gamma [29] image datasets, both publicly available, were used in this work. The Origa dataset comprises 650 fundus images, divided into two classes (482 non-glaucoma samples and 168 glaucoma samples. The gamma dataset comprises 100 fundus images, divided into three classes (50 non-glaucoma samples, 26 early glaucoma samples, and 24 progressive glaucoma samples). In this work, the training set with available labels was used. The GAMMA test set only has images, which prevents the use of supervised learning techniques and restricts the evaluation of results to challenge participants only.

3.2   Image Preprocessing and Data Augmentation

The pre-processing was carried out with the purpose of preparing the data that will be used in the following steps. Each sample was pre-processed, where the image pixels' normalization was performed, color channel standardization, and resizing to the 224×224 resolution due to hardware limitations.

Data Augmentation was used to improve the model's performance in which it was applied. Therefore, synthetic images were created to reduce the imbalance between existing classes. We used the Albumentations [3] library to apply two image transformations: GaussNoise and RandomGamma. Data augmentation was only applied to the Origa dataset. At the end of the data augmentation process, 336 synthetic images were generated, totaling 504 glaucoma samples.

3.3   Model Construction

In this step, the search for the best hyperparameters of a neural network that has its architecture based on the DenseNet and Inception networks was carried out. The proposed architecture has dense blocks, each containing convolutional blocks similar to those of the Inception network. The architecture is shown in Fig. 2. During the optimization process, a search was carried out by the number of dense blocks and the number of layers (Inception blocks) per block to find the best architecture to achieve the proposed objective. The complete hyperparameter search space is presented in Table 1. Models were trained for classifying fundus images in glaucoma and non-glaucoma using samples from the Origa dataset, which was divided into 70% for training, 10% for validation, and 20% for testing.

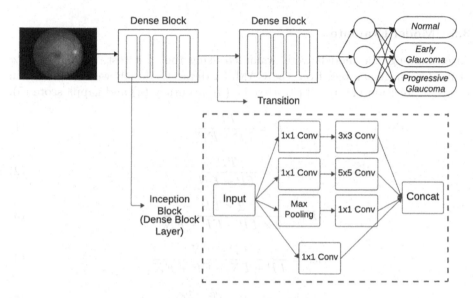

Fig. 2. Network Architecture.

Table 1. Hyperparameter Search Space.

Parameter	Search Space	Distribution
Number of Dense Blocks	[2, 3]	Categorical
Layer per Block	[2, 3]	Categorical
Growth Rate	[16, 32]	Categorical
Compress Factor	[0.5, 1]	Categorical
Dropout	[0.2, 0.3, 0.4]	Categorical

3.4   Model Tuning

In the previous step, models were trained using the samples from the ORIGA dataset [31], balanced after the data augmentation process. For the purpose of carrying out transfer learning, the model that achieved the best results in the classification of images in glaucoma and non-glaucoma was chosen to be adjusted for the classification of samples from the GAMMA dataset, which has samples from three classes, non-glaucoma, early-stage glaucoma, and progressive-stage glaucoma. At this stage, the chosen model has its classifier replaced by one adjusted for the three-class classification task. This classifier consists of two fully connected layers followed by one each of Global Average Pooling and a last layer composed of three neurons with softmax activation. A new training of the model was carried out, using 90% of the samples from the GAMMA dataset, with 10% of the samples being separated to evaluate the models.

3.5   Model Evaluate

After training, the models were evaluated using the split test, formed by 10% of fundus image samples from the GAMMA dataset. Models were evaluated in terms of precision (1), recall (2), f1-score (3), accuracy (4) and kappa score (5).

$$P = \frac{TP}{TP + FP} \tag{1}$$

$$S = \frac{TP}{TP + FN} \tag{2}$$

$$F1 = \frac{2 \times TP}{2 \times TP + FP + FN} \tag{3}$$

$$Acc = \frac{TP + TN}{TP + TN + FP + FN} \tag{4}$$

$$kappa = k = \frac{p_0 - p_e}{1 - p_e} \tag{5}$$

in which TP is the number of True Positive predictions; TN is the number of True Negative predictions; FP is the number of False Positive predictions; FN is the number of False Negative predictions; p_0 is accuracy and p_e is the sum of the products of the actual and predicted numbers corresponding to each category, divided by the square of the total number of samples.

4   Results and Discussion

This work proposes a method for grading the glaucoma stage using fundus images and transfer learning. In the model-building stage, the hyperparameters and architecture optimization of CNNs models for classifying fundus images in glaucoma and non-glaucoma was performed using samples from the ORIGA dataset. In the tuning step, models that achieved the highest metrics in the previous step were fine-tuned for classifying fundus images in early, progressive, and non-glaucoma using samples from the GAMMA dataset. The Hyperopt [2] framework was used to perform the hyperparameter search. The results achieved using CNN model DenseNet121 and the best results achieved using the optimized architecture in the split test are presented in Table 2. The confusion matrix is presented in Fig. 3.

Table 2. Best results from the methodology proposed in the GAMMA dataset.

Model	Precision	Recall	F1-Score	Accuracy	Kappa
Dense121	0.65	0.70	0.64	0.70	0.51
Proposed Method	0.90	0.90	0.89	0.90	0.83

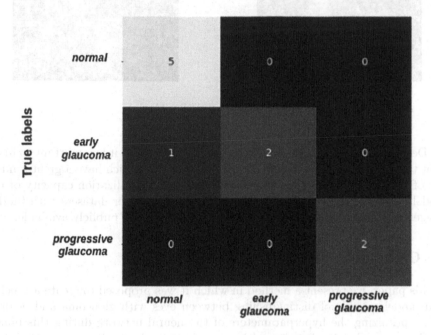

Fig. 3. Confusion matrix, glaucoma grading stage task using the optimized architecture.

The results show that the pre-trained model built with dense and inception blocks achieved promising results in classifying the stage of glaucoma using fundus images. Figure 4 presents an activation map created to visualize which regions of the images were decisive for the predictions made by the model. Through them, it is possible to see that the optic disc region was decisive for classification, which was expected due to the cup-to-disc ratio being a biological marker for detecting and classifying the glaucoma stage [25].

As the GAMMA dataset was released recently, few related works used the dataset. One of the factors that makes comparison difficult is the unavailability of the image labels that form the preliminary test dataset, which are only available to challenge participants. Furthermore, some of the studies aim to segment the disc and optical cup [15, 19], without presenting results on the glaucoma grading stage.

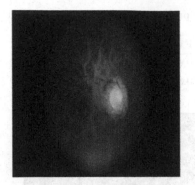 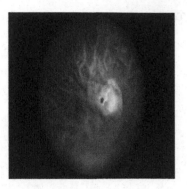

Fig. 4. Class Activation Map.

Despite the results achieved by the proposed method, it is important to highlight that it needs to be evaluated on other datasets, which have a greater number of images, making it possible to evaluate the generalization capacity of the models better. However, this is difficult because no other datasets with fundus images labeled early, progressive, and non-glaucoma are publicly available.

5   Conclusion

In this paper, we present a method in which it was proposed to create a specialized model capable of distinguishing between eyes with glaucoma and healthy eyes, optimizing the hyperparameters of the neural network during this phase. Furthermore, the developed model was subsequently used to grade the glaucoma stage using fundus image samples in non-glaucoma, early glaucoma, and advanced glaucoma.

The results show that the use of a network that combines dense and inception blocks achieved good results, enabling not only the detection of glaucoma but also the classification of stages of the disease, which allows more severe cases to be identified more quickly, and that interventions be made to stop the progress of the disease. Furthermore, it allows cases of early-stage glaucoma to be identified to begin treatment, avoiding permanent vision impairment.

This work evaluated a network that uses convolutional blocks from other CNNs widely used in image classification and segmentation tasks. To find an optimal architecture to achieve the proposed objective, a search for hyperparameters was carried out, with the main purpose of finding the number of dense blocks and layers per block to build the classification model. The results show that using dense blocks formed by Inception blocks increases the classification capacity of the models. However, since there were few images for training, only models with few blocks achieved good results. Deeper models with many blocks performed poorly, with gradient disappearance as the likely cause of overfitting. Despite results close to related works, new tests need to be carried out to analyze the robustness and generalization capacity of the models.

In future works, we intend to evaluate the use of multilevel architectures requiring optical disk capture, which would be used as input for a second level of feature extraction. It is also necessary to evaluate other convolutional blocks, such as VGG networks, which could be evaluated as layers of dense blocks.

References

1. An, G., et al.: Glaucoma diagnosis with machine learning based on optical coherence tomography and color fundus images. J. Healthc. Eng. **2019** (2019)
2. Bergstra, J., Komer, B., Eliasmith, C., Yamins, D., Cox, D.D.: Hyperopt: a python library for model selection and hyperparameter optimization. Comput. Sci. Discov. **8**(1), 014008 (2015). http://stacks.iop.org/1749-4699/8/i=1/a=014008
3. Buslaev, A., Iglovikov, V.I., Khvedchenya, E., Parinov, A., Druzhinin, M., Kalinin, A.A.: Albumentations: fast and flexible image augmentations. Information **11**(2) (2020). https://doi.org/10.3390/info11020125, https://www.mdpi.com/2078-2489/11/2/125
4. Cai, Z., Lin, L., He, H., Tang, X.: COROLLA: an efficient multi-modality fusion framework with supervised contrastive learning for glaucoma grading. In: 2022 IEEE 19th International Symposium on Biomedical Imaging (ISBI), pp. 1–4. IEEE (2022)
5. Camara, J., Neto, A., Pires, I.M., Villasana, M.V., Zdravevski, E., Cunha, A.: Literature review on artificial intelligence methods for glaucoma screening, segmentation, and classification. J. Imaging **8**(2), 19 (2022)
6. CBO: A importância de combater e prevenir a cegueira (2020). https://www.vejabem.org/noticia/a-importancia-de-combater-e-prevenir-a-cegueira1657730359
7. CBO: Casos de glaucoma aumentaram 26% no primeiro trimestre de 2022 (2022)
8. Coan, L., et al.: Automatic detection of glaucoma via fundus imaging and artificial intelligence: a review. Surv. Ophthalmol. (2022)
9. Dosovitskiy, A., et al.: An image is worth 16×16 words: transformers for image recognition at scale. arXiv preprint arXiv:2010.11929 (2020)
10. Elmoufidi, A., Skouta, A., Jai-Andaloussi, S., Ouchetto, O.: CNN with multiple inputs for automatic glaucoma assessment using fundus images. Int. J. Image Graph. 2350012 (2022)
11. Fan, R., et al.: Detecting glaucoma from fundus photographs using deep learning without convolutions: Transformer for improved generalization. Ophthalmol. Sci. **3**(1), 100233 (2023)
12. Fang, H., Shang, F., Fu, H., Li, F., Zhang, X., Xu, Y.: Multi-modality images analysis: a baseline for glaucoma grading via deep learning. In: Fu, H., Garvin, M.K., MacGillivray, T., Xu, Y., Zheng, Y. (eds.) OMIA 2021. LNCS, vol. 12970, pp. 139–147. Springer, Cham (2021). https://doi.org/10.1007/978-3-030-87000-3_15
13. Ferreira, M.M., Esteve, G.P., Junior, G.B., de Almeida, J.D.S., de Paiva, A.C., Veras, R.: Multilevel CNN for angle closure glaucoma detection using AS-OCT images. In: 2020 International Conference on Systems, Signals and Image Processing (IWSSIP), pp. 105–110. IEEE (2020)
14. Gonçalves, C., et al.: Computer vision in automatic visceral leishmaniasis diagnosis: a survey. IEEE Lat. Am. Trans. **21**(2), 310–319 (2022)
15. He, H., Lin, L., Cai, Z., Cheng, P., Tang, X.: JOINEDTrans: prior guided multi-task transformer for joint optic disc/cup segmentation and fovea detection. arXiv preprint arXiv:2305.11504 (2023)

16. Huang, G., Liu, Z., Weinberger, K.Q.: Densely connected convolutional networks. CoRR abs/1608.06993 (2016). http://arxiv.org/abs/1608.06993
17. Krishna, A., et al.: EffUnet-SpaGen: an efficient and spatial generative approach to glaucoma detection. J. Imaging **7**(6), 92 (2021)
18. Li, Y., et al.: Multimodal information fusion for glaucoma and diabetic retinopathy classification. In: Antony, B., Fu, H., Lee, C.S., MacGillivray, T., Xu, Y., Zheng, Y. (eds.) OMIA 2022. LNCS, vol. 13576, pp. 53–62. Springer, Cham (2022). https://doi.org/10.1007/978-3-031-16525-2_6
19. Li, Z., Lu, S., Li, H., Liu, H., Wang, N.: A pyramid spatial attention network for fovea localization. In: 2022 4th International Conference on Advances in Computer Technology, Information Science and Communications (CTISC), pp. 1–5. IEEE (2022)
20. Sarhan, A., Rokne, J., Alhajj, R.: Glaucoma detection using image processing techniques: a literature review. Comput. Med. Imaging Graph. 101657 (2019)
21. SBG: Pesquisa de opinião pública sobre glaucoma (2020)
22. Shanmugam, P., Raja, J., Pitchai, R.: An automatic recognition of glaucoma in fundus images using deep learning and random forest classifier. Appl. Soft Comput. **109**, 107512 (2021)
23. Szegedy, C., et al.: Going deeper with convolutions. In: Proceedings of the IEEE Conference on Computer Vision and Pattern Recognition, pp. 1–9 (2015)
24. Tham, Y.C., Li, X., Wong, T.Y., Quigley, H.A., Aung, T., Cheng, C.Y.: Global prevalence of glaucoma and projections of glaucoma burden through 2040: a systematic review and meta-analysis. Ophthalmology **121**(11), 2081–2090 (2014)
25. Tian, H., Lu, S., Sun, Y., Li, H.: GC-net: Global and class attention blocks for automated glaucoma classification. In: 2022 IEEE 17th Conference on Industrial Electronics and Applications (ICIEA), pp. 498–503 (2022). https://doi.org/10.1109/ICIEA54703.2022.10005946
26. Touvron, H., Cord, M., Douze, M., Massa, F., Sablayrolles, A., Jégou, H.: Training data-efficient image transformers & distillation through attention. In: International Conference on Machine Learning, pp. 10347–10357. PMLR (2021)
27. Valencia-Moreno, J.M., González-Fraga, J.Á., Febles-Rodríguez, J.P., Gutierrez-Lopez, E.: Review of intelligent algorithms for breast cancer control: a Latin America perspective. IEEE Lat. Am. Trans. **21**(2), 226–241 (2022)
28. WHO: World report on vision (2019). www.who.int
29. Wu, J., et al.: Gamma challenge: glaucoma grading from multi-modality images. arXiv preprint arXiv:2202.06511 (2022)
30. Zhang, Z., et al.: ORIGA(-light): An online retinal fundus image database for glaucoma analysis and research, vol. 2010, pp. 3065–3068 (2010). https://doi.org/10.1109/IEMBS.2010.5626137
31. Zhang, Z., et al.: ORIGA-light: an online retinal fundus image database for glaucoma analysis and research. In: 2010 Annual International Conference of the IEEE Engineering in Medicine and Biology, pp. 3065–3068. IEEE (2010)

Abnormality Detection in Wireless Capsule Endoscopy Images Using Deep Features

Daniel G. P. de Sá$^{(\boxtimes)}$, Giulia de A. Freulonx, Marcio P. Ferreira,
Alexandre C. P. Pessoa, Darlan B. P. Quintanilha, and Aristófanes C. Silva

Applied Computing Group (NCA - UFMA), Federal University of Maranhão,
São Luís, MA, Brazil
{daniel.piorsky,giulia.freulon}@discente.ufma.br,
{marcio.ferreira,alexandre.pessoa,dquintanilha,ari}@nca.ufma.br

Abstract. The capsule endoscopy examination is a common medical procedure used to diagnose and treat gastrointestinal tract diseases without the need for invasive procedures. Images captured during the examination can reveal a wide range of abnormalities, including lesions, inflammation, ulcers, bleeding, and tumors. However, interpreting these images can be a challenge for physicians since the videos contain a large number of frames (images) to be analyzed. To attempt to achieve an early diagnosis and reduce the lethality of gastrointestinal system pathologies, the use of artificial intelligence has been extensively studied to alleviate the workload of healthcare professionals, as the large number of images resulting from an examination makes manual categorization of each image challenging. This work studied the use of machine learning methods such as OneClassSVM and XGBoost based on features extracted from deep neural networks and compared them to traditional convolutional neural network methods, such as the ResNet152 network. The Kvasir-Capsule and ERS datasets were used to evaluate the proposed methods, focusing on classifying images as normal or abnormal. Among the evaluated methods, XGBoost showed the best results among others, with a weighted F1-score of 0.71 on the ERS dataset and 0.87 on the Kvasir-Capsule dataset. The class imbalance in both datasets proved to be a continuous challenge, adding to the challenge of the low quantity images in the ERS dataset.

Keywords: Endoscopy · Deep Features · One-Class · XGBoost

1 Introduction

A endoscopy represents one of the procedures used for the diagnosis of gastrointestinal diseases. Usually conducted through the ingestion of a tube equipped with a camera (endoscope), this method produces a sequence of images that experts in the field have the ability to classify as indicative of health or adverse conditions. Various forms of diseases can be identified through this technique [7].

A. Cunha et al. (Eds.): MobiHealth 2023, LNICST 578, pp. 173–184, 2024.
https://doi.org/10.1007/978-3-031-60665-6_13

In contrast, Wireless Capsule Endoscopy (WCE), a more recent innovation, offers a non-invasive, patient-friendly approach to meticulously visualizing the gastrointestinal tract. Compared to the traditional approach of endoscopy, which involves the insertion of a flexible tube through the mouth, capsule endoscopy offers several significant advantages. This includes reduced invasiveness, increased patient comfort, more comprehensive imaging, a reduced risk of complications, and the ability to access hard-to-reach areas [2, 28].

The capsule endoscope is a small capsule that contains a camera and is swallowed by the patient, allowing the doctor to visualize the gastrointestinal tract. During the examination, the capsule endoscope captures hundreds of images that are later reviewed by the physician to detect abnormalities. The result of this endoscopic examination is a long video of the entire gastrointestinal system of the patient. Such a video results in a relatively large number of images that can depict either normal tissue or tissue with some pathology [12].

The lethality of various diseases in the human gastrointestinal system can be significantly reduced with early diagnosis. That is, the earlier diseases such as colorectal cancer are detected, the lower the risk of mortality and permanent sequelae for patients [8].

Therefore, the use of machine learning techniques and deep neural networks to address the binary classification problem of pathologies becomes essential in assisting healthcare professionals in their work. Due to the large quantity of images generated by exams such as capsule endoscopy, manually verifying each image by a trained physician becomes slow and impractical. Thus, models created by these techniques serve to automate anomaly detection and achieve early diagnosis.

One approach to address this challenge is the application of artificial intelligence algorithms to assist in the identification of anomalies in capsule endoscopy videos, as manual analysis of these images by doctors can be exhaustive due to their large quantity. The use of these techniques to support healthcare professionals in early disease diagnosis is already widely explored by the scientific community, as highlighted in recent studies [15, 22]. As a result, several approaches and datasets have been proposed to achieve this goal.

Recent research has focused on the development of robust binary classification models for capsule endoscopy images. [11] utilized the Kvasir-Capsule database [27] in conjunction with deep learning techniques to reduce false negatives, a crucial aspect due to the severity associated with non-detection of gastrointestinal diseases. [13] utilizes fractal dimension for feature extraction and a random forest classifier to detect abnormal frames.

O WCENet [14], a deep convolutional neural network model, classifies and segments anomalous regions in WCE images into four categories (polyp, vascular, inflammatory, or normal). It achieves an accuracy of 98% and an area under the ROC curve of 99%, outperforming nine conventional machine learning and deep learning models on the KID dataset. This performance highlights its potential clinical use.

The performance of eight deep learning-based models for polyp detection and classification is compared in [16]: Faster RCNN [25], YOLOv3 [24], YOLOv4 [4],

SSD [20], RetinaNet [18], DetNet [17], RefineDet [30], and ATSS [29]. The results indicate that the RefineDet model achieved the best performance in polyp detection, with an F1-score of 88.6.

In the study by [21], an intelligent approach is proposed for classifying alimentary canal diseases such as Barrett's, Esophagitis, Hemorrhoids, Polyps, and Ulcerative colitis. The method involves image preprocessing, the application of Empirical Wavelet Transform (EWT) for extracting distinct patterns, and a two-stage classification using deep Convolutional Neural Networks (CNNs). The results show 96.65% accuracy in abnormal image detection and 94.25% accuracy in classifying these images into specific diseases.

Notably, the state-of-the-art works in this field have primarily focused on binary classification and have not evaluated anomaly detection through deep feature extraction or one-class classification methods. This study aims to develop a method for anomaly detection using video capsule endoscopy images by utilizing features extracted from convolutional neural networks and one-class classification method. The capsule endoscopy, coupled with machine learning techniques, plays a pivotal role in early diagnosis of gastrointestinal diseases, reducing their lethality and improving patient outcomes.

2   Materials and Methods

This section comprises the description of the procedures used in this study, including image acquisition, preprocessing, the machine learning techniques employed, loss function, and evaluation metrics.

2.1   Dataset

In the development of this study, two distinct datasets were used. The first one is the Kvasir-Capsule dataset [27], consisting of images captured by capsules ingested by patients. This dataset includes a total of 47,238 images from 117 videos. Out of the collected images, 34,338 were labeled as "Normal Clean Mucosa", referring to images with little or no fluid and mucosa with healthy villi and no pathological findings, representing the normal class. The remaining 12,900 images were labeled in the following categories: "Foreign Body", "Polyp", "Ulcer", "Erosion", "Blood - Hematin", "Blood - Fresh", "Angiectasia", "Erythema", "Lymphangiectasia", "Reduced Mucosal View", "Ileocecal Valve", "Ampulla of Vater", and 'Pylorus", representing the abnormal class.

The second dataset is the ERS dataset [6], also intended for multi-label classification. This dataset includes 123 labels divided into 5 categories: "Gastro", "Colono", "Healthy", "Blood", and "Quality", and these labels were assigned according to the Minimal Standard Terminology 3.0 (MST 3.0) standard [1]. The dataset consists of approximately 6,000 precisely labeled images and about 115,000 imprecise images, collected from 1,520 VCE videos of 1,135 patients. The precisely labeled images were classified by medical professionals from the Medical University of Gdańsk [6].

This study used only the precise images, with 1,019 labeled as normal and 2,494 labeled as abnormal. The low number of precise images poses a challenge for training, which adds to the challenge of class imbalance between the normal and abnormal classes.

2.2 Preprocessing

The images were resized to a size of 224×224 pixels, using their 3 RGB color channels. Subsequently, image normalization was performed using the Min-Max method to ensure that the pixel values ranged from 0 to 1.

2.3 Extraction of Deep Features

The analysis of medical images is a complex task due to the diversity and complexity of the information contained in these images. Visual features extracted from images play a crucial role in classification, anomaly detection, and disease diagnosis. However, in many cases, low-level features are not sufficient to capture the complexity of medical information [19].

To address this limitation, deep learning features, also known as "deep features", emerge as a solution. These features are intermediate representations learned by deep neural networks during training on extensive datasets. They encode hierarchical and abstract information about the objects present in the images, making them more discriminative and informative when compared to traditional features [10].

In this context, the ResNet152 network [9] was chosen for deep feature extraction. Despite its extensive depth with 152 layers, which can typically result in performance degradation issues, the residual connections embedded in the architecture, allowing for the direct passage of information between convolutional layers, help mitigate this problem. The choice of ResNet152 in this study is based on its superior performance compared to other evaluated architectures, making it the ideal choice for deep feature extraction.

Additionally, to address class imbalance, the "Binary Focal Loss" loss function was used. This function was specially designed for binary classification tasks, offering an effective solution for situations where classes are not equally distributed, i.e., one class occurs more frequently compared to the other. It adjusts the training focus to the most challenging examples, considering the correct class probability (p_t), an adjustment factor (α_t) to balance the classes, and a modulation parameter (γ). These elements together allow the model to prioritize examples that are more difficult to classify correctly, improving its ability to deal with class imbalance and, consequently, enhancing the accuracy of the final classification. The "Binary Focal Loss" equation is given by:

$$\text{Binary Focal Loss}(p_t) = -\alpha_t \cdot (1 - p_t)^{\gamma} \cdot \log(p_t) \tag{1}$$

2.4   Anomaly Detection

One-Class methods are a class of machine learning algorithms specifically designed to address problems where there is a predominant class (normal class) and a minority class of interest (anomalies). They play a crucial role in situations where identifying uncommon patterns is essential, such as in the analysis of medical images for early disease detection and anomaly identification.

The fundamental concept of One-Class methods is to create a model that learns only from examples of the normal class. This approach is based on the assumption that the normal class is well represented in the dataset and that anomalies are rare and different from this class. The main objective is to establish a boundary or threshold that encompasses the normal class, identifying any examples that fall outside this threshold as anomalies [23].

In this work, the One-Class Support Vector Machine (One-Class SVM) method was used [26]. Its operation involves creating a hyperplane that separates the data of the class of interest from regions considered not to belong to that class.

Given a training dataset $X = x_1, x_2, \ldots, x_n$, where x_i represents an example, the goal is to find a separation hyperplane that maximizes the margin around the positive class. Training examples are mapped to a high-dimensional space using a kernel function. The most common kernel used in OC-SVM is the Gaussian kernel (RBF - Radial Basis Function). The One-Class SVM solves the following optimization problem [26]:

$$\min \frac{1}{2}|w|^2 - \nu \sum_{i=1}^{n} \xi_i \qquad (2)$$

subject to $\langle w, \phi(x_i) \rangle \geq \rho - \xi_i$ for $i = 1, 2, \ldots, n$, where:

- w is a weight vector defining the separation hyperplane;
- ν is a hyperparameter that controls the amount of data that can fall into the margin region;
- ξ_i are slack variables that allow some examples to be within the margin;
- $\phi(x_i)$ represents the transformation of data into the high-dimensional space;
- ρ is the distance from the hyperplane to the nearest point of the positive class.

Consequently, the One-Class SVM detects any deviation from the "normal" class trained as belonging to an "abnormal" class. This makes it a valuable tool in real-world scenarios where completely new images not present in the training dataset need to be analyzed, enabling effective anomaly identification.

For the purpose of comparing the results of the One-Class method, which exclusively trains with the normal class, with another machine learning approach that uses two classes during the training process, XGBoost algorithm was employed. This choice will allow for the evaluation of performance differences between these two methods regarding the specific task at hand.

XGBoost [5] is a machine learning algorithm based on decision trees that excels in medical image classification. Unlike traditional approaches that use

CNNs, XGBoost employs a set of decision trees to predict an image's class. It can capture complex patterns and nonlinear interactions in the data, making it a powerful option for identifying discriminative features in images. XGBoost is particularly effective in cases where the dataset is unbalanced among its classes and is also known for its interpretability, allowing medical professionals to understand how the model arrives at its decisions.

3   Results

This section presents and discusses the results obtained with the proposed method for abnormality detection using video capsule endoscopy images. For evaluation, the datasets described were divided into three sets: training, validation, and test, ensuring that images from the same video captured from a patient were present in only one of the sets. Tables 1 and 2 present the proportion of images in the three sets for the Kvasir Capsule and ERS datasets, respectively.

Table 1. Division of the Kvasir Capsule dataset for evaluating the proposed method.

Pathology	Total	Training	Validation	Test
Normal	34338	18130	8315	7893
Abnormal	6659	3259	2461	939

Table 2. Division of the ERS dataset for evaluating the proposed method.

Pathology	Total	Training	Validation	Test
Normal	1019	761	125	133
Abnormal	2494	1590	384	520

The results here shown come from in-dataset scenarios, with no cross-dataset scenarios happening.

3.1   Deep Feature Extraction

The extraction of deep features was conducted using the ResNet152 architecture, which was initially pre-trained with ImageNet dataset weights. This pre-training provides the network with the ability to acquire useful representations of general visual features, making it valuable for computer vision tasks. After this pre-training step with the ImageNet dataset, ResNet152 was fine-tuned using the Kvasir-Capsule and ERS datasets with the goal of classifying images as normal or abnormal.

During the training process, Data Augmentation was employed to regularize the model, preventing overfitting. Various transformations such as rotation, translation, flipping, shearing, and scaling were applied to enrich the variety and robustness of the training data.

To optimize the model's hyperparameters, the Hyperopt optimizer was used to maximize the F1-score metric. For the Kvasir-Capsule dataset, the best hyperparameters for the Binary Focal Loss were set to $\alpha = 0.35$ and $\gamma = 2.0$. For the ERS dataset, the optimal hyperparameters were set to $\alpha = 0.2$ and $\gamma = 2.6$. In both implementations, the Adam optimizer was used, with a learning rate of 1×10^{-6}. This approach played a crucial role in effectively fine-tuning the model according to the specific characteristics of each dataset, resulting in the maximization of its performance.

Tables 3 and 4 display the classification results of images into normal and abnormal categories using the ResNet152 architecture on two distinct image datasets. In both sets of results, remarkable accuracy is observed in the classification of classes that contain a larger volume of images. This means that the model performed well on classes for which it received more examples during training, namely the "normal" class in the Kvasir-Capsule dataset and the "abnormal" class in the ERS dataset.

Table 3. Results of standard training of ResNet152 with the test split of the Kvasir-Capsule dataset.

Class	F1-Score	Precision	Recall
Normal	0.87	0.89	0.85
Abnormal	0.11	0.10	0.14
Average	0.49	0.50	0.49
Weighted Average	0.79	0.81	0.78

Table 4. Results of standard training of ResNet152 with the test split of the ERS dataset.

Class	F1-Score	Precision	Recall
Normal	0.25	0.25	0.25
Abnormal	0.81	0.81	0.81
Average	0.53	0.53	0.53
Weighted Average	0.69	0.69	0.69

Once the best models were defined for each dataset, the classification layer of the ResNet152 architecture was removed, allowing for the exclusive extraction of deep features.

3.2 Abnormality Detection

In the Kvasir-Capsule dataset, the hyperparameters used in the OneClassSVM method remained consistent with those used during standard training.

However, when applying the XGBoost algorithm, hyperparameters were tuned to `max_depth` = 6, `learning_rate` = 0.25, and `n_estimators` = 5000.

In the ERS dataset, the hyperparameters used in the OneClassSVM method remained consistent with those used during standard training. However, when applying the XGBoost algorithm, hyperparameters were tuned to `max_depth` = 6, `learning_rate` = 0.2, and `n_estimators` = 3560.

All the hyperparameters discussed in the implementations were obtained through the use of the Hyperopt hyperparameter optimizer [3]. It is worth noting that the hyperparameters used in the OneClassSVM method for both datasets remained unchanged. This behavior is related to the fact that the model does not correctly classify the two classes but instead assumes that all images belong to only one category.

Tables 5 and 6 display the best results obtained with the application of the OneClassSVM method on both datasets. However, it is important to highlight that the result in the ERS dataset suggests that the model is essentially classifying all images as belonging to the abnormal class. One of the reasons for this situation may be the class imbalance, with a larger number of abnormal images compared to normal images, which can affect the model's ability to correctly identify normal images.

Table 5. Results of applying the OneClassSVM with the test split of the Kvasir-Capsule dataset.

Class	F1-Score	Precision	Recall
Normal	0.61	0.82	0.49
Abnormal	0.38	0.28	0.64
Average	0.50	0.55	0.56
Weighted Average	0.56	0.69	0.52

Table 6. Results of applying the OneClassSVM with the test split of the ERS dataset.

Class	F1-Score	Precision	Recall
Normal	0.00	0.00	0.00
Abnormal	0.89	0.80	1.00
Average	0.44	0.40	0.50
Weighted Average	0.71	0.63	0.80

Tables 7 and 8 present the best results obtained with the application of the XGBoost method on both datasets. It is observed that, contrary to the problem identified in the application of the OneClassSVM method with the ERS dataset, XGBoost does not exhibit the same behavior of labeling all images as belonging to the majority class in the training set. However, there is still a noticeable tendency for the model to assume that images belong to the majority class during prediction. In the Kvasir-Capsule dataset, the model tends to classify more images as normal, while in the ERS dataset, it tends to classify more images as abnormal.

Table 7. Results of applying XGBoost with the test split of the Kvasir-Capsule dataset.

Class	F1-Score	Precision	Recall
Normal	0.94	0.90	0.99
Abnormal	0.20	0.55	0.12
Average	0.57	0.73	0.56
Weighted Average	0.87	0.87	0.90

Table 8. Results of applying XGBoost with the test split of the ERS dataset.

Class	F1-Score	Precision	Recall
Normal	0.15	0.23	0.11
Abnormal	0.85	0.80	0.90
Average	0.50	0.51	0.51
Weighted Average	0.71	0.68	0.74

The analysis of the results of the three methods - ResNet152, OneClassSVM, and XGBoost - reveals that XGBoost achieved the best performance among them. Therefore, it is evident that, for the task of abnormality detection in video capsule endoscopy images, the combination of XGBoost with deep feature extraction is the most robust and effective approach for addressing this specific problem.

4 Conclusion

In this study, we evaluated the performance of ResNet152 in the binary classification task and explored the use of OneClassSVM and XGBoost methods in an attempt to improve the final results. When employing the Kvasir-Capsule dataset, it became evident that the methods used were impacted by the class imbalance issue, where there was an unequal distribution of images between classes. In the case of the ERS dataset, this class imbalance problem was compounded by the limitation of a low overall quantity of images. As a result, the ResNet152 and XGBoost methods proved to be more effective in correctly classifying images belonging to the class they were predominantly trained on. It is expected that, with the refinement of the techniques used and, most importantly, with better-balanced datasets, more acceptable results can be achieved in the overall context of the classes.

It is also essential to highlight the importance of the patient-based data splitting strategy, which ensures the validity of the obtained results for analysis. One of the main challenges encountered in this work was the use of invalid data splits. This means that, in certain cases, the splits allowed for the sharing of images from the same patient across the training, validation, and test stages. Initially, the results obtained were very promising, but when the infeasibility of these invalid splits was realized, these results had to be discarded. This aspect underscores the critical importance of the patient-based data splitting approach to ensure the reliability of the results in any analysis or experiment.

Although the obtained results did not reach the desired level of performance, the analysis of the challenges encountered here has become essential for understanding them and future improvements.

For future research and the continuation of this work, it would be highly beneficial to investigate ways to improve class balance in the datasets used. Additionally, exploring the possibility of incorporating some or all of the images labeled as "uncertain" in the ERS dataset could be a promising strategy to significantly enhance the final results. These measures have the potential to considerably improve the performance of abnormality detection methods in video capsule endoscopy images.

References

1. Aabakken, L., et al.: Minimal standard terminology for gastrointestinal endoscopy-MST 3.0. Endoscopy **41**(08), 727–728 (2009)
2. Alaskar, H., Hussain, A., Al-Aseem, N., Liatsis, P., Al-Jumeily, D.: Application of convolutional neural networks for automated ulcer detection in wireless capsule endoscopy images. Sensors **19**(6), 1265 (2019)
3. Bergstra, J., et al.: Hyperopt: a python library for optimizing the hyperparameters of machine learning algorithms. In: Proceedings of the 12th Python in Science Conference, vol. 13, p. 20. Citeseer (2013)
4. Bochkovskiy, A., Wang, C.Y., Liao, H.Y.M.: Yolov4: optimal speed and accuracy of object detection. arXiv preprint: arXiv:2004.10934 (2020)
5. Chen, T., et al.: XGBoost: extreme gradient boosting. R Package Version 0.4-2 **1**(4), 1–4 (2015)
6. Cychnerski, J., Dziubich, T., Brzeski, A.: ERS: a novel comprehensive endoscopy image dataset for machine learning, compliant with the MST 3.0 specification (2022)
7. Du, W., et al.: Review on the applications of deep learning in the analysis of gastrointestinal endoscopy images. IEEE Access **7**, 142053–142069 (2019)
8. Hawkes, N.: Cancer survival data emphasise importance of early diagnosis. BMJ **364** (2019). https://doi.org/10.1136/bmj.l408
9. He, K., Zhang, X., Ren, S., Sun, J.: Deep residual learning for image recognition. CoRR **abs/1512.03385** (2015). http://arxiv.org/abs/1512.03385
10. He, K., Zhang, X., Ren, S., Sun, J.: Deep residual learning for image recognition. In: Proceedings of the IEEE Conference on Computer Vision and Pattern Recognition, pp. 770–778 (2016)

11. Hollstensson, M.: Detecting gastrointestinal abnormalities with binary classification of the Kvasir-Capsule dataset: a TensorFlow deep learning study (2022)
12. Iddan, G., Meron, G., Glukhovsky, A., Swain, P.: Wireless capsule endoscopy. Nature **405**(6785), 417 (2000). https://doi.org/10.1038/35013140
13. Jain, S., et al.: Detection of abnormality in wireless capsule endoscopy images using fractal features. Comput. Biol. Med. **127**, 104094 (2020) https://doi.org/10.1016/j.compbiomed.2020.104094, https://www.sciencedirect.com/science/article/pii/S001048252030425X
14. Jain, S., et al.: A deep CNN model for anomaly detection and localization in wireless capsule endoscopy images. Comput. Biol. Med. **137**, 104789 (2021) https://doi.org/10.1016/j.compbiomed.2021.104789, https://www.sciencedirect.com/science/article/pii/S0010482521005837
15. Lee, Y., Kang, P.: AnoViT: unsupervised anomaly detection and localization with vision transformer-based encoder-decoder. IEEE Access **10**, 46717–46724 (2022)
16. Li, K., et al.: Colonoscopy polyp detection and classification: dataset creation and comparative evaluations. PLOS ONE **16**(8), 1–26 (2021). https://doi.org/10.1371/journal.pone.0255809
17. Li, Z., Peng, C., Yu, G., Zhang, X., Deng, Y., Sun, J.: DetNet: a backbone network for object detection. arXiv preprint: arXiv:1804.06215 (2018)
18. Lin, T.Y., Goyal, P., Girshick, R., He, K., Dollár, P.: Focal loss for dense object detection. In: Proceedings of the IEEE International Conference on Computer Vision, pp. 2980–2988 (2017)
19. Litjens, G., et al.: A survey on deep learning in medical image analysis. Med. Image Anal. **42**, 60–88 (2017)
20. Liu, W., et al.: SSD: single shot multibox detector. In: Leibe, B., Matas, J., Sebe, N., Welling, M. (eds.) Computer Vision - ECCV 2016. Lecture Notes in Computer Science(), vol. 9905, pp. 21–37. Springer, Cham (2016). https://doi.org/10.1007/978-3-319-46448-0_2
21. Mohapatra, S., Kumar Pati, G., Mishra, M., Swarnkar, T.: Gastrointestinal abnormality detection and classification using empirical wavelet transform and deep convolutional neural network from endoscopic images. Ain Shams Eng. J. **14**(4), 101942 (2023). https://doi.org/10.1016/j.asej.2022.101942, https://www.sciencedirect.com/science/article/pii/S2090447922002532
22. Mukherjee, P., Roy, C.K., Roy, S.K.: OcFormer: one-class transformer network for image classification. arXiv preprint: arXiv:2204.11449 (2022)
23. Perera, P., Oza, P., Patel, V.M.: One-class classification: a survey (2021)
24. Redmon, J., Farhadi, A.: Yolov3: an incremental improvement. arXiv preprint: arXiv:1804.02767 (2018)
25. Ren, S., He, K., Girshick, R., Sun, J.: Faster R-CNN: towards real-time object detection with region proposal networks. In: Advances in Neural Information Processing Systems, vol. 28 (2015)
26. Shin, H.J., Eom, D.H., Kim, S.S.: One-class support vector machines-an application in machine fault detection and classification. Comput. Ind. Eng. **48**(2), 395–408 (2005) https://doi.org/10.1016/j.cie.2005.01.009, https://www.sciencedirect.com/science/article/pii/S0360835205000100
27. Smedsrud, P.H., et al.: Kvasir-capsule, a video capsule endoscopy dataset. Sci. Data **8**(1), 142 (2021)
28. Wang, S., Xing, Y., Zhang, L., Gao, H., Zhang, H.: Deep convolutional neural network for ulcer recognition in wireless capsule endoscopy: experimental feasibility and optimization. Comput. Math. Methods Med. **2019** (2019)

29. Zhang, S., Chi, C., Yao, Y., Lei, Z., Li, S.Z.: Bridging the gap between anchor-based and anchor-free detection via adaptive training sample selection. In: Proceedings of the IEEE/CVF Conference on Computer Vision and Pattern Recognition, pp. 9759–9768 (2020)
30. Zhang, S., Wen, L., Bian, X., Lei, Z., Li, S.Z.: Single-shot refinement neural network for object detection. In: Proceedings of the IEEE Conference on Computer Vision and Pattern Recognition, pp. 4203–4212 (2018)

Polyp Segmentation in Colonoscopy Images

Marcio P. Ferreira(✉) ⓘ, Giulia de A. Freulon, Daniel G. Piorsky,
Alexandre C. P. Pessoa, Darlan B. P. Quintanilha, and Aristófanes C. Silva

Applied Computing Group (NCA - UFMA), Federal University of Maranhão,
São Luís, MA, Brazil
{marcio.ferreira,alexandre.pessoa,dquintanilha,ari}@nca.ufma.br,
{giulia.freulon,daniel.piorky}@discente.ufma.br

Abstract. Colorectal cancer is a prevalent form of cancer, often detectable through polyps in the gastrointestinal tract. Unfortunately, these polyps typically do not display noticeable symptoms, making early detection challenging. While procedures like colonoscopy and endoscopy can identify polyps, they can miss some, leading to the need for a more automated approach. One innovative solution is capsule endoscopy, which records detailed images of the gastrointestinal tract over an extended period. However, the massive volume of data generated necessitates automation for efficient analysis. Artificial intelligence, particularly convolutional neural networks (CNNs) like TransUNet, can be crucial in quickly and accurately identifying suspicious areas in capsule endoscopy images. This study focuses on automating polyp detection using TransUNet and aims to enhance the early detection of colorectal cancer. The research utilizes the Kvasir-SEG database, containing polyp images and annotated segmentation masks. Various CNN architectures, like UNet, ResUNet, and ResUNet++, are employed, with metrics like Dice Loss and Tversky Loss used for performance evaluation through techniques like cross-validation. Results demonstrate that the TransUNet approach, leveraging transformers in its encoding layers, achieved 66% Dice Score, outperforming other architectures like UNet and ResUNet in this metric, however it did not surpass the ResUNet++ network. In conclusion, the TransUNet model shows potential for automating polyp detection in gastrointestinal images, offering a valuable tool in the fight against colorectal cancer. Integrating advanced technology into medicine promises more accurate and efficient gastrointestinal care.

Keywords: Video Capsule Endoscopy · Transformers · Polyp Segmentation

A. Cunha et al. (Eds.): MobiHealth 2023, LNICST 578, pp. 185–194, 2024.
https://doi.org/10.1007/978-3-031-60665-6_14

1 Introduction

Colorectal cancer, a disease of significant impact, ranks second most prevalent cancer among women and the third most common among men [6]. In its early stages, this form of cancer often originates as polyps, abnormal tissue growths on the mucous membrane lining the interior of the digestive system. Sadly, these polyps tend not to exhibit discernible symptoms, complicating their detection. However, screening procedures such as colonoscopy and endoscopy can usually identify these formations. It is concerning to note that studies point to a tendency to overlook the presence of polyps during these examinations, with detection failure rates ranging from 14 to 30%, depending on the size of the polyp [6].

Colonoscopy and endoscopy are highly invasive examinations that can potentially lead to undesirable side effects such as nausea, vomiting, intestinal pain, and even minor bleeding. These effects result from the procedure involving the endoscope. An alternative to these approaches is the adoption of capsule endoscopes, which incorporate cameras inside them. Patients swallow these capsules, and they naturally traverse the entire path that would be explored by the endoscope. During this journey, the capsule continuously records images and videos of the digestive tract, which are transmitted to a receiving device attached to the patient's waist throughout the procedure.

The advantages of using capsules in examinations are that they avoid the side effects commonly associated with colonoscopy and endoscopy procedures, and they are considerably less invasive. However, a significant drawback of using capsules is that the procedure generates a large number of images or a very long video since the capsule naturally travels through the entire digestive tract, which takes around 8 to 12 h [4].

Given the general challenge of detection error rates and the need to analyze a large amount of material from capsule examinations, one solution is the automation of polyp detection, such as the use of image segmentation techniques. Image segmentation is a technique that aims to highlight an area of interest in an image, with the area, in this case, being the polyp itself.

Improving the efficiency of polyp detection implies a decrease in colorectal cancer rates. Thus, finding ways to enhance the identification rate of these structures and automate this process emerges as an achievement of immeasurable value for people's health and quality of life. An approach with potential for this automation lies in the application of computer vision techniques, particularly in the field of image segmentation. Image segmentation, a sophisticated technique, aims to isolate relevant information within an image in this context, explicitly highlighting the area of interest of the polyps. This approach facilitates the interpretation of results and signals a promising path for optimizing the early detection of these anomalies [6]. The objective of this study is to evaluate the effectiveness of computer vision and neural network approaches in automating the process of detecting polyps in images of the gastrointestinal system. Through extensive testing and analysis, this research aims to contribute valuable insights into the performance, strengths and limitations of the proposed methods. The following sections will delve deeper into the experimental setup, dataset, and evaluation of results, clarifying practical implications and advances achieved through comprehensive testing.

2   Related Work

Research involving technologies such as machine learning and CNN for medical image analysis is widely conducted by researchers from various public and private institutions. Given this large number of researchers, it is possible to find a wide variety of research and different techniques in the field. In Table 1, a selection of related works and their respective techniques are presented.

Table 1. Related works with datasets and techniques used.

Work	Dice	Dataset	Technique
JHA et al. [7]	81.33%	Kvasir-SEG	ResUNet and modifications
TOMAR et a. [10]	85.76%	Kvasir-SEG	DDANet
SRIVASTAVA et al. [8]	92.17%	Kvasir-SEG	MSRF-Net
YEUNG et al. [11]	91%	Kvasir-SEG	Focus U-Net
JHA et al. [5]	92.93%	CVC-ClinicDB	ResUNet++ with CRF and TTA

In a study conducted by [7], ResUNet and its enhanced variations were employed for the segmentation of polyps in the Kvasir-SEG dataset. In this context, the more refined iteration of the network, known as ResUNet++, achieved an impressive Dice score of 81.33%.

DDANet is an architecture based on a dual-attention decoder, and in experiments conducted by [10], it achieved a remarkable Dice score of 85.76% when applied to the Kvasir-SEG dataset.

In the work by [8], the MSRF-Net was introduced as an innovative approach to medical image segmentation in [8], utilizing DSDF (Dual-Scale Dense Fusion) blocks. The results demonstrated a Dice score of 92.17% when applied to the Kvasir-SEG dataset.

The Focus U-Net [11], a network that incorporates the Focus Gate, a model that combines channel-based and spatial-based attention mechanisms. This approach achieved a Dice score of 91% when evaluated on the Kvasir-SEG dataset.

A study conducted by [5] employed the ResUNet++ architecture and improved its performance through the integration of techniques such as Conditional Random Field (CRF) and Test-Time Augmentation (TTA). As a result of these optimizations, a remarkable Dice score of 92.93% was achieved on the CVC-ClinicDB dataset using ResUNet++ in conjunction with the CRF approach.

This work contributes to tests of Kvasir-SEG on TransUNet Network and several tests carried out with this network, and comparison of its performance with UNet and other networks used in medical image segmentation.

3   Materials and Methods

3.1   Dataset

The dataset used was Kvasir-SEG. This dataset consists of 1,000 images of polyps and their respective masks annotated by professionals in the field. The images range from 332×487 to 1920×1072 pixels. Kvasir-SEG was created to be a public dataset that researchers could use in their studies, as obtaining such a dataset for research purposes is challenging.

3.2   Pre-processing

Initially, tests were conducted using the Kvasir-SEG dataset, using the images at their original resolutions. Subsequently, new experiments were carried out after resizing the images to a resolution of 512×512 pixels while preserving their proportions. Based on these initial tests, superior performance was observed with the resized images. Based on these results, it was decided to adopt the resized images as the standard for the subsequent research steps.

3.3   Method

UNet. UNet is a Convolutional Neural Network (CNN) originally developed for medical image segmentation. Its main objective was to achieve highly accurate segmentation while efficiently using computational resources. The term "UNet" derives from its "U"-shaped architecture. This characteristic design of the architecture is responsible for its nomenclature.

The UNet architecture can be divided into two main parts: the downsampling layers and the upsampling layers. In the downsampling phase, the input image goes through a series of operations. First, consecutive convolutions with 3×3 filters are applied, followed by Rectified Linear Activation (ReLU) activation, which solves gradient problems by mapping positive values to themselves and negative values to zero. Next, the downsampling layers incorporate Max Pooling operations with 2×2 filters. Max Pooling is a common technique in CNNs to reduce the dimensionality of feature maps.

In the upsampling layers, the outputs of the downsampling layers go through a sequence of Upsampling operations with 2×2 filters. At each Upsampling step, the output is concatenated with the corresponding output from the downsampling layer. Finally, the last layer performs a convolution with a 1×1 filter, which maps the image's features. This final layer is followed by a sigmoid function, which generates a binary segmentation mask.

TransUNet. TransUNet is a neural network architecture based on transformers, designed to overcome the limitations inherent to CNNs. CNNs often exhibit poor performance on target structures that display wide inter-patient variations in terms of texture, shape, and size due to the nature of multiple convolution operations. While convolutions are effective at identifying local features, they do not excel at capturing long-range information or global context.

As a solution to this challenge, [1] proposed incorporating self-attention mechanisms, akin to transformers. By adopting this approach, TransUNet aims to address the need to capture long-range relationships between image elements effectively, allowing for a more effective understanding of contextual and global information. This contributes to improving the segmentation and understanding of complex and variable structures among different medical images.

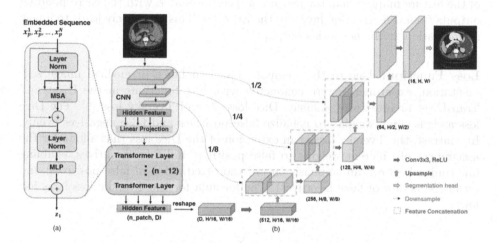

Fig. 1. TransUNet structure [10].

As we can see in Fig. 1, TransUNet adopts a structure similar to U-Net, however, its fundamental distinction lies in the addition of transformer layers, which are not present in the conventional UNet. These transformer layers can establish long-range connections between different regions of the image.

The operation of TransUNet consists of the image initially passing through convolution layers to extract relevant features from the input image. Subsequently, these features are passed to the transformer layers, whose purpose is to capture relationships that extend over a significant distance between different regions of the image.

Within the transformer layers, the following operations take place:

- Layer Normalization: Normalizes input values for each channel of the layer, which helps regularize and normalize activations, making the learning process more stable;
- Multi-Head Self-Attention (MSA): Applies multiple self-attention, where the input is projected into various attention dimensions, allowing the network to focus on relevant information at different positions and scales. This allows the network to capture long-range relationships and broader contexts;

- Layer Normalization: A second layer of normalization is applied after the self-attention operation for the output of that layer;
- Multi-Layer Perceptron (MLP): A layer for learning complex relationships between input features. This helps transform and merge information obtained from the previous operation, allowing the network to capture non-linear relationships.

After obtaining the hidden features from the output of the transformer layers, they are passed through a set of Upsampling layers, which expand the resolution of the feature maps. Then, the features are concatenated with the corresponding outputs from the attention layers in the Encoder. This ultimately leads to image segmentation at the network's output.

Loss Function. Due to the common class imbalance in medical image segmentation, experiments were conducted with loss functions in the UNet and TransUNet architectures, namely, Dice loss [2] and Tversky loss [9]. The Dice loss assigns equal weights to penalize false positives and false negatives evenly. In contrast, the Tversky loss is an extension of the Dice loss that allows for the assignment of different weights to false positives and false negatives, enabling fine-tuning between an emphasis on precision (reduction of false positives) and recall (reduction of false negatives). The formula for the Tversky loss is as follows:

$$T(\alpha, \beta) = 1 - \frac{\sum_{i,j} p_{ij} \times t_{ij}}{\sum_{i,j} p_{ij} \times t_{ij} + \alpha \times \sum_{i,j} p_{ij} \times (1 - t_{ij}) + \beta \times \sum_{i,j} (1 - p_{ij}) \times t_{ij}}$$

where p_{ij} represents the model's prediction probability for the pixel or element at position (i, j), and t_{ij} is the true (label) value of the pixel or element at position (i, j). The parameters α and β adjust the weight assigned to false positives and false negatives, respectively.

In the experiments with both the UNet and TransUNet architectures, the Tversky loss proved to be more effective.

3.4   Evaluation of Results

The evaluation metrics used in the proposed method were Dice score, Precision, Recall, and Mean Intersection over Union (mIOU). The calculations for these metrics were based on the following formulas:

- Dice Score = 2 * (Precision * Recall)/(Precision + Recall)
- Precision = TP/(TP + FP)
- Recall = TP/(TP + FN)
- mIOU = TP/(TP + FP + FN)

where TP stands for true positives, TN for true negatives, FP for false positives, and FN for false negatives [3].

4 Results

In this section, the results of the performance evaluation of segmentation on the Kvasir-SEG dataset (resized while maintaining proportions) using the TransUNet network are presented. A comparison is conducted between the ADAM (Adaptive Moment Estimation) and SGD (Stochastic Gradient Descent) optimizers in various configurations.

Initially, hyperparameter optimization tests were conducted with HyperOpt library. These tests consisted of 20 evaluations, each involving training for 100 epochs using the Tversky Loss function. The data split for training was 70% for training, 15% for validation, and 15% for testing.

Based on the results obtained in this optimization phase, a new training was conducted using these values. The initial tests revealed better performance with the SGD optimizer compared to ADAM. Table 2 summarizes the performance metric results for each optimizer.

Table 2. Comparative Test between ADAM and SGD optimizers in the TransUNet network.

Optimizer	Dice	mIOU	Recall	Precision
ADAM	0.4058	**0.6346**	**0.7236**	0.2820
SGD	**0.7020**	0.4358	0.6519	**0.7605**

Based on this preliminary analysis, the choice of the SGD optimizer was made to proceed with further tests. The next step involved conducting a cross-validation with 5 folds, each containing 200 images. In each cross-validation run, 3 folds were used for training, 1 for validation, and 1 for testing, ensuring that each fold was used once for testing and once for validation. The configurations obtained in the hyperparameter optimization stage for the SGD optimizer were used. The results of this process can be seen in Table 3.

Table 3. Cross-validation in TransUNet.

Fold	Dice	mIOU	Recall	Precision
1	**0.7217**	**0.4805**	**0.7212**	0.7222
2	0.6364	0.3521	0.6530	0.6207
3	0.6795	0.3047	0.6397	0.7245
4	0.6844	0.4752	0.6560	0.7153
5	0.6191	0.1189	0.5317	**0.7409**
Average	0.6682	0.3467	0.6403	0.7047
Standard Deviation	0.0412	0.1327	0.0700	0.0469

Additionally, cross-validation was conducted with the UNet network after preliminary hyperparameter tuning to make a comparison between the methods. The results of this evaluation are summarized in Table 4.

Table 4. Cross-validation in UNet.

Fold	Dice	mIOU	Recall	Precision
1	0.5639	0.0571	0.5649	0.5785
2	0.5836	0.0576	0.5424	0.6584
3	**0.6190**	0.0579	0.5784	**0.6797**
4	0.5439	0.0559	**0.6207**	0.5042
5	0.5530	**0.0580**	0.5218	0.5915
Average	0.5726	0.0573	0.5656	0.6026
Standard Deviation	0.0275	0.0007	0.0363	0.0615

When comparing the results, it becomes evident that the utilization of transformers in the encoding (encoder) phase of the TransUNet network demonstrates superiority over the UNet approach.

Furthermore, to have a more robust comparison we performed a cross-validation of the ResUNet and ResUNet++ networks from the work of Jha et al. [7] for comparison purposes only, following preliminary hyperparameter adjustments. The results obtained from this evaluation can be seen in Table 5 and Table 6.

Table 5. Cross-validation in ResUNet.

Fold	Dice	mIOU	Recall	Precision
1	**0.7099**	0.4380	0.6520	0.0469
2	0.6198	0.4407	0.6227	**0.7964**
3	0.6560	0.4376	0.6577	0.7914
4	0.6941	**0.4485**	**0.7095**	0.6963
5	0.6254	0.4394	0.5778	0.7824
Average	0.6610	0.4408	0.6439	0.7768
Standard Deviation	0.0368	0.0040	0.0467	0.0439

Table 7 compares the average cross-validation results of the networks. While TransUNet achieved a superior Dice score compared to ResUNet, it couldn't surpass ResUNet++ in any evaluation metric.

Table 6. Cross-validation in ResUNet++.

Fold	Dice	mIOU	Recall	Precision
1	0.7927	0.7656	0.6165	**0.9456**
2	0.7836	0.7728	0.6806	0.9001
3	**0.8611**	**0.8124**	**0.7241**	0.9347
4	0.7914	0.7771	0.6729	0.8743
5	0.7205	0.7180	0.5653	0.8912
Average	0.7898	0.7692	0.6519	0.9092
Standard Deviation	0.0548	0.0317	0.0531	0.0287

Table 7. Comparison of cross-validations

Network	Dice	mIOU	Recall	Precision
TransUNet	0.6682	0.3467	0.6403	0.7047
UNet	0.5726	0.0573	0.5656	0.6026
ResUNet	0.6610	0.4408	0.6439	0.7768
ResUNet++	**0.7898**	**0.7692**	**0.6519**	**0.9092**

5   Conclusion

Based on experiments conducted with different networks using the Kvasir-SEG dataset, it can be concluded that the TransUNet network's approach, which incorporates transformers into the encoding layers, demonstrated superior performance in terms of the Dice score compared to the UNet and ResUNet architectures, although it did not surpass the results of ResUNet++. The results obtained indicated significant improvements in TransUNet in evaluation metrics such as Dice score, recall, and precision, and, even though it did not surpass ResUNet++, it effectively extracts relevant features from medical images.

Furthermore, the additional use of cross-validation methods on the networks, as applied in the work of Jha et al. [7], contributed to obtaining more consistent and robust results. This approach allowed for a more comprehensive validation of the networks, providing a more reliable view of real performance in different scenarios.

In light of the foregoing, it becomes apparent that the outcomes of this study yield valuable insights pertinent to the choice of neural network architectures in the context of medical image segmentation tasks. These findings underscore the transformative potential inherent in the employment of the transformer-based approach, exemplified by TransUNet. Nevertheless, it is essential to underscore that further research and experimentation remain imperative in the pursuit of enhanced network performance. This includes the exploration of alternative loss functions and the incorporation of post-processing techniques to attain superior results.

Moreover, given the promising trajectory outlined by this study, several opportunities for future research emerge. One possible direction would be the exploration of hybrid strategies that combine the advantages of the TransUNet approach with other cutting-edge architectures, such as Generative Adversarial Networks (GANs), aiming to further improve the accuracy and fidelity of segmentations obtained. Additionally, it would be interesting to explore modifications to the base UNet architecture, such as the incorporation of multi-scale attention mechanisms to enrich the network's contextualization capability, which could yield interesting results. Finally, expanding to more diverse and challenging datasets, as well as applying the TransUNet approach to other areas of medical image analysis, would open up new research frontiers and solidify its potential impact on clinical practice and the advancement of medical science.

References

1. Chen, J., et al.: TransUNet: transformers make strong encoders for medical image segmentation. arXiv preprint: arXiv:2102.04306 (2021)
2. Dice, L.R.: Measures of the amount of ecologic association between species. Ecology 26(3), 297–302 (1945). http://www.jstor.org/stable/1932409
3. Diniz, J., et al.: Detecção de covid-19 em imagens de raio-x de tórax através de seleção automática de pré-processamento e de rede neural convolucional. In: Anais do XXIII Simpósio Brasileiro de Computação Aplicada à Saúde. pp. 162–173. SBC, Porto Alegre, RS, Brasil (2023). https://doi.org/10.5753/sbcas.2023.229576, https://sol.sbc.org.br/index.php/sbcas/article/view/25286
4. Gupta, A., Singh, A., Shah, D.: Capsule endoscopy. StatPearls [Internet] (2023). https://doi.org/10.1001/jamanetworkopen.2022.29881, https://www.ncbi.nlm.nih.gov/books/NBK546951/
5. Jha, D., et al.: A comprehensive study on colorectal polyp segmentation with ResUNet++, conditional random field and test-time augmentation. IEEE J. Biomed. Health Inform. 25(6), 2029–2040 (2021)
6. Jha, D., et al.: Kvasir-SEG: a segmented polyp dataset. In: Ro, Y., et al. (eds.) MultiMedia Modeling. Lecture Notes in Computer Science(), vol. 11962, pp. 451–462. Springer, Cham (2020). https://doi.org/10.1007/978-3-030-37734-2_37
7. Jha, D., et al.: ResUNet++: an advanced architecture for medical image segmentation. In: 2019 IEEE International Symposium on Multimedia (ISM), pp. 225–2255. IEEE (2019)
8. Srivastava, A., et al.: MSRF-Net: a multi-scale residual fusion network for biomedical image segmentation. IEEE J. Biomed. Health Inform. 26(5), 2252–2263 (2021)
9. Terven, J., Cordova-Esparza, D.M., Ramirez-Pedraza, A., Chavez-Urbiola, E.A.: Loss functions and metrics in deep learning. a review. arXiv preprint: arXiv:2307.02694 (2023)
10. Tomar, N.K., et al.: DDANet: dual decoder attention network for automatic polyp segmentation. In: Del Bimbo, A., et al. (eds.) Pattern Recognition. ICPR International Workshops and Challenges. Lecture Notes in Computer Science(), vol. 12668, pp. 307–314. Springer, Cham (2021). https://doi.org/10.1007/978-3-030-68793-9_23
11. Yeung, M., Sala, E., Schönlieb, C.B., Rundo, L.: Focus U-Net: a novel dual attention-gated CNN for polyp segmentation during colonoscopy. Comput. Biol. Med. 137, 104815 (2021)

Automating the Annotation of Medical Images in Capsule Endoscopy Through Convolutional Neural Networks and CBIR

Rodrigo Fernandes[1,2]([📧]), Marta Salgado[3], Ishak Paçal[4], and António Cunha[1,2]

[1] UTAD—University of Trás-os-Montes and Alto Douro, 5001-801 Vila Real, Portugal
acunha@utad.pt

[2] INESC TEC—Institute for Systems and Computer Engineering, Technology and Science,
4200-465 Porto, Portugal
rodrigo.c.fernandes@inesctec.pt

[3] Centro Hospitalar Universitário de Santo António, 4099-001 Porto, Portugal
martasalgado.gastro@chporto.min-saude.pt

[4] Igdir University, Iğdır, Turkey
ishak.pacal@igdir.edu.tr

Abstract. This research addresses the significant challenge of automating the annotation of medical images, with a focus on capsule endoscopy videos. The study introduces a novel approach that synergistically combines Deep Learning and Content-Based Image Retrieval (CBIR) techniques to streamline the annotation process. Two pre-trained Convolutional Neural Networks (CNNs), MobileNet and VGG16, were employed to extract and compare visual features from medical images. The methodology underwent rigorous validation using various performance metrics such as accuracy, AUC, precision, and recall. The MobileNet model demonstrated exceptional performance with a test accuracy of 98.4%, an AUC of 99.9%, a precision of 98.2%, and a recall of 98.6%.

On the other hand, the VGG16 model achieved a test accuracy of 95.4%, an AUC of 99.2%, a precision of 97.3%, and a recall of 93.5%. These results indicate the high efficacy of the proposed method in the automated annotation of medical images, establishing it as a promising tool for medical applications. The study also highlights potential avenues for future research, including expanding the image retrieval scope to encompass entire endoscopy video databases.

Keywords: Automatic Medical Image Annotation · Convolutional Neural Networks · Content-Based Image Retrieval

1 Introduction

Capsule endoscopy, a recent innovation in gastroenterology, offers a non-invasive visualisation of the gastrointestinal tract, paving the way for improved diagnoses and interventions [1]. However, this advancement brings challenges. The vast amount of video data each examination generates demands extensive manual interpretation, introducing risks of omissions and errors.

A. Cunha et al. (Eds.): MobiHealth 2023, LNICST 578, pp. 195–207, 2024.
https://doi.org/10.1007/978-3-031-60665-6_15

Artificial intelligence, particularly machine learning, presents a promising solution to these challenges. CNNs, having been applied in various medical contexts from image diagnosis [2, 3] to genomic analysis [4, 5], can automate the identification and categorisation of critical areas in capsule endoscopy, optimising analysis time and accuracy [6].

Our research group has been dedicated to advancements in wireless capsule endoscopy and its automated analysis. In [7], utilising the DenseNet-161 model, we tackled the challenge of manual analysis, achieving significant precision and recall rates in lesion detection. Our work in [8] provided a comprehensive overview of endoscopic capsule technology's evolution, emphasising its advantages over traditional endoscopic procedures. Meanwhile, [9] explored the challenges of abnormality detection in endoscopy videos. We demonstrated effective classification even with limited video capsule endoscopy data by leveraging deep learning and transfer learning.

The efficacy of CNNs largely rests on the availability of vast annotated datasets. Acquiring such datasets in many medical areas, including gastroenterology, poses difficulties due to ethical dilemmas, patient confidentiality, and the data's specialised nature.

The central challenge addressed in this research is the time-consuming and potentially inconsistent nature of manual medical image annotation, particularly in capsule endoscopy. Manual annotation demands expertise and is often subjective, leading to professional variability. Ethical and privacy concerns further constrain the availability of manually annotated datasets.

Traditional content-based image retrieval (CBIR) methods serve as a cornerstone in the quest to search for images within databases based on their inherent visual attributes like colour, shape, and texture, reliant on low-level features, and struggle to grasp the detailed nuances of medical images. This necessitates a novel method to automate the annotation process, integrating deep learning with CBIR to bridge this semantic gap.

The main objective of this study is to develop an automated method for annotating medical images, focusing specifically on capsule endoscopy videos. The research aims to extract and compare visual features from medical images by taking advantage of the capabilities of pre-trained Convolutional Neural Networks (CNN), such as MobileNet and VGG16. Combining deep learning techniques with CBIR methods, this study seeks to eliminate the need for manually annotated datasets, often scarce in medical contexts due to ethical and privacy restrictions. Through rigorous validation involving various performance metrics such as accuracy, AUC, precision and retrieval, the study aims to establish the effectiveness of the proposed methodology for the automatic annotation of medical images.

2   Related Work

Over recent years, CBIR has witnessed exponential growth in theoretical frameworks and practical applications [10, 11]. Despite these advances, the state-of-the-art in CBIR is far from perfect and presents limitations. Some of the most relevant contributions on this topic are highlighted below.

One of the most challenging barriers in the evolution of CBIR systems is the semantic gap disconnect between low-level visual descriptors and the high-level semantic meaning that humans associate with images [12]. Various strategies have been proposed to mitigate this issue. Djeraba [13], for instance, championed a knowledge-content-based retrieval system that leverages insights gleaned from image repositories, offering a fresh avenue for CBIR systems.

Douze et al. [14] explored the idea of using attribute vectors for image retrieval to further bridge the semantic gap. Their work yielded performance metrics on par with contemporary state-of-the-art methods, suggesting that attribute-based techniques could be valuable to CBIR systems.

In medical imaging, CBIR encounters unique hurdles. Medical images encapsulate spatial and intricate structural data, often poorly represented by traditional, low-level CBIR methods [15]. This highlights an urgent need for CBIR frameworks that can incorporate high-level structural nuances and the spatial relationships between different regions of an image.

The incorporation of machine learning techniques into CBIR has been a game-changing development. Ali & Sharma [16] developed a CBIR system combining feature extraction with machine learning, aiming to improve retrieval accuracy and efficacy.

Efficient indexing mechanisms and relevance feedback are indispensable for optimising CBIR performance. In this context, Jeyasekhar & Mostefai [17] expounded on the importance of state-of-the-art indexing methodologies, such as R-trees and KDB trees, in augmenting the retrieval efficiency of CBIR systems.

Despite the progress of CBIR, the method continues to grapple with issues related to scalability, efficiency, and accuracy. Ouni et al. [18] recently proposed a novel CBIR framework that merges semantic segmentation networks with swift spatial binary encoding, aiming to achieve rapid retrieval at a reduced computational cost.

Despite significant advances in the field of CBIR, there are still gaps that need attention. While many works have focused on mitigating the semantic gap problem, the ideal combination of techniques that can effectively overcome this challenge is still a topic of investigation. Additionally, the application of CBIR in the context of medical imaging, and more specifically capsule endoscopy, presents unique challenges due to the complexity and variety of the data. Automating the annotation of these images is crucial to improving clinical efficiency and diagnostic accuracy. Our work stands out by introducing an innovative approach that combines deep learning and CBIR techniques using convolutional neural networks for the automated annotation of capsule endoscopy images.

3   Methodology

The study's methodology unfolds in several phases, as illustrated in the provided image (Fig. 1):

The images extracted from the original capsule endoscopy dataset undergo a meticulous 'Frame Selection' process to identify pertinent frames based on specific criteria as described in the "Frame Selection Process" section. Subsequently, these frames are adapted and structured during the 'Data Preprocessing' phase, optimising them for enhanced machine learning model performance. Leveraging Convolutional Neural Networks (CNNs), the classifier discerns between similar and non-similar frames, utilising

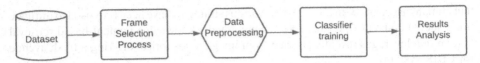

Fig. 1. Flowchart of the experiment.

intrinsic visual features and inter-frame distances. The classifier's proficiency is then rigorously assessed using performance metrics such as accuracy, AUC, precision, and recall, offering a holistic evaluation of the model's capabilities.

3.1 Dataset

This study used a dataset made up of 320 capsule endoscopy videos in GVF format, acquired from a private medical source. All the videos feature patients with various abnormalities detected in the gastrointestinal tract, such as polyps, bleeding, ulcers, among others. These abnormalities were duly noted by medical experts during the review of the videos. It is important to mention that although the images are annotated, they are not categorised into specific classes. The dataset has been anonymised to respect patient privacy and includes 2896 annotated frames with a resolution of 320 × 320 pixels. To guarantee the quality of the data, the videos went through cleaning and validation processes. During pre-processing, the images were cleaned to remove a black band introduced during extraction, and they were also resized to 224 × 224 pixels to fit pre-trained networks. In addition, a validation stage was carried out to ensure the correct correspondence between the annotated frames and the originals, enabling accurate annotation of abnormalities.

3.2 Frame Selection Process

For each video in our dataset, we focus on frames annotated by medical experts, referred to as 'target frames'. A pre-trained CNN model first processes these target frames to extract feature vectors. Subsequently, every frame in a video is individually processed to create its feature vector.

We define an interval of 100 frames before and after each target frame to establish a probable correspondence zone. Frames outside this interval are classified as 'not similar'. Using Euclidean distance as a similarity metric, we compare each frame's feature vector with the target frame's.

This generates a ranking of each class's top 10 most similar frames ('similar' or 'not similar'). The procedure is repeated for each target frame across all videos in the dataset. This process is exemplified in Fig. 2 for a more straightforward perception.

Frames Preprocessing

To efficiently integrate the frames with the Convolutional Neural Networks (CNN) models used in this study, it was necessary to implement a preprocessing stage focused on resizing the images. This step is essential, as the CNN models were originally trained

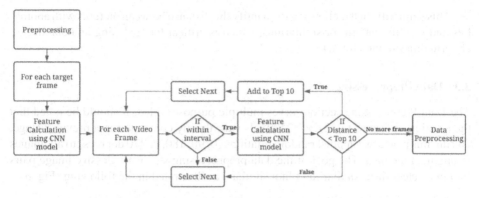

Fig. 2. Flowchart of the proposed frame selection algorithm.

with inputs of specific dimensions. We, therefore, adapted each frame to a standard size of 224 × 224 pixels, thus ensuring compatibility with the neural network architectures.

CNN Models
The previous study used the 25 pre-trained CNN models in the TensorFlow library as feature extractors for localising frames in wireless endoscopic (WCE) capsule videos. These models, which include MobileNet, MobileNetV2, MobileNetV3, ResNet50, ResNet101, ResNet152, ResNet50V2, ResNet101V2, ResNet152V2, ResNet200V2, VGG16, VGG19, DenseNet121, DenseNet169, DenseNet201, InceptionV3, InceptionResNetV2, NASNetMobile, NASNetLarge, EfficientNetB0 to EfficientNetB7, and Xception, have different architectures, providing unique extraction characteristics. Through rigorous preliminary evaluations, considering both accuracy and computational efficiency, eight models were selected for in-depth experimentation: MobileNet, ResNet152v2, VGG19, VGG16, DenseNet121, InceptionResNetv2, ResNet50v2 and ResNet101v2.For the current study, we focused solely on the pre-trained MobileNet model, which demonstrated superior performance in our previous research.

Similarity Metric
A similarity metric quantifies the similarity or dissimilarity between two objects or datasets. In this project, we use the Euclidean distance as the similarity metric.

The Euclidean distance is a widely used metric for calculating the distance between two points in an Euclidean space. It is calculated as the square root of the sum of the squares of the differences between the coordinates of the points. The Euclidean distance Eq. 1 for the two points $\mathbf{p}$ and $\mathbf{q}$, in a space of n dimensions, is given by:

$$dist(p, q) = \sqrt{\sum_{i=1}^{n} (q_i - p_i)^2} \tag{1}$$

where p_i and q_i represent the coordinates of the points $\mathbf{p}$ and $\mathbf{q}$ in the dimension i, respectively.

The Euclidean distance measures the magnitude of the vector connecting the two points and is used to evaluate their closeness or similarity. The smaller the Euclidean distance, the more similar the points are.

This similarity metric allows us to quantify the distance between pictures with anomalies and identify patterns or similarities, which is critical for analysing and classifying abnormalities in the GI tract.

3.3 Data Preprocessing

The Data Preprocessing section serves multiple purposes. First, it should be noted that the resizing of frames to 224 × 224 pixels was already completed in a previous stage. During this phase, we applied random rotations (0, 90, 180, or 270 degrees) to all images to augment the data. The goal of the data preprocessing step is to classify image pairs into two categories: 'similar' and 'not similar', as illustrated in the following (Fig. 3).

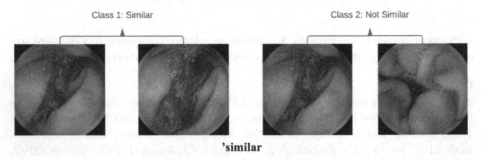

'similar

Fig. 3. Data Preprocessing Workflow.

The dataset at this stage contains 57,565 image pairs, comprising 28,885 in the 'similar' category (Class 1) and 28,680 in the 'not similar' category (Class 2). In Class 1, each target frame is paired with one of the top 10 most similar frames, based on the interval of 100 frames defined in the Frame Selection Process section. Conversely, in Class 2, each target frame is paired with one of the top 10 most similar frames but from an interval of 100 frames away from the target frame. This classification process is repeated for each of the top 10 most similar frames for all target frames across the dataset. The dataset was then split into 70%, 15%, and 15% for training, validation, and testing. This classification process defines the classes for the classifier's training.

3.4 Classifier Training

The Classifier Training section outlines a meticulous process for processing each 'image pair. This process is shown in Fig. 4.' Initially, each image in the pair is individually fed into a pre-trained Convolutional Neural Network (CNN) model. Stripped of its original classification layers, this model serves as a feature extractor and generates a feature vector for each image.

After extraction, we concatenate the feature vectors of the two images, creating a composite vector that embodies the image pair's features. Next, this composite vector is flattened, converting it into a one-dimensional array, making it more manageable for the upcoming neural network layers.

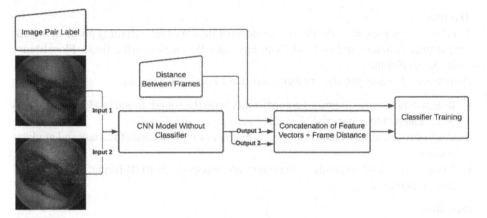

Fig. 4. Classifier Training Flowchart

An additional metric, the frame distance between the two images, is added to the beginning of this one-dimensional vector. Expressed as the difference in the number of frames between the two images (for example, a difference of 10 frames would be represented as 999–989 = 10), this serves as an extra feature for the classifier.

This enriched vector, which now includes both the intrinsic features of the images and the relative frame distance between them, is then provided to the classifier for training, along with a corresponding label indicating their 'similarity' or 'non-similarity.' This comprehensive method ensures the classifier is trained with a rich, multidimensional representation of each image pair, maximising the model's effectiveness and accuracy in the classification tasks.

It's important to note that the classifier's output represents how well the model discerns the degree of similarity sufficient for categorising an image pair within the interval of interest for similarity. This output is vital for the learning objective, empowering the classifier to distinguish between similar and non-similar image pairs effectively.

CNN Models
In this subsection, we conduct experiments with both CNN models, VGG16 [19] and MobileNet [20], to provide a solid basis for comparison. These two models were selected from the eight we tested in our previous study based on their exceptional performance in preliminary tests. Both have been stripped of their original classifier layers and are used exclusively for feature extraction. Using both networks allows for a more robust comparative analysis, reinforcing the validity of our findings.

The VGG16 model, known for its deep and robust architecture, offers the advantage of capturing high-level features, making it highly effective for complex classification tasks. On the other hand, the MobileNet model is known for its computational efficiency, making it an ideal choice for applications that require real-time processing or computational resource limitations. Both models serve as robust feature extractors and complement each other in different aspects, making the analysis more comprehensive.

Training

This subsection presents a detailed description of the classifier's training process, including parameter choices and the model's architecture. We employed the TensorFlow library for code development.

Parameters. Several parameters were adjusted to optimise training:

- Image dimensions: To ensure compatibility with the foundational models, the images were adjusted to a size of 224 × 224 pixels.
- Batch size: We used a batch size of 32 to balance computational efficiency and gradient quality.
- Number of colour channels: The images are processed in RGB format, resulting in 3 colour channels.

Base Model

The base model chosen can be MobileNet or VGG16, both with weights pre-trained on the ImageNet dataset. The layers of this model have been frozen to prevent training during this phase, allowing us to use the features learned in previous tasks.

Additional Layers and Concatenation

After processing by the convolutional layers of the base model, the outputs corresponding to the two input images are concatenated. The result is then flattened to form a one-dimensional vector, adding the distance between the image frames (in number of frames) at the beginning of the vector.

Dense Layers and Activation

The concatenated and flattened vector is passed through a dense layer of 256 units with ReLU activation, which is used to learn more complex representations. Subsequently, a dense layer with a single unit and sigmoidal activation is used for binary classification.

Compilation and Metrics

The model is compiled using the binary cross entropy loss function and the Adam optimiser. Several metrics are monitored during training to evaluate performance, including accuracy, AUC(Area Under the ROC Curve), precision and recall.

Training

The training step is performed over 100 epochs and incorporates an early stopping mechanism to closely monitor the validation loss. If the validation loss does not improve for ten consecutive epochs, training is stopped, and the model weights are restored to the epoch state with the lowest validation loss. We use a custom data generator to provide batches of data to the model during training.

4   Results and Discussion

This section presents the experimental results obtained by applying Convolutional Neural Networks (CNN) in content-based image retrieval (CBIR) for medical images. The "Results" subsection provides a quantitative analysis of the performance metrics achieved by the models, while the "Discussion" delves into the implications and complexities of these results. Together, they offer a cohesive understanding of the study's findings and their relevance in the broader context of medical image analysis.

4.1 Results

This section details the experimental results obtained using the MobileNet and VGG16 models. Both models were evaluated based on five crucial metrics: Test Loss, Test Accuracy, Test AUC, Test Precision and Test Recall.

Table 1 shows the results obtained from training the model as described in the classifier training section:

Table 1. Models result with the distance between frames.

	MobileNet	VGG16
Loss	0.042	0.123
Accuracy	0.984	0.954
AUC	0.999	0.992
Precision	0.982	0.973
Recall	0.986	0.935

The results in Table 1 indicate that MobileNet outperformed VGG16 in all the metrics evaluated. MobileNet recorded a loss of 0.042, an accuracy of 98.4%, an AUC of 0.999, a precision of 98.2% and a recall of 98.6%. On the other hand, VGG16 showed a loss of 0.123, accuracy of 95.4%, AUC of 0.992, precision of 97.3% and recall of 93.5%.

To ensure that the model was not relying excessively on the distance between frames metric, a test was conducted without supplying this metric to the model. Table 2 shows the results of this test:

Table 2. Models result without distance between frames.

	MobileNet	VGG16
Loss	0.581	0.641
Accuracy	0.705	0.680
AUC	0.715	0.700
Precision	0.717	0.697
Recall	0.810	0.793

Analysing Table 2, we see that MobileNet obtained a loss of 0.581, accuracy of 70.5%, AUC of 0.715, precision of 71.7% and recall of 81.0%. In turn, VGG16 showed a loss of 0.641, accuracy of 68.0%, AUC of 0.700, precision of 69.7% and recall of 79.3%. These results indicate a reduction in performance compared to the results where the distance metric was provided but still demonstrate the models' ability to identify similarities between frames based on the extracted visual characteristics.

4.2 Discussion

The main aim of this study was to develop an automated method for identifying similar frames within a specific range using content-based image retrieval (CBIR) techniques. This is a significant step towards reducing reliance on manually annotated datasets, often scarce in clinical settings due to ethical and privacy concerns.

The results show that by using convolutional neural networks (CNNs) such as MobileNet and VGG16 for visual feature extraction, it is possible to achieve high accuracy in identifying similar frames. Notably, the MobileNet model outperformed VGG16 in all the metrics evaluated, highlighting its effectiveness and efficiency in CBIR.

A crucial observation from the results is the impact of the distance between frames metric. When this information was removed during the model's training and testing, a performance reduction was observed, but the metrics remained at acceptable levels. This suggests that although distance information contributes to the model's accuracy, the visual characteristics extracted by the CNN also play a crucial role in determining the similarity between frames.

However, it is worth emphasising that the reduction in performance without the distance metric highlights the importance of combining multiple features and metrics for robust and accurate classification. Combining various features can be the key to achieving reliable and clinically relevant results in medical scenarios where accuracy is critical.

Analysing the following image provides insight into the complexity of identifying similar frames in endoscopy videos (Fig. 5).

The "target frame" represents a specific example of an image in search of matches. We have ten images from each class to the right of this target image. The images in Class 1, identified as similar, were selected based on the smallest Euclidean distance to the reference frame within a specific range. However, not all images in Class 1 manifest the pathology present in the target image, even if they show remarkable visual similarities in terms of texture, colour and shape. This contradiction has significant implications. Without the aid of distance metrics, the model may face challenges when trying to discern between visually similar frames but differ in clinical terms.

On the other hand, images in Class 2, although categorised as different, are not radically different in appearance. Some of these images display visual structures remarkably similar to the target image, even though the overall colour tone may be lighter. This subtle feature can confuse the model, especially when trying to differentiate between frames based on visual characteristics alone, without additional distance information.

Thus, visualising this arrangement of images reiterates the intricate nature of the problem and the need for a model that can consider multiple features and metrics to make sound classification decisions.

4.3 Limitations and Future Work

One limitation is the size and diversity of the data set used. Although we have achieved promising results, exploring how this approach behaves with more extensive and diverse datasets is necessary. In addition, the CBIR technique still needs to be compared

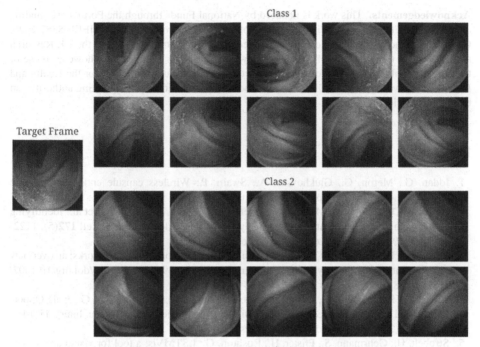

Fig. 5. Comparison between target frame and both class matches.

directly with traditional annotation methods to evaluate its effectiveness and efficiency comprehensively.

In future research, we plan to expand the application of this approach to search for similar images throughout the video, not just in a specific time interval. The aim will be to identify frames that may represent the same medical condition, even if these frames have not been previously annotated. This can reveal undetected cases of similar diseases, thus providing an even more robust tool for automated annotation and diagnosis.

Future research could also explore different network architectures and similarity metrics to improve the method's effectiveness further. Evaluating this method in a natural clinical setting would also be helpful to validate its applicability and effectiveness.

5 Conclusion

This study introduces a novel technique for identifying similar frames in endoscopic capsule videos using content-based image retrieval (CBIR). The approach aims to reduce reliance on manually annotated datasets, a challenge in medical environments due to ethical and privacy concerns. Image features were extracted using the CNN models MobileNet and VGG16, and a classifier was trained, with MobileNet outperforming VGG16 on all metrics.

The implications of this work are vast for automated annotation in medicine. Future plans include expanding this technique to identify similar images throughout the video, which could enhance the detection of unannotated cases of similar medical conditions.

Acknowledgements. This work is financed by National Funds through the Portuguese funding agency,FCT Fundacäo para a Ciéncia e a Tecnologia, within project PTDC/EEIEEE/5557/2020. Co funded by the European Union (grant number 101095359) and supported by the UK Research and Innovation (grant number 10058099). Views and opinions expressed are however those of the author(s) only and do not necessarily reflect those of the European Union or the Health and Digital Executive Agency (HaDEA). Neither the European Union nor the granting authority can be held responsible for them.

References

1. Iddan, G., Meron, G., Glukhovsky, A., Swain, P.: Wireless capsule endoscopy. Nature **405**(6785), 417 (2000). https://doi.org/10.1038/35013140
2. Kermany, D., Goldbaum, M., Cai, W., Valentim, C., Liang, H., Baxter, S., et al.: Identifying medical diagnoses and treatable diseases by image-based deep learning. Cell **172**(5), 1122–1131.e9 (2018). https://doi.org/10.1016/j.cell.2018.02.010
3. Yamashita, R., Nishio, M., Gian, R., Togashi, K.: Convolutional neural networks: an overview and application in radiology. Insights Imaging **9**(4), 611–629 (2018). https://doi.org/10.1007/s13244-018-0639-9
4. Ching, T., Himmelstein, D., Beaulieu-Jones, B., Kalinin, A., Brian, T., Way, G., et al.: Opportunities and obstacles for deep learning in biology and medicine. J. Roy. Soc. Interf. **15**(141), 20170387 (2018). https://doi.org/10.1098/rsif.2017.0387
5. Strobelt, H., Gehrmann, S., Pfister, H., Rushton, G.: LSTMVis: a tool for visual analysis of hidden state dynamics in recurrent neural networks. IEEE Trans. Vis. Comput. Graph. **24**(1), 667–676 (2018). https://doi.org/10.1109/tvcg.2017.2744158
6. Xie, S., Yu, Z., Lv, Z.: Multi-disease prediction based on deep learning: a survey. Comput. Model. Eng. Sci. **128**(2), 489–522 (2021). https://doi.org/10.32604/cmes.2021.016728
7. Lesions multiclass classification in endoscopic capsule frames. Proc. Comput. Sci. **164**, 637–645 (2019). https://doi.org/10.1016/j.procs.2019.12.230
8. Libório, A., Couto, S., Cunha, A., Coelho, P.: Endoscopy—Brief historical survey, developments and therapeutics. In: 2011 IEEE 1st International Conference on Serious Games and Applications for Health (SeGAH), pp. 1–4, November 2011. https://doi.org/10.1109/SeGAH.2011.6165440
9. Fonseca, F., Nunes, B., Salgado, M., Cunha, A.: Abnormality classification in small datasets of capsule endoscopy images. Proc. Comput. Sci. **196**, 469–476 (2022). https://doi.org/10.1016/j.procs.2021.12.038
10. Rui, Y., Huang, T.S., Chang, S.-F.: Image retrieval: current techniques, promising directions, and open issues. J. Vis. Commun. Image Represent. **10**(1), 39–62 (1999)
11. Sugamya, K., et al.: CBIR using SIFT & FDCT with relevance feedback mechanism. Int. J. Innov. Technol. Explor. Eng. **8**(11), 1103–1108 (2019). https://doi.org/10.35940/ijitee.j1193.0981119
12. Khodaskar, A., Ladhake, A.: New-fangled alignment of ontologies for content based semantic image retrieval
13. Djeraba, C.: Association and content-based retrieval. IEEE Trans. Knowl. Data Eng. **15**(1), 118–135 (2003)
14. Douze, M., Ramisa, A., Schmid, C.: Combining attributes and fisher vectors for efficient image retrieval. In: CVPR 2011. IEEE (2011)
15. Sharma, H., et al.: Determining similarity in histological images using graph-theoretic description and matching methods for content-based image retrieval in medical diagnostics. Diagn. Pathol. **7**(1), 1–20 (2012)

16. Ali, A., Sharma, S.: Content based image retrieval using feature extraction with machine learning. In: 2017 International Conference on Intelligent Computing and Control Systems (ICICCS). IEEE (2017)
17. Jeyasekhar, S., Mostefai, S.: Towards effective relevance feedback methods in content-based image retrieval systems. Int. J. Innov. Manag. Technol. **5**(1) (2014)
18. Ouni, A., Chateau, T., Royer, E., Chevaldonné, M., Dhome, M.: A new CBIR model using semantic segmentation and fast spatial binary encoding. In: Nguyen, N.T., Manolopoulos, Y., Chbeir, R., Kozierkiewicz, A., Trawiński, B. (eds.) ICCCI 2022. LNCS, vol. 13501, pp. 437–449. Springer, Cham (2022). https://doi.org/10.1007/978-3-031-16014-1_35
19. Simonyan, K., Zisserman, A.: Very deep convolutional networks for large-scale image recognition, 10 April 2015. https://doi.org/10.48550/arXiv.1409.1556
20. Howard, A.G., et al.: MobileNets: efficient convolutional neural networks for mobile vision applications, 16 April 2017. http://arxiv.org/abs/1704.04861. Accessed 25 Sept 2023

Similarity-Based Explanations for Deep Interpretation of Capsule Endoscopy Images

Miguel Fontes[1,2]([✉]), Danilo Leite[2], João Dallyson[3], and António Cunha[1,2]

[1] UTAD—University of Trás-os-Montes and Alto Douro, 5001-801 Vila Real, Portugal
[2] INESC TEC—Institute for Systems and Computer Engineering, Technology and Science,
4200-465 Porto, Portugal
`miguel.f.fontes@inesctec.pt, {danilol,acunha}@utad.pt`
[3] UFMA—Federal University of Maranhão, São Luís, Brazil
`jdallyson@nca.ufma.br`

Abstract. Artificial intelligence (AI) is playing a growing role today in several areas, especially in health, where understanding AI models and their predictions is extremely important for health professionals. In this context, Explainable AI (XAI) plays a crucial role in seeking to provide understandable explanations for these models.

This article analyzes two different XAI approaches applied to analyzing gastric endoscopy images. The first, more conventional approach uses Grad CAM, while the second, even less explored but with great potential, is based on "similarity-based explanations". This example-based XAI technique aims to provide representative examples to support the decisions of AI models.

In this study, we compare these two techniques applied to two different models: one based on the VGG16 architecture and the other based on ResNet50, designed to classify images from the KVASIR-capsule database. The results reveal that Grad-CAM provided intuitive explanations only for the VGG16 model, while the "similarity-based explanations" technique provided consistent explanations for both models. We conclude that exploring other XAI techniques can be a significant asset in improving the understanding of the various AI models.

Keywords: XAI · Example-based · Similarity-based explanations · endoscopy

1 Introduction

Deep learning has gained increasing importance in medical image processing, significantly influencing areas such as detection, recognition, segmentation and computer-aided diagnosis [1]. Deep learning models have demonstrated outstanding performance in tasks such as classification, lesion detection and segmentation [2]. However, the complexity of medical decisions requires a deep understanding and proper interpretation of the models in use.

Explainable Artificial Intelligence (XAI) refers to the development of Artificial Intelligence (AI) models and techniques that are able to offer transparent and interpretable

© ICST Institute for Computer Sciences, Social Informatics and Telecommunications Engineering 2024
Published by Springer Nature Switzerland AG 2024. All Rights Reserved
A. Cunha et al. (Eds.): MobiHealth 2023, LNICST 578, pp. 208–222, 2024.
https://doi.org/10.1007/978-3-031-60665-6_16

explanations for their decisions and predictions [3]. In medical imaging, XAI plays an essential role in providing information about the reasoning behind the model's predictions and thus earning the trust of doctors and patients [4]. Several XAI techniques are employed in medical imaging, including model interpretation, which involves understanding learned features, and interpretation of model results, which includes attribution-based methods such as saliency maps and class activation maps [4]. An exciting approach to XAI is example-based explanation, which consists of providing specific examples or instances to illustrate how the AI model arrived at a decision [5]. These example-based explanations can improve the interpretability of AI models, especially in medical diagnostic imaging, where the "black box" nature of deep learning models has hindered their adoption in clinical workflows [5].

1.1 Related Work

In medical image analysis using deep learning techniques, several recent studies have contributed to significant advances, incorporating XAI techniques to improve the interpretability of models.

One of these studies focused on developing an architecture called HAnet, applying deep convolutional neural networks (CNNs) to recognize ulcers in images of endoscopic capsules (WCE). In addition, the Class Activation Mapping (CAM) technique was used to visualize and interpret the network's activation regions, making CNN's decision-making process more transparent [6]. Another study proposed an explainable machine learning tool to support the interpretation of gastric images in vivo. Using convolutional neural networks and visual explanations, this research sought to provide understandable insights for healthcare professionals, highlighting the potential of these XAI approaches in medical contexts [7]. In addition, another study focused on the application of Convolutional Neural Networks (CNNs) in the segmentation of polyps in colonoscopy images, enhancing Fully Convolutional Networks (FCNs) architectures to achieve meaningful results, also using XAI techniques to interpret the results [8].

These investigations illustrate the growing importance of deep learning and XAI techniques, such as CAM, in improving the analysis of medical images and supporting clinical decision-making, making models more transparent and reliable for healthcare professionals.

Our research group has maintained a significant focus on the analysis of capsule endoscopy images. One of the group's papers [9] demonstrated success in using a Visual Transformers model to analyze capsule endoscopy images, achieving exceptionally high accuracy and sensitivity rates. Another relevant work [10] explored the challenge of classifying abnormalities in small, unbalanced data sets, highlighting the potential of using transfer learning even with a limited number of samples. In addition, the group also developed an unsupervised method for estimating homography in capsule endoscopy frames [11], which has the potential to considerably improve the precise localization of the endoscopic capsule. The cumulative contributions of these studies reflect the group's commitment to promoting innovative solutions to the persistent challenges associated with capsule endoscopy image analysis, excelling in the advancement of effective diagnosis of conditions related to the gastrointestinal tract.

1.2 Objective

Given that most XAI techniques applied to medical images are based on visual explanations, such as Grad-CAM and LIME, this article aims to introduce an example-based XAI approach called "similarity-based explanations". In addition, it seeks to compare the explanations generated by this approach with the explanations of a more conventional technique, Grad-CAM. This research aims to provide valuable insights into the effectiveness and applicability of these techniques in interpreting results in medical images. Importantly, our focus extends beyond merely optimizing image classification accuracy, encompassing a broader understanding of the interpretative value of XAI in medical contexts.

2 Methodology

The methodology, in Fig. 1, adopted in this study follows a well-defined pipeline. Initially, the images contained in the database go through a pre-processing process. The data set is then divided into three parts: a training set, a validation set and a test set. The training and validation sets are used to train the models created to address the problem in question, while the test set is reserved exclusively for evaluating the model's performance.

Two XAI techniques are applied once the model's predictions have been obtained on the test set. These techniques are used to analyze and interpret the model predictions and provide a deeper understanding of the functioning and performance of the XAI techniques used. Finally, the results generated by both XAI techniques are analyzed, contributing to a deeper understanding of the problem under study and the methods employed.

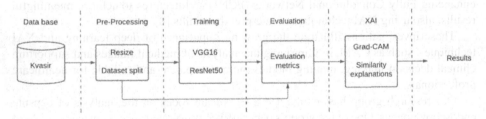

Fig. 1. Methodology Pipeline.

2.1 Database

The Kvasir-Capsule database is the only source of data for this study. It consists of 117 capsule endoscopy videos, which can be divided into 4,741,504 image frames. This database includes various information covering anatomical landmarks such as the Z-line, pylorus, and caecum and pathological findings, such as esophagitis, polyps and ulcerative colitis [12].

For this research, we used only part of the dataset, selecting 4,000 images from 8 specific medical classes within this database, which is represented in Fig. 2. This careful selection allowed us to focus on the classes relevant to the research.

This database is remarkable not only for the amount of data available but also for the quality of the medical annotations. A total of 47,238 image frames were meticulously annotated and reviewed by specialist doctors, providing a valuable labelled dataset.

In addition, the database includes a vast collection of 4,694,266 unlabeled frames, which represent a significant opportunity to explore advanced deep learning approaches.

This combination of labelled and unlabeled data provides a solid basis for investigating the interpretability of deep learning models in medical applications while seeing to achieve high classification performance.

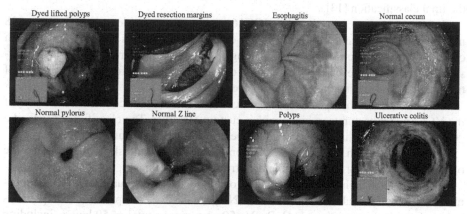

Fig. 2. Examples of images from the different classes.

2.2 Pre-Processing

To use the images from the Kvasir-capsule database in this study, it was necessary to carry out appropriate pre-processing in line with the models employed. Since this study demonstrates two different XAI approaches, we opted to simplify the pre-processing rather than achieve high classification accuracy.

Pre-processing mainly consisted of resizing the images to make them compatible with the input format of the classification model. The images were resized to a dimension of 224 pixels high, 224 pixels wide and 3 color channels (RGB). This transformation allowed the images to be processed uniformly by the classification model, facilitating integration with XAI techniques.

It is important to note that this pre-processing was carried out in a minimalist manner since the main focus was evaluating the XAI approaches, and not optimizing the classification accuracy of the images.

At this stage, the database was also divided into training, validation and test datasets. 2240 images were allocated to the training set, 960 images to the validation set and 800 images to the test set. This division was carried out to ensure the robustness of the experiments and to allow proper evaluation of the XAI techniques on different datasets.

2.3 Training Models

To classify the images after the pre-processing stage, two models were developed.

Model selection

With regard to the models developed, the first adopts the VGG16 architecture, while the second is based on ResNet50.

The VGG16 architecture is a deep convolutional network (CNN) that is widely recognized and used in various research domains. This architecture consists of a total of 16 layers, of which 13 are convolutional layers, and 3 are fully connected layers. In the convolutional layers, 3 × 3 filters are used, making it possible to extract detailed and deep features from the images. In addition, the architecture incorporates pooling layers to reduce the dimensionality of the data, followed by fully connected layers to perform the final classification [13].

It is important to note that the VGG16 architecture provides approximately 138 million trainable parameters. This wealth of parameters allows the network to learn complex representations of images, making it capable of performing high-level classification tasks. However, this advantage comes with the need for an extensive set of training data and substantial computing resources [13].

In the context of this specific study, we chose to use only the convolutional layers of the VGG16 architecture combined with a custom classifier. The classifier consists of a "Global Average Pooling 2D" layer, followed by 5 dense layers and 2 dropout layers.

This configuration was chosen based on the needs of the task in question and the objective of extracting significant features from the input images.

The ResNet50 architecture, a variation of the ResNet (Residual Network) architecture, is a Convolutional Neural Network (CNN) notable for its depth and the implementation of residual connections [14]. ResNet50 comprises a total of 50 layers, including convolutional layers, pooling layers and dense layers. The distinctive feature of this network is the use of so-called "residual layers," in which the input of a block is added to the output of the previous block. This allows information to be transmitted directly between layers, minimizing information loss.

The residual connections approach is a fundamental innovation that solves the challenge of performance degradation in deep networks by allowing the network to learn deeper and more complex representations of image characteristics [14].

The ResNet50 architecture has been widely adopted in a number of computer vision applications in various fields, and its characteristics make it a popular choice for tasks that require deep neural networks with high performance.

In this study, we chose to use the ResNet50 architecture up to the last convolutional layer, connecting it to the same classifier employed in the VGG16-based model.

Optimizer and loss function

In both models developed in this study, the parameters related to the optimizer and loss function were kept consistent to ensure a fair and rigorous comparison. The configurations of these elements are detailed below:

Optimizer: We chose to use the "Stochastic Gradient Descent (SGD)" optimizer in both models. This choice was motivated by its effectiveness in supervised learning tasks and its ability to adjust the weights of the neural network iteratively, which is especially relevant for training complex models.

Loss function: Given that both tasks involved classifying data into several classes, we selected the "Categorical Crossentropy" loss function. This loss function is appropriate for multi-class classification tasks, helping the model to calculate the discrepancy between the predicted probabilities and the actual data labels.

Standardizing these elements in the configuration of both models ensured a solid basis for comparing results and a consistent approach throughout the study. These methodological choices were aimed at obtaining robust and reliable conclusions regarding the performance of the models in multi-class classification tasks.

Callbacks

In this study, three callback techniques were used during model training. These techniques were selected to optimize model performance, avoid overfitting and efficiently manage the available computing resources. The three Callback techniques used are described below:

ModelCheckpoint: We used the ModelCheckpoint Callback to save the model weights in temporary files during training. This procedure was triggered whenever the model reached its best performance in relation to the defined evaluation metrics. This allowed us to retain the weights corresponding to the model's best performance, guaranteeing the ability to restore it later if necessary.

Reduce Learning Rate on Plateau: We implemented the Reduce Learning Rate on Plateau Callback to monitor the model's performance over training epochs. This Callback automatically adjusts the learning rate if the model's performance does not show significant improvements after a specified number of consecutive epochs. We started training with a learning rate of 0.001, and the Callback configuration was set to reduce it by a factor of 0.01 after three epochs of no improvement in 'val_loss', with a minimum learning rate set at 1e−5. This adaptive approach allows the model to adjust its learning rate according to fluctuations in performance, increasing the likelihood of effective convergence.

EarlyStopping: We integrated Callback EarlyStopping to stop training the model if it was no longer able to improve its performance. This was based on a defined stop metric. The inclusion of EarlyStopping helped to avoid excessively long training runs and unnecessary computational resources by ensuring that the model was only trained as long as it continued to improve at its specific task.

Epochs and batch size

When training the neural network, we adopted a batch size of 64 images per batch, and the training process was conducted over 100 epochs. These configurations were selected with the aim of balancing computational efficiency and the model's ability to converge on an optimal solution. It is important to note that, although the training was programmed for 100 epochs, we frequently observed the activation of the Early Stopping mechanism, which interrupted the training around epochs 30 to 35.

2.4 Evaluation

After training the model, we tested the model on the test dataset in order to obtain the model's predictions and used the following evaluation metrics:

Precision: Precision quantifies the proportion of correct predictions of a positive class in relation to the total number of positive predictions made by the model.

Recall: Recall measures the model's ability to effectively identify all samples belonging to a positive class, expressing the proportion of true positives (TP) in relation to the sum of true positives and false negatives (FN). Rev is relevant when you want to avoid losing positive samples.

F1-Score: The F1-Score is a metric that harmonizes Precision and Recall in a single measure. The F1-Score provides a balanced assessment of the model when there is a need to balance the ability to identify true positives and avoid false negatives and false positives.

Accuracy: Accuracy represents the proportion of correct predictions in relation to the total number of samples. It is calculated as the sum of TP and true negatives (TN) divided by the sum of TP, TN, false positives (FP) and FN. Accuracy provides an overview of the model's ability to classify all samples correctly but can be misleading in scenarios with class imbalance.

Macro and Weighted Average: The macro and weighted average provide aggregate summaries of the metrics (Precision, Recall and F1-Score) calculated for all classes. The macro average calculates a simple average, while the weighted average takes class imbalance into account, assigning weight based on the support of each class. These averages are useful for evaluating the overall performance of the model, taking all classes into account and adjusting for class imbalance where applicable.

These evaluation metrics are crucial for assessing the performance of machine learning models in classification tasks, providing valuable insights into the model's ability to make accurate predictions and correctly identify relevant samples.

2.5 Explainable Artificial Intelligence (XAI)

XAI is an area of research that seeks to make machine learning models understandable by revealing how models make decisions, highlight important features and reduce uncertainties, which is fundamental in critical applications. In this study, we used XAI techniques to understand how our model makes decisions and highlights features in images, improving our analysis by employing two different approaches.

Grad-CAM

Grad-CAM is an XAI technique that aims to reveal which regions of an image are most influential in the decision-making of a deep learning model during classification. Unlike other techniques that focus only on the last convolutional layer of a neural network, Grad-CAM analyzes activation gradients in intermediate layers [15].

It works by calculating gradients of the class of interest in relation to the activations of the intermediate layer of the neural network. These weighted gradients are then aggregated to create an activation map that highlights the most critical areas of the image for classification. Grad-CAM offers a valuable visual interpretation, allowing researchers and practitioners to better understand how the model makes decisions and to identify which image features are relevant to a given class [15].

This technique has been widely adopted in Machine Learning Explainability studies to improve the interpretability of deep learning models, making it a valuable tool for analyzing and understanding the behaviour of neural networks in computer vision and image classification tasks.

Similarity-based explanations

Similarity-based explanations are an approach that seeks to make the workings of machine learning models more understandable. This technique focuses on presenting examples of training data that are similar to the current data input, with the aim of explaining why the model made a certain prediction.

This explanation follows intuitive logic, where the model states something like, "This prediction is valid because similar examples in the training set also resulted in similar predictions". This approach is analogous to the way humans make decisions based on past experiences. The main benefit of similarity-based explanations is their high comprehensibility. They make it easier for users to understand the reasoning behind the model's predictions, which is particularly important in critical applications [16, 17].

However, it is important to note that this technique has its limitations, such as the reliance on high-quality training data and the need for similar instances in the training set. Furthermore, it may not be suitable for extremely complex models that are not based on direct similarities between instances.

In this context, we chose to use cosine distance as the main similarity metric. Cosine distance is a widely recognized metric applied in data analysis and machine learning. It measures the similarity between two feature vectors, taking into account their relative orientation in the feature space, rather than calculating a direct measure of the Euclidean distance between these vectors [16].

In simple terms, the cosine distance ranges from -1 to 1, where 1 indicates that the vectors have an identical direction (i.e. maximum similarity), 0 indicates that they are orthogonal (neutrality), and -1 indicates that they have opposite directions (i.e. maximum dissimilarity). This metric is particularly useful when dealing with vector data and is known for its interpretability, making it a suitable choice for explaining model predictions based on the intuitive logic that predictions are valid when similar examples have resulted in similar predictions in the training set.

Cosine distance offers an effective way of quantifying the similarity or dissimilarity between data instances, which contributes significantly to making our similarity-based explanations more understandable and accessible to users.

3 Results

3.1 Evaluation Metrics

The results of the evaluation metrics for the two models can be seen in Tables 1 and 2.
VGG16:

Table 1. Evaluation metrics of the VGG16 model.

	Precision	Recall	F1-Score	Number of images
Class 0	0.94	0.84	0.89	100
Class 1	0.88	0.96	0.92	100
Class 2	0.88	0.81	0.84	100
Class 3	0.92	0.98	0.95	100
Class 4	0.97	1.00	0.99	100
Class 5	0.83	0.89	0.86	100
Class 6	0.94	0.90	0.92	100
Class 7	0.97	0.95	0.96	100
Total accuracy	0.92			800
Macro avg	0.92	0.92	0.92	800
Weighted avg	0.92	0.92	0.92	800

ResNet50:

Table 2. Evaluation metrics of the ResNet50 model.

	Precision	Recall	F1-Score	Number of images
Class 0	0.88	0.82	0.85	100
Class 1	0.84	0.87	0.85	100
Class 2	0.86	0.80	0.83	100
Class 3	0.98	0.99	0.99	100
Class 4	0.98	0.95	0.96	100
Class 5	0.79	0.86	0.82	100
Class 6	0.92	0.98	0.95	100
Class 7	0.98	0.95	0.96	100
Total accuracy	0.90			800
Macro avg	0.90	0.90	0.90	800
Weighted avg	0.90	0.90	0.90	800

3.2 Explainable Artificial Intelligence (XAI)

The results of applying XAI techniques are as follows.

Grad-CAM

The results of the Grad-CAM technique show that it was applied to four images from the test set that were correctly classified by both models, as shown in Figs. 3 and 5. In addition, the technique was applied to four images from the test set that were incorrectly classified, as shown in Figs. 4 and 6.

VGG16:

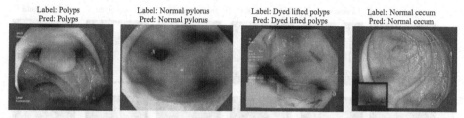

Fig. 3. Grad-CAM results on images correctly classified by the VGG16 model.

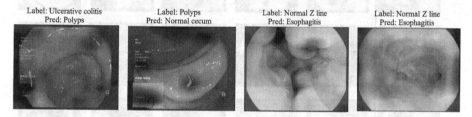

Fig. 4. Grad-CAM results on images incorrectly classified by the VGG16 model.

ResNet50:

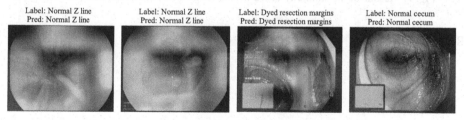

Fig. 5. Grad-CAM results on images correctly classified by the ResNet50 model.

Similarity-based explanations

In the results of the similarity-based explanation technique, it was possible to see four images from the test set for each model. For each of these images, the five most similar images found in the training set were displayed. Figure 7 shows the technique applied to the VGG16 model, while Fig. 8 shows the technique applied to the ResNet50 model.

VGG16:

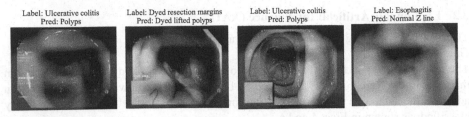

Fig. 6. Grad-CAM results on images incorrectly classified by the ResNet50 model.

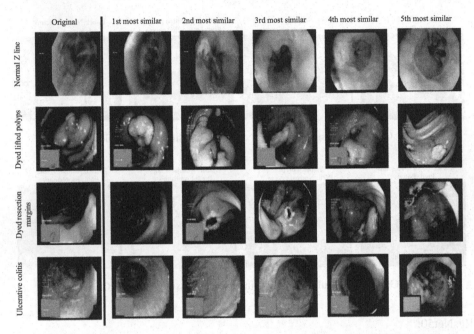

Fig. 7. Results of the similarity-based explanations technique of the VGG16 model.

ResNet50:

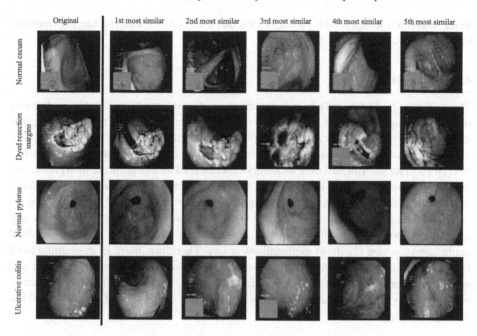

Fig. 8. Results of the similarity-based explanations technique of the ResNet50 model.

4 Discussion

4.1 Analysis of the Results of Evaluation Metrics and XAI Techniques

When analyzing the evaluation metrics presented in the tables for each model, it is clear that, although the main focus of this study was not training the models, both showed satisfactory performance in classifying the various classes present in the database. However, there were some notable difficulties in classifying images from the "dyed resection margins", "esophagitis", and "normal z-line" classes. These difficulties can be attributed to the existence of images in different classes that share similar characteristics, such as color and structure.

When applying the Grad-CAM technique to understand the predictions of each model, we observed a significant difference. The VGG16 model provided more intuitive explanations, focusing on features that are easily understood by humans. On the other hand, the explanations provided by ResNet50 seem to follow a less intuitive pattern for all the images in the database, not focusing on the specific structures of each class.

Due to this inconsistency in the explanations generated by the previous technique, we opted to implement the similarity-based explanations approach. This technique follows the logic of "This prediction is valid because similar examples in the training set also resulted in similar predictions." As a result, this approach provided the 5 most similar images from the training set for each image classified by the model. The results of this technique proved to be highly intuitive for both the VGG16 model and the ResNet50 model. It was able to present images from the training set that were remarkably similar to the classified images, with identical structures and colors, making the explanations highly understandable and informative.

4.2 Limitations

The technique of similarity-based explanations for interpreting capsule endoscopy images, although innovative, has some significant limitations, mainly related to the quality and quantity of the data and the complexity of the deep learning models used. The effectiveness of the technique is strongly influenced by the diversity and representativeness of the data set. Limited or low-quality sets can lead to less accurate interpretations, while the presence of noise or artifacts in the images can compromise the generation of useful explanations. In addition, the complexity of the models used is another crucial factor. More complex models may offer greater precision, but their transparency and ease of interpretation are often reduced, a particularly challenging aspect in medical applications, where clarity of explanations is key. Therefore, there is an ongoing need for research to improve datasets and develop methods capable of providing clear and accurate explanations, even in highly complex models. The balance between accuracy, interpretability and practical applicability is a constant challenge in the field of XAI in medical imaging.

4.3 Perspectives and Future Work

After a thorough analysis and comparison of the results of this study, the exploration of various XAI techniques is of great importance, especially in the context of the rapid advancement of AI in various areas. It is essential to provide intuitive explanations for professionals in different sectors, given the growing adoption of complex AI models in various applications.

As part of future research, it would be highly beneficial to further explore example-based XAI techniques, such as the similarity-based explanation approach. These techniques have the potential to offer significant levels of explainability in a variety of applications, making them accessible to a wide audience. In addition, the development of new algorithms and approaches to further improve the effectiveness of these techniques can be a valuable contribution in several fields, most notably healthcare. Considering the combination of algorithms could also be a promising direction, as it could provide additional benefits in terms of the explainability and interpretability of machine learning models.

5 Conclusion

In this research, we presented an example-based XAI approach, called "similarity-based explanations," and compared it with the widely used Grad-CAM in medical image analysis. Our results show that the example-based XAI approach offers a valuable alternative perspective on the interpretation of deep learning models. The ability to explain decisions based on examples provides a more accessible and practical understanding for healthcare professionals, improving the transparency and reliability of predictions. This research contributes to the evolution of the field of XAI in medical imaging, highlighting the importance of interpretability in clinical applications. As deep learning models gain ground in medicine, approaches such as "similarity-based explanations" will play a crucial role in confidence and informed decision-making in key clinical scenarios.

Acknowledgements. This work is financed by National Funds through the Portuguese funding agency,FCT Fundacăo para a Ciéncia e a Tecnologia, within project PTDC/EEIEEE/5557/2020. Co funded by the European Union (grant number 101095359) and supported by the UK Research and Innovation (grant number 10058099). Views and opinions expressed are however those of the author(s) only and do not necessarily reflect those of the European Union or the Health and Digital Executive Agency (HaDEA). Neither the European Union nor the granting authority can be held responsible for them.

References

1. Maier, A., Syben, C., Lasser, T., Riess, C.: A gentle introduction to deep learning in medical image processing (2019). https://doi.org/10.1016/j.zemedi.2018.12.003
2. Do, S., Song, K.D., Chung, J.W.: Basics of deep learning: a radiologist's guide to understanding published radiology articles on deep learning (2020). https://doi.org/10.3348/kjr.2019.0312
3. Barredo Arrieta, A., et al.: Explainable Artificial Intelligence (XAI): concepts, taxonomies, opportunities and challenges toward responsible AI (2020). https://doi.org/10.1016/j.inffus.2019.12.012
4. Huff, D.T., Weisman, A.J., Jeraj, R.: Interpretation and visualization techniques for deep learning models in medical imaging (2021). https://doi.org/10.1088/1361-6560/abcd17
5. Patrício, C., Neves, J.C., Teixeira, L.F.: Explainable deep learning methods in medical imaging diagnosis: a survey (2022). https://doi.org/10.48550/arxiv.2205.04766
6. Wang, S., Xing, Y., Zhang, L., Gao, H., Zhang, H.: Deep convolutional neural network for ulcer recognition in wireless capsule endoscopy: experimental feasibility and optimization (2019). https://doi.org/10.1155/2019/7546215
7. Malhi, A., Kampik, T., Pannu, H., Madhikermi, M., Framling, K.: Explaining machine learning-based classifications of in-vivo gastral images (2019). https://doi.org/10.1109/dicta47822.2019.8945986
8. Wickstrom, K., Kampffmeyer, M., Jenssen, R.: Uncertainty modeling and interpretability in convolutional neural networks for polyp segmentation (2018). https://doi.org/10.1109/mlsp.2018.8516998
9. Lima, D.L.S., Pessoa, A.C.P., De Paiva, A.C., da Silva Cunha, A.M.T., Júnior, G.B., De Almeida, J.D.S.: Classification of video capsule endoscopy images using visual transformers. In: 2022 IEEE-EMBS International Conference on Biomedical and Health Informatics (BHI), pp. 1–4 (2022). https://doi.org/10.1109/BHI56158.2022.9926791
10. Fonseca, F., Nunes, B., Salgado, M., Cunha, A.: Abnormality classification in small datasets of capsule endoscopy images. Proc. Comput. Sci. **196**, 469–476 (2022). https://doi.org/10.1016/j.procs.2021.12.038
11. Gomes, S., Valério, M.T., Salgado, M., Oliveira, H.P., Cunha, A.: Unsupervised neural network for homography estimation in capsule endoscopy frames. Proc. Comput. Sci. **164**, 602–609 (2019). https://doi.org/10.1016/j.procs.2019.12.226
12. Smedsrud, P.H., et al.: Kvasir-capsule, a video capsule endoscopy dataset (2021). https://doi.org/10.1038/s41597-021-00920-z

13. Simonyan, K., Zisserman, A.: Very Deep Convolutional Networks for Large-Scale Image Recognition (2014). https://doi.org/10.48550/arxiv.1409.1556

14. He, K., Zhang, X., Ren, S., Sun, J.: Deep Residual Learning for Image Recognition (2016). https://doi.org/10.1109/cvpr.2016.90

15. Selvaraju, R.R., Cogswell, M., Das, A., Vedantam, R., Parikh, D., Batra, D.: Grad-CAM: Visual Explanations From Deep Networks via Gradient-Based Localization (2017). https://doi.org/10.1109/iccv.2017.74

16. Hanawa, K., Yokoi, S., Hara, S., Inui, K.: Evaluation of Similarity-Based Explanations (2020). https://doi.org/10.48550/arxiv.2006.04528

17. Charpiat, G., Girard, N., Felardos, L., Tarabalka, Y.: Input Similarity From the Neural Network Perspective (2021). https://doi.org/10.48550/arxiv.2102.05262

Deep Learning Applications in Histopathological Images

Luis Felipe Rocha Pereira[1]([✉]) [ID], Anselmo Cardoso de Paiva[2,3] [ID],
Alexandre de Carvalho Araújo[3] [ID], Geraldo Braz Junior[3] [ID],
Joao Dallyson Sousa de Almeida[1,2,3] [ID], and Aristófanes Corrêa Silva[1,2,3] [ID]

[1] Universidade Federal do Maranhão, UFMA, Av. dos Portugueses, 1966 - Vila
Bacanga, São Luís, MA 65080-805, Brazil
luisfrp741@gmail.com, {jdallyson,ari}@nca.ufma.br
[2] Núcleo de Computação Aplicada, NCA, Av. dos Portugueses, 1966 - Vila Bacanga,
São Luís, MA 65080-805, Brazil
[3] Departamento de Informática, Deinf, Campus Dom Delgado, UFMA, Av. dos
Portugueses, 1966 - Vila Bacanga, São Luís, MA 65080-805, Brazil
{paiva,alexandrearaujo,geraldo}@nca.ufma.br

Abstract. Breast cancer is a neoplasm that mainly affects women above
the age of 45. However, an increase in the incidence of this disease among
young women has been observed. Although it is considered a cancer
with a good prognosis when diagnosed early, early detection remains
a challenge. In Brazil, the mortality rate due to breast cancer remains
high, which is directly related to the late diagnosis of the disease. To
contribute to the reduction of this rate, the development of effective
early detection techniques is essential. These techniques can assist in
diagnosing the disease at its initial stages, enabling quicker treatment
and thereby increasing the chances of a cure. Computer-aided detection and diagnosis systems have been developed and improved in the
field of computing. These systems base their accuracy and reasoning
on data obtained through a combination of computer vision techniques,
such as pattern recognition and machine learning. When applied, these
techniques assist doctors and specialists in data analysis to provide diagnostic support and treatment planning. This significantly enhances a
patient's chances of recovery. More recently, within the machine learning
field, Deep Learning has become a prevalent focus of research due to its
ability to automatically extract relevant features for the target task. In
this work, the methodology proposed employs Convolutional Neural Networks for machine learning. While the results obtained are not superior
to those in the literature, they are close and generally require fewer com-

Supported by PIBIC - This work was carried out with the support of the Coordination
for the Improvement of Higher Education Personnel - Brazil (CAPES) - Financing
Code 001, Maranhão Research Foundation (FAPEMA), National Council for Scientific
and Technological Development (CNPq).

A. Cunha et al. (Eds.): MobiHealth 2023, LNICST 578, pp. 223–238, 2024.
https://doi.org/10.1007/978-3-031-60665-6_17

putational resources for training the selected networks after the selection process.

Keywords: Classification · Breast Cancer · Deep Learning

1 Introduction

1.1 Motivation

Cancer is the generic term for a set of more than a hundred diseases that share two basic characteristics: the ability of neoplastic (cancerous) cells to reproduce uncontrollably, forming tumors and potentially invading adjacent organs and tissues, and the ability to spread to distant organs and tissues from the original tumor, a process known as metastasis.

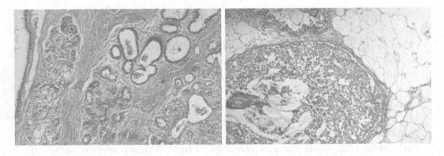

Fig. 1. Image of Benign and Malignant Cancer Cells, adapted from [32]

Breast carcinoma is a diverse disease, displaying wide variation in both its morphological and molecular characteristics, as well as responding variably to clinical treatment [19]. Early diagnosis and timely treatment are essential for a good prognosis and patient recovery. The earlier the diagnosis, the more effective the treatment.

The final diagnosis present in the anatomopathological report is issued by the pathologist through the microscopic analysis of tissue samples obtained by biopsy, also known as histopathological imaging, and additionally, from the surgical specimen. Examples of histopathological images can be seen in Fig. 1. This report should contain essential information, such as the histological subtype and the degree of tumor differentiation [18]. One of the main challenges during the analysis of histopathological examinations is related to the high demand for diagnoses, which is exacerbated by the limited availability of specialized doctors to perform this task. This scenario contributes to delays in diagnoses, as the process requires concentrated effort and can lead to professional fatigue, resulting in potential errors.

Biopsy is a procedure used to acquire histopathological images, and the process involves collecting a tissue sample from the affected area of the breast [4]. Subsequently, this collected sample is carefully examined under a microscope to identify and classify the nature of the tumor. Although it is a relatively invasive procedure, and there are different methods for breast cancer detection, biopsy is the only way to confidently diagnose whether cancer is truly present. For this reason, histopathological diagnosis is considered the gold standard for the clinical diagnosis of cancer [1]. Among biopsy techniques, the most common ones are fine-needle aspiration, core needle biopsy, vacuum-assisted biopsy, and open surgical biopsy (SOB) [32].

1.2   State-of-the-Art

Deep learning is a subfield of artificial intelligence that has revolutionized the ability of machines to learn and understand complex patterns. It utilizes deep neural networks to perform sophisticated tasks in analysis and decision-making. Authors such as Srinidhi et al. [33] and Van der Laak et al. [21] discuss the impact of these techniques and how they have become the most popular area in histopathological image analysis in recent years due to their high capacity for automatic feature extraction. In general, both works categorize deep learning networks based on the type of learning they rely on, which includes supervised learning, weakly supervised learning, unsupervised learning, and transfer learning. In this section, we will focus on supervised learning and transfer learning techniques.

In supervised learning, learning occurs in the form of a function that learns to map an input to an output based on pairs of input-output examples [25]. Typically, classification techniques for this type of learning will either work with classifying patches, small pieces of images, to classify the entire image, or they will work with the whole image for classification. These techniques can range from simple Convolutional Neural Network (CNN) architectures [7] to more complex models [22]. The models traditionally used for image classification can be seen in the field of histopathological images, such as VGGNet [31], InceptionNet [35], ResNet [38], and MobileNet [14].

The main objective of transfer learning is to transfer knowledge from a source domain to a target domain. This strategy relaxes the assumption that the test and training groups must be autonomous and evenly distributed. In the field of histopathology, knowledge transfer is often performed using pre-trained models from the ImageNet dataset, and notable works include [11], [17] and [20].

Several researchers have explored methodologies to enhance feature extraction quality in neural networks. For example, Umer et al. [39] employ transfer learning and machine learning techniques to validate a feature vector. In another study, Ibraheem et al. [16] propose the 3PCNNB-Net, a network comprising three parallel CNN branches designed to optimize information extraction and feature fusion. In Chhipa et al. [5], an unsupervised approach called MPCS is used for representation learning in histopathological images, resulting in high cancer classification accuracy on the BreakHis dataset. In Seo et al. [29], a more image processing and feature extraction-based approach combined with the Support Vector Machine (SVM) classifier is proposed. The proposed method involves dividing histopathological images into patches, and for each magnification level, Parameter Free Threshold Statistics (PFTS) features are extracted and classified by the pdMISVM (Primal-Dual Multi-Instance Support Vector Machine) classifier. The reported accuracy on the BreakHis dataset in the cited works is respectively 97.14%, 92.70%, 92.15%, and 89.8%.

Finally, Saini et al. [26] propose a Deep Learning architecture involving transfer learning based on VGGNet. The proposed architecture adds dense, batch normalization, dropout, and flattened layers to VGGNet, as well as an Inception block. The network is pre-trained on the ImageNet dataset, and a refinement step, similar to that done by [5], is performed on the BreakHis dataset. The reported accuracy on the dataset is 96.81%.

2 Deep Learning Models

In this section, we will briefly discuss the architectures that have achieved the best performance in the proposed methodology. MobileNetV2 [27] is an evolution of the MobileNet architecture [14], improved for better efficiency and representation capacity. It introduces enhancements such as the Bottleneck Residual Block, inspired by ResNet [12], which captures residual information, and the Inverted Residual Blocks, which effectively expand and reduce the dimensions of intermediate representations, as seen in Fig. 2.

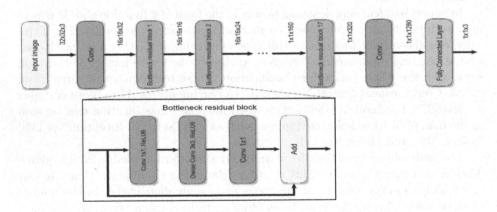

Fig. 2. Architecture of mobileNetV2 adapted from [28].

The network also uses Linear Bottleneck layers to increase flexibility and non-linearity, along with Squeeze and Excitation (SE) Activation Filters, which are used to enhance crucial information by modeling dependencies between feature channels.

The central idea of EfficientNetV2 [37] is to improve training speed while maintaining parameter efficiency, which is associated with the ability to achieve good results with a smaller number of parameters. The EfficientNetV2 introduces several modifications compared to EfficientNet [36], as seen in Fig. 3, including the use of new types of blocks, a combination of MBconv and fused-MBConv [10] adjustments in expansion rates and kernel sizes, and the removal of the stride-1 step. These changes are made to enhance the efficiency and performance of the architecture [37]. We can see the structure of MBConv and FusedConv in Fig. 4.

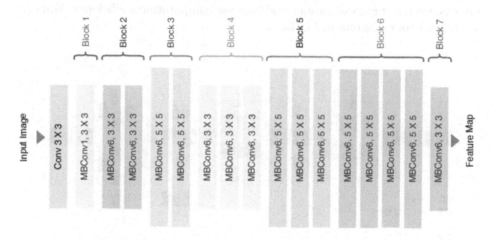

Fig. 3. Architecture of EfficientNet-B0 with MBConv as Basic building blocks, adapted from [2].

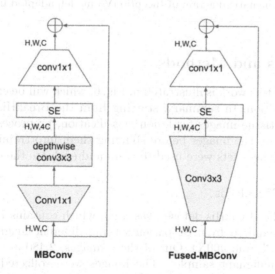

Fig. 4. Architecture of MBConv and FusedConv, adapted from [37].

Inception-v3 [34] is a variant of Inception-v2 that incorporates the concept of BN-auxiliary. This term refers to the version where the fully connected layer of the auxiliary classifier is also normalized, extending beyond just the convolutions. In this context, the combination of Inception-v2 with BN-auxiliary is called Inception-v3, representing an evolution in the original architecture. Additionally, Inception-v3 also incorporates the idea of Reduction Modules between these Inception modules. The reduction modules employ larger convolutions, such as 3×3 with increased stride, followed by 1×1 convolutions, to reduce the dimensionality of representations and increase computational efficiency. You can see the network diagram in Fig. 5.

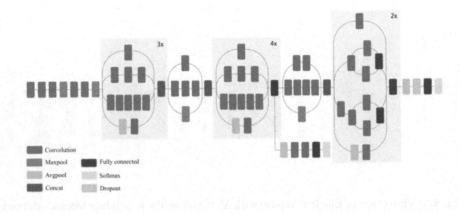

Fig. 5. Schematic diagram of InceptionV3 model, adapted from [23].

3   Materials and Methods

The flowchart of this work is illustrated in Fig. 6, which will be explained in more detail in this section. In summary, starting from the BreakHis dataset, which contains breast tissue images for lesion classification, preprocessing procedures were performed on the images before splitting them into training, testing, and validation sets. These sets were used to train and evaluate the different models.

3.1   Dataset BreakHis

For this work, the BreakHis dataset was used, which contains 7,909 histopathological images acquired from 82 patients using different magnification factors (40X, 100X, 200X, and 400X). Out of these images, 2,480 are benign samples, and 5,429 are malignant samples. The images were collected using the SOB method, have a resolution of 700×460 pixels, and consist of 3 channels of 8-bit color (RGB). A complete description of the sample count for each magnification level in the dataset can be seen in Table 1. The associated task with this dataset is the automated classification of these images [32].

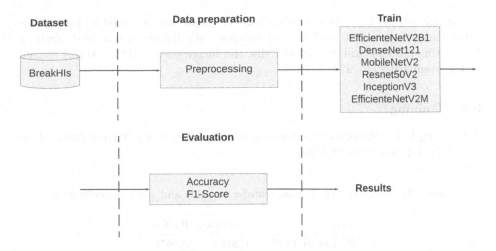

Fig. 6. Pipeline of the developed work.

Table 1. Description of the number of images in the BreakHis dataset by classes and magnification, adapted from [32]

Magnification	Benign	Malignant	Total
40X	652	1,370	1,995
100X	644	1,437	2,081
200X	623	1,390	2,013
400X	588	1,232	1,820
Total number of images	2,480	5,429	7,909

3.2 Data Preparation

In the preprocessing step of the images, data augmentation techniques were used, applying various transformations to each training instance while preserving the relationship with the annotations, with the aim of artificially expanding the amount of information for improved network learning [24].

The techniques applied for data augmentation were: Horizontal Flip, used to horizontally flip the image; Vertical Flip, used to vertically flip the image; Rotation, used to rotate the image; and Brightness, responsible for adjusting the brightness level in the images. All data augmentation techniques were conditioned to a factor of 0.2.

To reduce discrepancies among various images, a technique known as stain normalization [8] essentially transfers the average color from the source of one image to other images. Although deep learning (DL) algorithms may be able to partially reduce color variations through data augmentation, the performance of the results deteriorates due to the limited amount of data.

In this work, the stain normalization technique was adopted to reduce the color variability in histopathological images, establishing a standard, thereby facilitating model learning. Additionally, the image size of 460×700 was resized to the standard 224×224.

3.3   Training

After completing the preprocessing step of the images using stain normalization and data augmentation techniques,

Table 2. Results obtained using transfer learning and stain normalization.

Model	Accuracy	F1-Score
EfficienteNetV2B1	0,8581	0,8971
DenseNet121	0,8551	0,8940
MobileNetV2	0,8739	0,9090
Resnet50V2	0,8406	0,8877
InceptionResNetV2	0,8365	0,8846
InceptionV3	0,8710	0,9067
VGG16	0,7994	0,8564
EfficientNetV2M	0,8427	0,8852

The fitness function is responsible for evaluating the performance of a neural network with the aim of enhancing and seeking an improvement in results with each generation [30]. For this work, the optimizer used was Adam with a learning rate of 5e-4. The loss function employed was BinaryCrossentropy, which aims to minimize the discrepancies towards the desired class value. Training was conducted for 100 epochs, and the networks used were Resnet50V2 [13], DenseNet121 [15], MobileNetV2 [27], VGG16 [31], InceptionResNetV2 [34], InceptionV3 [35], EfficienteNetV2B1 [37] and EfficientNetV2M [37].

After training all the networks, the top 3 networks with the highest accuracy were selected, as shown in Table 2. This allowed for the selection of the network ensemble that will be used in the next phase.

Ensemble. Ensemble learning [40] is a method in which multiple models are combined to enhance the performance of a final model in machine learning tasks. Ensemble methods provide a powerful way to improve the generalization capability and accuracy of machine learning models. For the purpose of this binary classification task, the adopted method was voting, as it is the most common and yields good results [40].

Voting is a common method of combination, which can be implemented in various ways, including majority voting. Thus, majority voting is a method of combining predictions from multiple base models in an ensemble. Majority voting counts how many models predict each class and then makes the final prediction based on the class that receives the majority of votes [9].

After selecting the three networks with the best performance, we combined their predictions using a voting approach. Since we are dealing with a binary classification task where classes are represented as 0 (benign) or 1 (malignant), we applied the following criterion: if a class received an equal or greater number of votes than 2, it is considered to belong to the malignant class; otherwise, if it received 1 vote or none, it is classified as benign. This process results in the creation of an array of consolidated predictions through this voting process.

3.4 Evaluation

In this section, we will discuss the definition of the metric used in this work: Accuracy and F1-Score.

Accuracy is the ratio of the number of correctly classified samples to the total number of samples. We can understand it as follows, as per Eq. 1: True Positive (TP) represents the number of true positive cases. True Negative (TN) is the number of true negative cases. False Positive (FP) is the number of false positives, and False Negative (FN) is the number of false negatives. All of these values are derived from the confusion matrix [6].

$$acc = \frac{TP + TN}{TP + TN + FP + FN} \tag{1}$$

The F1-Score is the harmonic mean of Precision and Recall [6], as seen in Eq. 2. Therefore, when the F1-Score is low, it indicates that either Precision or Recall is low.

$$f1 = 2\frac{precision \times recall}{precision + recall} \tag{2}$$

Recall is the number of relevant items retrieved as a proportion of all relevant items [3]. We can describe Recall as the ratio of the number of true positives to the sum of true positives and false negatives. In this way, Recall is used to assess the percentage of data classified as positive compared to the actual quantity of positives in the sample [3].

$$recall = \frac{TP}{TP + FN} \tag{3}$$

Precision is a measure of purity used to assess the performance of Recall, as it gauges the effectiveness in excluding irrelevant items from the retrieved set. Therefore, both high Precision and high Recall are desirable [3].

$$precision = \frac{TP}{TP + FP} \tag{4}$$

4   Results

In this section, the results obtained in different experiments will be presented. Additionally, the evaluations were conducted using accuracy as the metric.

Table 3. Results obtained with the original dataset.

Model	Accuracy	F1-Score
EfficienteNetV2B1	0,8177	0,8756
DenseNet121	0,8023	0,8629
MobileNetV2	0,7965	0,8563
ResNet50V2	0,7827	0,8464
InceptionResNetV2	0,6987	0,8226
InceptionV3	0,6987	0,8226
VGG16	0,7827	0,8464
EfficientNetV2M	0,7553	0,8354

When conducting tests with the original dataset, we observed that the EfficientNetV2B1 network demonstrated superior performance compared to other architectures, as highlighted in Table 3. Therefore, we chose to use this network to obtain the images that will be used as a reference when applying the stain normalization technique. To do this, we analyze the predictions in the training set, prioritizing those with the highest associated confidence. This procedure allows us to identify which malignant or benign images contributed most significantly to the learning of the neural network.

Table 4. Results of the accuracies obtained using benign and malignant targets.

Model	Target benign	Target malignant
EfficienteNetV2B1	0,8054	0,8581
DenseNet121	0,8410	0,8551
MobileNetV2	0,8280	0,8739
Resnet50V2	0,8236	0,8406
InceptionResNetV2	0,8262	0,8365
InceptionV3	0,8245	0,8710
VGG16	0,7072	0,7072
EfficientNetV2M	0,8315	0,8427

After selecting the benign image with the best performance and the malignant image, we conducted an additional experiment to assess which of the two would stand out after being subjected to the stain normalization process, as shown in Table 4. Due to the substantial computational cost associated with training on the complete image set, the decision was made to exclusively train using magnifications of 200x and 400x. In this context, the training set consisted of a total of 2,682 images, with 804 images allocated for validation purposes (30%), 1,878 images for the actual training (70%), and finally, 1,151 images for the test set.

Table 5. Comparison of the accuracies obtained using stain normalization alone and using stain normalization with transfer learning.

Model	Stain Normalization	Stain Normalization + Transfer Learning
EfficienteNetV2B1	0,7611	0,8581
DenseNet121	0,6987	0,8551
MobileNetV2	0,6987	0,8739
Resnet50V2	0,7499	0,8426
InceptionResNetV2	0,6987	0,8365
InceptionV3	0,6987	0,8710
VGG16	0,6987	0,6987
EfficientNetV2M	0,7387	0,8427

After verifying that using the malignant image as a reference for stain normalization in the dataset, along with techniques like data augmentation and transfer learning, resulted in improved model performance, we expanded this approach to the entire set of images. We can observe how the use of transfer learning affected the learning of the networks, as seen in Table 5. Additionally, data augmentation was applied in both experiments.

Table 6. Result obtained and compared to the literature.

Method	Accuracy	F1-Score
pdMISVM [29]	0,8960	0,9112
Feature-level fusion-based FS framework [39]	0,9270	–
MPC [5]	0,9223	–
3PCNNB [16]	0,9180	–
VGG16 Modified with Inception block and dense layer [26]	0,9681	0,9387
Proposed	0,8847	0,9169

When analyzing Table 6, it becomes evident that the proposed methodology did not manage to surpass the accuracy of the works in the same area. However, it is crucial to highlight that all of these methods employ custom feature extraction processes, as mentioned in [29]. Furthermore, although the computational cost for training the complete set of networks to select the top three was higher compared to the analyzed works, the total training cost for these three top-performing networks ends up being lower than that of the compared works.

This occurs, in part, due to the lower complexity of the chosen networks compared to those mentioned in [31] and [26], which have a higher number of parameters. This difference in the number of parameters may require more substantial computational resources and can lead to overfitting issues.

In this study, the networks selected for the ensemble were InceptionV3, MobileNetV2, and EfficientNetV2B1, containing 23.9, 3.5, and 8.2 million parameters, respectively, totaling 38.8 million parameters. This approach of combining models aims to explore their complementarities and mitigate their individual limitations, thereby seeking a more robust result.

5   Discussion

Overall, the results obtained individually by the top three networks are quite similar. However, when we employ the voting technique, we can observe a modest improvement in the model's accuracy. Below, we present the model's predictions based on a small sample of the test set, as illustrated in Fig. 7.

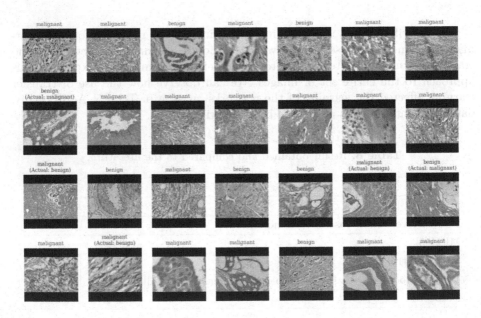

Fig. 7. Predictions of the proposed method

We can also analyze the results from the perspective of the confusion matrix, which provides a visualization of the balance between correct predictions and errors of the final model, as demonstrated in the Fig. 8.

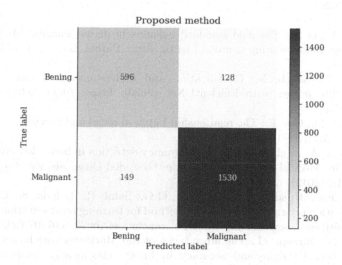

Fig. 8. Confusion matrix of the proposed method

When examining the confusion matrix, we notice that despite the imbalance present in the dataset, we were able to achieve a satisfactory number of correct predictions. Out of the 724 benign images in the set, the model correctly predicted 596, which corresponds to an accuracy rate of approximately 82%. Regarding the 1679 malignant images, the model correctly predicted 1530, resulting in an accuracy rate of around 91%.

These results demonstrate the model's ability to make accurate predictions, even in a scenario where the classes are unbalanced.

6   Conclusion

The improvement in disease detection in breast tissue through feature extraction and computational methods for the analysis of histopathological exams, using image processing, is of fundamental importance for both physicians and patients. This study presents the development of an image classification method using machine learning techniques, specifically in the field of Deep Learning, for the detection of breast cancer in histopathological images. Although the proposed methodology did not manage to surpass the accuracy of works in the same area, the results obtained are satisfactory, even when compared to the literature. The computational cost for training the complete set of networks to select the top 3 is higher compared to the analyzed works. However, the training of the top 3 networks ends up being more cost-effective than in the comparative works.

The study employs InceptionV3, MobileNetV2, and EfficientNetV2B1 in the ensemble, totaling 38.8 million parameters.

References

1. Aeffner, F., et al.: The gold standard paradox in digital image analysis: manual versus automated scoring as ground truth. Arch. Pathol. Lab. Med. **141**(9), 1267–1275 (2017)
2. Ahmed, T., Sabab, N.: Classification and understanding of cloud structures via satellite images with EfficientUNet (2020). https://doi.org/10.1002/essoar.10507423.1
3. Buckland, M., Gey, F.: The relationship between recall and precision. J. Am. Soc. Inf. Sci. **45**(1), 12–19 (1994)
4. Chekkoury, A., et al.: Automated malignancy detection in breast histopathological images. In: Medical Imaging 2012: Computer-Aided Diagnosis, vol. 8315, pp. 332–344. SPIE (2012)
5. Chhipa, P.C., Upadhyay, R., Pihlgren, G.G., Saini, R., Uchida, S., Liwicki, M.: Magnification prior: a self-supervised method for learning representations on breast cancer histopathological images. arXiv preprint: arXiv:2203.07707 (2022)
6. Chicco, D., Jurman, G.: The advantages of the Matthews correlation coefficient (MCC) over F1 score and accuracy in binary classification evaluation. BMC Genomics **21**(1), 1–13 (2020)
7. Cruz-Roa, A., et al.: Automatic detection of invasive ductal carcinoma in whole slide images with convolutional neural networks. In: Medical Imaging 2014: Digital Pathology, vol. 9041, p. 904103. SPIE (2014)
8. Deng, S., et al.: Deep learning in digital pathology image analysis: a survey. Front. Med. **14**, 470–487 (2020)
9. Ganaie, M.A., Hu, M., Malik, A., Tanveer, M., Suganthan, P.: Ensemble deep learning: a review. Eng. Appl. Artif. Intell. **115**, 105151 (2022)
10. Gupta, S., Tan, M.: Efficientnet-EdgeTPU: creating accelerator-optimized neural networks with AutoML. Google AI Blog **2**(1) (2019)
11. Hassan, A.M., El-Mashade, M.B., Aboshosha, A.: Deep learning for cancer tumor classification using transfer learning and feature concatenation. Int. J. Electr. Comput. Eng. **12**(6), 6736 (2022)
12. He, K., Zhang, X., Ren, S., Sun, J.: Deep residual learning for image recognition. In: Proceedings of the IEEE Conference on Computer Vision and Pattern Recognition, pp. 770–778 (2016)
13. He, K., Zhang, X., Ren, S., Sun, J.: Identity mappings in deep residual networks (2016)
14. Howard, A.G., et al.: MobileNets: efficient convolutional neural networks for mobile vision applications. arXiv preprint: arXiv:1704.04861 (2017)
15. Huang, G., Liu, Z., van der Maaten, L., Weinberger, K.Q.: Densely connected convolutional networks (2018)
16. Ibraheem, A.M., Rahouma, K.H., Hamed, H.F.: 3pcnnb-net: Three parallel CNN branches for breast cancer classification through histopathological images. J. Med. Bio. Eng. **41**(4), 494–503 (2021)
17. Ijaz, A., et al.: Modality specific CBAM-VGGNet model for the classification of breast histopathology images via transfer learning. IEEE Access **11**, 15750–15762 (2023)

18. INCA: Estimativa 2020, incidência de câncer no brasil (2020). https://www.inca.gov.br/estimativa/introducao#:~:text=Nas%20mulheres%2C%20exceto%20o%20c%C3%A2ncer,%25

19. INCA: Detecção precoce do câncer (2021b), referência completa: *Instituto Nacional de Câncer José Alencar Gomes da Silva. Detecção precoce do câncer.* Rio de Janeiro: INCA, 2021b. Disponível em: https://www.inca.gov.br/publicacoes/livros/deteccao-precoce-do-cancer. Acesso em: 16 ago. 2023

20. Joshi, S.A., Bongale, A.M., Olsson, P.O., Urolagin, S., Dharrao, D., Bongale, A.: Enhanced pre-trained Xception model transfer learned for breast cancer detection. Computation **11**(3), 59 (2023)

21. Van der Laak, J., Litjens, G., Ciompi, F.: Deep learning in histopathology: the path to the clinic. Nat. Med. **27**(5), 775–784 (2021)

22. Liu, J., et al.: An end-to-end deep learning histochemical scoring system for breast cancer TMA. IEEE Trans. Med. Imaging **38**(2), 617–628 (2018)

23. Mahdianpari, M., Salehi, B., Rezaee, M., Mohammadimanesh, F., Zhang, Y.: Very deep convolutional neural networks for complex land cover mapping using multi-spectral remote sensing imagery. Remote Sens. **10**(7), 1119 (2018)

24. Pérez-García, F., Sparks, R., Ourselin, S.: Torchio: A python library for efficient loading, preprocessing, augmentation and patch-based sampling of medical images in deep learning. Comput. Methods Programs Biomed. **208**, 106236 (2021). https://doi.org/10.1016/j.cmpb.2021.106236, https://www.sciencedirect.com/science/article/pii/S0169260721003102

25. Russell, S.J.: Artificial Intelligence a Modern Approach. Pearson Education Inc., London (2010)

26. Saini, M., Susan, S.: VGGIN-Net: deep transfer network for imbalanced breast cancer dataset. IEEE/ACM Trans. Comput. Biol. Bioinform. **20**, 752–762 (2022)

27. Sandler, M., Howard, A., Zhu, M., Zhmoginov, A., Chen, L.C.: MobileNetV2: inverted residuals and linear bottlenecks. In: Proceedings of the IEEE Conference on Computer Vision and Pattern Recognition, pp. 4510–4520 (2018)

28. Seidaliyeva, U., Akhmetov, D., Ilipbayeva, L., Matson, E.: Real-time and accurate drone detection in a video with a static background. Sensors **20**, 3856 (2020). https://doi.org/10.3390/s20143856

29. Seo, H., Brand, L., Barco, L.S., Wang, H.: Scaling multi-instance support vector machine to breast cancer detection on the BreaKHis dataset. Bioinformatics **38**(Supplement_1), i92–i100 (2022)

30. Silva, D.A., et al.: Otimização da função de fitness para a evolução de redes neurais com o uso de análise envoltória de dados aplicada à previsão de séries temporais (2011)

31. Simonyan, K., Zisserman, A.: Very deep convolutional networks for large-scale image recognition. arXiv preprint: arXiv:1409.1556 (2015)

32. Spanhol, F.A., Oliveira, L.S., Petitjean, C., Heutte, L.: A dataset for breast cancer histopathological image classification. IEEE Trans. Biomed. Eng. **63**(7), 1455–1462 (2016). https://doi.org/10.1109/TBME.2015.2496264

33. Srinidhi, C.L., Ciga, O., Martel, A.L.: Deep neural network models for computational histopathology: a survey. Med. Image Anal. **67**, 101813 (2021)

34. Szegedy, C., Ioffe, S., Vanhoucke, V., Alemi, A.: Inception-v4, inception-ResNet and the impact of residual connections on learning (2016)

35. Szegedy, C., Vanhoucke, V., Ioffe, S., Shlens, J., Wojna, Z.: Rethinking the inception architecture for computer vision. In: Proceedings of the IEEE Conference on Computer Vision and Pattern Recognition, pp. 2818–2826 (2015)

36. Tan, M., Le, Q.: EfficientNet: rethinking model scaling for convolutional neural networks. In: International Conference on Machine Learning, pp. 6105–6114. PMLR (2019)
37. Tan, M., Le, Q.V.: EfficientNetV2: smaller models and faster training (2021)
38. Targ, S., Almeida, D., Lyman, K.: ResNet in ResNet: generalizing residual architectures. arXiv preprint: arXiv:1603.08029 (2016)
39. Umer, M.J., Sharif, M., Alhaisoni, M., Tariq, U., Kim, Y.J., Chang, B.: A framework of deep learning and selection-based breast cancer detection from histopathology images. Comput. Syst. Sci. Eng. **45**(2) (2023)
40. Zheng, Y., et al.: Application of transfer learning and ensemble learning in image-level classification for breast histopathology. Intell. Med. **3**(02), 115–128 (2023)

Tooth Detection and Numbering in Panoramic Radiographs Using YOLOv8-Based Approach

Felipe Rogério Silva Teles[1]([✉])(iD), Alison Corrêa Mendes[1](iD),
Anselmo Cardoso de Paiva[1](iD), João Dallyson Sousa de Almeida[1](iD),
Geraldo Braz Junior[1](iD), Aristófanes Corrêa Silva[1](iD),
and Pedro De Alcantara Dos Santos Neto[2](iD)

[1] Núcleo de Computacão Aplicada - Universidade Federal do Maranhão (UFMA),
Caixa Postal 65.085-580, São Luís, MA, Brazil
frs.teles@discente.ufma.br, {alison.mendes,paiva}@nca.ufma.br,
{joao.dallyson,geraldo.braz,ac.silva}@ufma.br
[2] Departamento de Computação, Universidade Federal do Piauí, Teresina, Brazil
pasn@ufpi.edu.br

Abstract. Before a dental professional performs any procedure or diagnosis, they need to know the patient's dental arch. For that, it is common
for them to ask the patient to take a panoramic radiograph. The use of
neural networks to assist this professional in this stage is not recent, and
most studies use segmentation networks to solve the problem. However,
the segmentation result does not make explicit the specific position of
the tooth and its numbering according to the international system (FDI),
presenting only more specific details. In this study, we aimed to use a
powerful and efficient detection neural network called You Only Look
Once v8 to perform automated tooth detection and numbering based
on FDI, using a dataset that contains 166 anonymized and deidentified
panoramic dental radiographs of patients from Noor Medical Imaging
Center, Qom, Iran, and are public. Labels were created using an online
tool for production in the YOLO standard. The metrics used to evaluate
the trained model were precision, recall, and mAP50. The results of each
were 0.95818, 0.95505, and 0.97384. The conclusion of the study uses
the model training generated a weight to test the model in a real-world
scenario.

Keywords: tooth detection · panoramic radiography · deep learning ·
dental image

1 Introduction

One of the most important exams for dental professionals is the panoramic radiograph, and it's the most popular screening test prescribed in dentistry too [6].
It is also a util and necessary tool in several areas of dentistry, mainly in the

A. Cunha et al. (Eds.): MobiHealth 2023, LNICST 578, pp. 239–253, 2024.
https://doi.org/10.1007/978-3-031-60665-6_18

diagnosis and treatment of oral diseases such as caries, periodontal diseases, and oral pathologies [12,23]. It is noteworthy that in addition to being a low-cost exam, those who perform are not so exposed to radiation. Radiograph also provides images of the dental arch and the mandibular and maxillary region. They recommended that not all patients must be tested and those who do be limited to areas necessary for proper diagnosis and treatment based on the good exercise of professional judgment [26].

When the dentist has images of the examination, he can examine it and then diagnose it. To increase the accuracy of diagnosis, tooth type, and teeth numbering should be identified and determined based on their anatomy and location [5]. When discussing a small number of exams, it is possible to do the procedure manually and carefully. But in practice, a dentist has several patients, and the amount of exams he has to analyze is large [18], which causes more errors to occur because of fatigue and the fact that factors such as subjectivity and experience influence the analysis [16].

The use of computers and systems is increasing more and more in the health area, and dentistry is no different because it facilitates diagnosis and, consequently, simplifies treatment planning [4]. That being said, one of the main technologies that have been used is Artificial Intelligence (AI), which over time has become frequent in many areas. They make the computer mathematically imitate how the human brain thinks and makes decisions [25]. Recently, AIs have experienced accelerated development and have become one of the most influential innovations worldwide, and AI-based methods are beginning to be used to assist dentists in interpreting radiographic results [29]. These methods help to make the identification and classification faster and reduce the errors from fatigue. Moreover, the increase of AIs could provide fully automated dental chart filling and treatment planning, giving more time to the dentist to perform treatments [5].

Artificial intelligence is a broad area, so the focus of this study was on Deep Learning(DL), which is a computer-assisted framework and a subarea of Machine Learning (ML) [30]. Deep Learning (DL) is considered the most cost-effective and time-efficient ML approach [8]. An advantage of DL is processing large amounts of data, such as text, sound, and images [20]. One of the basic types of architecture that works well in DL is the Convolutional Neural Network (CNN). For color and boundary detection functions, CNNs prove very accurate in image detection. Besides, they have several emerging applications in medical image analysis due to the advent of computing hardware algorithms and expansion in the amount of data [4].

This study aims to carry out the automated detection of tooth numbering in panoramic radiography exams using the most modern version of the YOLO v8 model, which allows training with more quality and less data [9], to evaluate its performance using precision, recall, and mean average precision (map) as metrics. After obtaining the results, we hope it can serve as an alternative to assist dental professionals in detecting and numbering teeth accurately and quickly.

2   Related Works

Miscellaneous previous studies have used Deep Learning techniques for the task of numbering teeth in radiographs using CNN-based architecture and various methods. Al-Sarem et al. [2] used different networks to try to find the position and number of the missing teeth. For this task, they used a dataset with 120 images, and the best results for segmentation and classification were using, respectively, a U-Net and DenseNet169 pre-trained model. The best result for segmentation was an accuracy of 90.81%, and for classification, the precision was 0.88 and recall 0.98. Görürgöz et al. [10] was designed based on R-CNN inception architecture that automatically detect and number the teeth on periapical images. They used a dataset with 660 images, and the results of F1 score, precision, and sensitivity were 0.8720, 0.7812, and 0.9867, respectively. The study of Alam et al. [3] consists of segmenting teeth into two modules, the first module designed to identify teeth and the second module designed to number teeth. For tooth numbering, they trained the VGG16 convolution architecture using 1300 images and evaluated the model using 200 images (1500 in total). Results obtained for teeth diagnosis were 89.8% and, for teeth numbering, precision of 86.5%.

In dental radiology, You Only Look Once(YOLO) v4 has already been used in detecting tooth numbering. Putra et al. [20] used YoloV4 and trained a dataset that contained 500 images, 400 for training and 100 for testing, and reached a result of 88.5% accuracy and 87.70% precision. Astuti et al. [5] also used YOLOv4 with the same amount of images to train and validate the model. However, they used other metrics to evaluate the model, and they achieved a sensitivity of 99.42% and a specificity of 87.06%.

This study experiments with an update of these approaches using a more up-to-date convolutional neural network called YOLOv8, which is a continuation of You Only Look Once v4 and has more precision and less need for data, which directly affects processing [11]. The obtained results were promising and demonstrated that YOLOv8 applied to the problem of automatic tooth detection performs well.

3   You only Look once

You Only Look Once (YOLO) is a potent object detection algorithm that detects objects in real-time using CNN16. The YOLO system treats object detection as a single regression problem, which makes it possible to discover which classes are present and where they are [21]. Currently, YOLO has eight versions, and its effectiveness is evidenced through a comparative analysis carried out in Terven et al. [27] that proves its efficiency and makes a comparative analysis of each version released in their work.

The annotation format used by the YOLO model consists of five params, and there are, respectively, the class of the object, the X and Y of the bounding box center, and the width and height of the bounding box as seen below:

$$(ObjectId - class)(Xcenter)(Ycenter)(Width)(Height) \qquad (1)$$

The initial convolutional layers of the network resize the image according to the chosen input size and extract features, while the fully connected layers predict the output probabilities and coordinates [21]. The input image is split into s × s grid cells (default = 7 × 7), with each cell predicting (B) bounding boxes, each containing five parameters and sharing prediction probabilities of classes (C) [11]. How appears in Fig. 1.

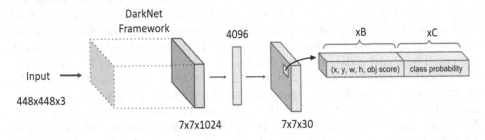

Fig. 1. General architecture of YOLO using a input size of 448 × 448 and 3 classes [11].

3.1 Bag of Freebies

Bag of Freebies (BoF) is the set of low computational cost techniques that YOLO has improved to improve YOLO training performance as they avoid overfitting and improve model generalization [32]. Examples of these techniques is Data augmentation.

Data Augmentation. Expanding the training dataset with variations of the original data using random geometry transformation and random color flickering [32]. This technique allows the YOLO model to learn efficiently with a much smaller number of images than a pure neural network would need [9].

3.2 YOLO V8

YOLO's latest version, YOLO v8, was officially released in January 2023 by Ultralytics, and even though it is considered incomplete about the level of functionality of previous versions, comparisons demonstrate its superiority as the new YOLO state-of-the-art[18]. The Fig. 2 shows a comparison between previous versions. YOLOv8, unlike YOLOv4, features an anchor-free system that allows data to be processed independently of objectivity, classification, and regression tasks. This design allows each branch to focus on its labor and improves the overall accuracy of the model [27]. Furthermore, YOLOv8 uses CIoU [33] and DFL [15] loss functions for bounding box loss and binary cross-entropy for classification that directly leads to improved object detection performance, especially when dealing with smaller objects [27].

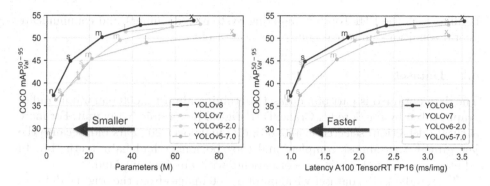

Fig. 2. Comparison chart between latest versions of yolo. [13]

4   Matherial and Methods

4.1   Tooth Numering

Tooth numbering is the most commonly used practice in dentistry to identify specific teeth in a patient's mouth and is an excellent way to perform a pre-diagnosis.

The Fédération Dentaire Internationale (FDI) Tooth Numbering System, officially developed by the World Dental Federation [19], divides the mouth into four quadrants: Upper Right (UR), Upper Left (UL), Lower Left (LL), Lower Right (LR), and divides each quadrant into eight teeth: Central Incisor (1), Lateral Incisor (2), Canine (3), First Premolar (4), Second Premolar (5), First Molar (6), Second Molar (7), Third Molar (8). In this way, the identification of the tooth occurs through two numbers, the first referring to the quadrant and the second referring to the tooth itself, as shown in Fig. 3.

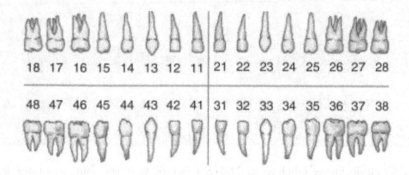

Fig. 3. Tooth numbering by FDI system [17]

This standardized numbering system simplifies communication between dental professionals and ensures that everyone, regardless of teeth location, can easily understand and reference specific teeth [28]. The practitioner needs to be familiar with the FDI Tooth Numbering System to document and communicate dental conditions and treatment plans accurately.

4.2 Dataset

The data obtained is part of a dataset containing almost 2,000 panoramic radiographs taken by the Soredex CranexD [1] digital panoramic X-ray unit. For more accurate detection, selected exams of individuals over 20 years old because the jaw growth was almost complete and they no longer had baby teeth [14]. In addition, we did not use images of patients with any implant kind.

This study used a dataset with, in total, 166 images from the original dataset, where 150 and their respective labels were used in the stage of training and validation of the model, and 16 non-labeled images were used to test the trained model in a real-world context.

4.3 Labeling Dataset

The labels were obtained manually through the free-to-use tool MakeSense (SkalskiP from GitHub) [24], and each tooth represented its respective tooth numbering class. The classes used following the numbering indicated in the international numbering system was 32 [19] and how it showed in the Fig. 3. There is an example of marking the bounding box in Fig. 4.

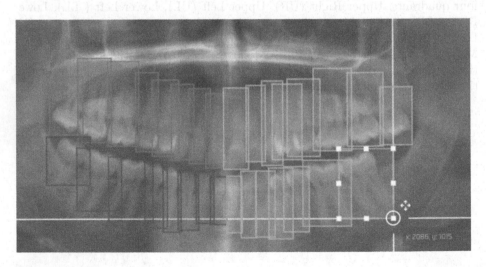

Fig. 4. Example image labeling on MakeSense tool that the four quadrants labels separated by color.

The total number of edentulous areas found was 4210, and the quantity of each one is present at Table 1. Not all patients had all their teeth. Therefore, the number of edentulous areas was not equal for all classes.

Table 1. On the right of the table you can see the amount of the teeth in the mandible region, and on the left you can see the amount of the teeth in the inferior jaw.

Maxillary Tooth	Labels Amount	Mandibular Tooth	Labels Amount
11	148	31	150
12	144	32	147
13	150	33	147
14	136	34	145
15	128	35	131
16	132	36	121
17	140	37	134
18	79	38	86
21	149	41	147
22	145	42	145
23	141	43	142
24	135	44	144
25	126	45	134
26	136	46	116
27	134	47	128
28	80	48	90

4.4   Training

With the notes completed, the training process begins. To carry out the study, the cloud development environment, Google Collaboratory, also called Google Colab, was used, which provides functional resources such as the Graphics Processing Unit (GPU), which reduces training time [7]. Google Colab proved efficient in training and saving memory on the local machine, as it allows integration with Google Drive. The model chosen for the train was YOLOv8x [13]. For training, 150 images of varying sizes were used. As seen in Sect. 3, the YOLO architecture resizes the image according to the size chosen in the training input. After a series of training attempts, it was concluded that the best input size for the problem was 640×640, and due to the low amount of data, training was carried out with batch size 6, requiring 100 epochs to reach the presented result.

4.5   Evaluating the Model

To evaluate the model presented, the metrics used were accuracy, precision, and mean Average Precision (mAP). However, before explaining each of the metrics, it is necessary to explain some basic concepts of variables used in the evaluation calculation of results, namely False Positives (FP), False Negatives (FN), and True Positives (TP).

False positives (FP) are the objects that the model detected wrongly. So, there are cases in which the model predicted an object, but there is no corresponding truth object. False Negatives (FN) are objects that the detection model was unable to detect despite representing instances where there are real objects in the image, which means that the model did not predict the bounding boxes accurately. True Positives (TP) are the objects that the model correctly detected. In other words, TP represents cases where the model's predicted bounding boxes almost right overlap the ground truth bounding boxes and are classified correctly.

Recall. Is the fraction of relevant instances that were retrieved, and it can be calculated using the following operation:

$$Recall = \frac{TP}{TP + FN} \tag{2}$$

Precision. As a result of calculating the precision, a measure of how many of the positive predictions made are correct is obtained, and it can be represented as follows:

$$Precision = \frac{TP}{TP + FP} \tag{3}$$

Intersection over Union. In order to grasp the concept of Mean Average Precision, which is the principal metric used to evaluate the quality of a detection model, it is essential to have a clear understanding of Intersection over Union (IoU). IoU is the most popular evaluation metric used in object detection benchmarks [22]. The bounding box referring to the labels presented in the input is known as the ground truth. Calculating the IoU is necessary to determine the gap between the bounding box demarcated by the model and the ground truth.

Mean Average Precision. It is calculated by finding Average Precision(AP) for each class and then averaging over several classes. Average precision (AP) is how the precision recovery curve is summarized as a single value representing the average of all precisions. Below is the Mean Average Precision calculation:

$$mAP = \frac{1}{n} \sum_{i=1}^{n} AP_i \tag{4}$$

For this study, map50 and map95 were used, and they refer to two different mAP calculations based on different IoU thresholds. The mAP50 uses an IoU threshold of 0.5 and is the most important evaluation indicator [31]. While mAP95 is using an IoU threshold of 0.95.

4.6   Testing

To test the model, we chose to use the 16 images that do not have a label, and we used the prediction function based on the weights obtained after training. It consists of the YOLO model analyzing the input image using its learned parameters and producing bounding boxes around the detected objects, corresponding class labels, and confidence scores. Contributing directly to evaluating the model in a practical scenario, that is, in the real world.

5 Results

Several training sessions were carried out to achieve the most promising result, carried out with 120 images and validated with 30. After one hundred epochs in a batch of six, we arrived at the results that will be presented in this session.

5.1 Confusion Matrix

It's workable to see the model's performance in a confusion matrix. The confusion matrix is a table with the number of rows and columns varying according to the number of classes and which reports the number of false positives, false negatives, true positives, and true negatives. It allows you to have more detailed information than just calculating metrics. As our experiment has many classes, the confusion matrix focuses on the diagonal, the number of negative verities we obtained. The plotted confusion matrix is in the Fig. 5.

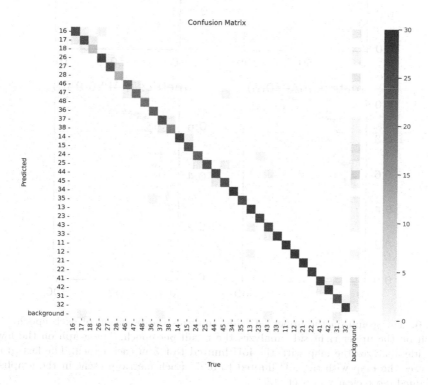

Fig. 5. Quantitative indicator of TP and FP for each class in a confusion matrix.

5.2   Qualitative Results

After knowing the number of false negatives, false positives, true negatives, and true positives, YOLO automatically generates the result in a CSV format, where each column has a metric, and each row represents an epoch. The best results obtained at different times and the precision, recall, and mAP50 were respectively 0.95818, 0.95505, and 0.97384. In addition to the CSV file with results, we also have graphs relating the times and the results obtained, as shown in Fig. 6. Map95 was also used, and the best result was 0.67214, but it is less relevant than map50 [31].

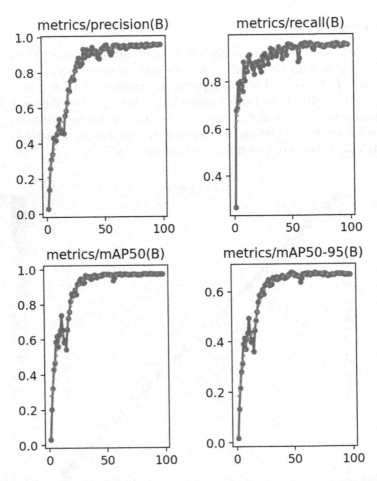

Fig. 6. The graph on the upper left side analyzes the precision of each epoch. The graph on the upper right side analyzes the recall per epoch. The graph on the lower left side analyzes the map with the IoU limited to 0.5 in each epoch. The last graph analyzes the map with the IoU limited to 0.95. Each metric present in the graphs is explained more clearly in Sect. 4.5

Analysis of the graphs shows stability in the main metrics from epoch 50 onwards, which proves the robustness of the model and the training process. This phenomenon indicates that the model has converged to a stable solution and that increasing the number of epochs is not a guarantee of improvement in the model's performance.

This stability is usual in deep learning models. It indicates that the model has learned patterns in the data well and has reached a point where additional training does not improve model performance. Therefore, it is worth a thorough analysis to ensure that the model hits a good level of generalization, that is, the model's ability to recognize tooth patterns learned from radiography images that were not present during training.

In summary, stabilization suggests that the model has reached a good level of training, and it is prepared for validation and testing to evaluate its concrete generalization performance in tooth numbering.

5.3 Quantitative Results

To carry out a more precise analysis, we evaluated the individual performance of each class according to tooth number. This step helps to identify whether the number of instances of each class influences the result. The application of metrics to each tooth class is shown in Table 2

Table 2. On the right of the table, you can see the results of the teeth in the mandible region, and on the left, you can see the results of the teeth in the inferior jaw.

Maxillary Tooth	Precision	Recall	Mandibular Tooth	Precision	Recall
11	0.981	1	31	0.962	0.846
12	0.975	1	32	0.967	0.983
13	0.994	0.968	33	0.953	1
14	0.965	0.976	34	0.989	1
15	0.918	1	35	0.913	1
16	0.943	0.959	36	1	0.985
17	0.881	0.964	37	0.927	0.91
18	0.794	0.862	38	0.907	0.979
21	0.988	1	41	0.829	0.97
22	0.979	1	42	0.941	0.967
23	0.985	1	43	0.993	0.933
24	0.94	1	44	0.977	0.966
25	0.899	1	45	0.937	0.929
26	0.966	0.989	46	0.881	0.913
27	0.859	0.939	47	0.867	0.917
28	0.884	0.895	48	0.951	0.909

With the individual analysis of each class, we came to the conclusion that the trained model presented a satisfactory result in the tooth numbering and detection task and is ready to perform the test. To check the model's generalization performance, we separated 16 images not present in the training stage and applied the generated weights.

5.4   Testing the Model

At the end of the training, the model-generated weights were used in this study to evaluate the model in a real-world application, that is, in a practical way and with images unknown to the model. This step contributes to automating the tooth detection and numbering process, as new training is unnecessary.

To test the model, we used 16 panoramic radiograph images that were not present in the training to evaluate the model in a real-use situation in an automated way and how the model behaves with generalization. In the Fig. 7, one of the images used to test the trained model.

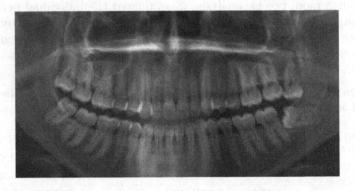

Fig. 7. Example of an image used to test the prediction of the model.

The prediction mode allows us to use the weights generated during training to carry out detection automatically, that is, without having to train the model again. Figure 8 has an example of successfully performed multi-object detection on panoramic radiographs with complete dentition and an edentulous area by YOLO v8.

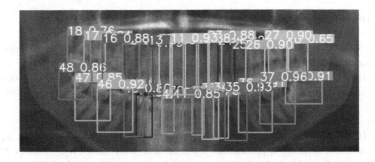

Fig. 8. Result of tooth numbering predict using You Only Look Once v8 on panoramic radiograph.

6 Conclusion

This work used a modern detection neural network based on deep learning methods to automatically execute the task of detecting each of the 32 teeth in panoramic radiographic images. To develop the model proposed in this study, we used 100 teeth images and extracted 2718 teeth, implant, and crown data. The model can number each tooth. The experimental results showed a high accuracy in tooth numbering using YOLO v8. As a result, the precision, recall, and mAP50 were respectively 0.95818, 0.95505, and 0.9738.

Through the weights obtained with the training, it is possible to perform the detection automatically using the prediction method of YOLO. It also allows the weights to carry out new models in future studies. Therefore, we consider the model presented as scalable.

Finally, it is expected that this system be used as decision support to help dentists as a way of helping them to save diagnosis time, using in practice only one computer in the clinic to improve the oral health system and increase the capacity of people that a professional can meet, and contribute to the development of radiology-related algorithms.

Acknowledgements. This work was carried out with the support of the Coordination for the Improvement of Higher Education Personnel - Brazil (CAPES) - Financing Code 001, Maranhão Research Support Foundation (FAPEMA), National Council for Scientific and Technological Development (CNPq) and Brazilian Company of Hospital Services (Ebserh) Brazil (Proc. 409593/2021-4).

The results presented in this paper were obtained through research carried out at the "CENTRO DE REFERÊNCIA EM INTELIGÊNCIA ARTIFICIAL - CEREIA", based at the Federal University of Ceará in partnership with the Hapvida NotreDame Intermédica Group and supported by the Grant 2020/09706-7, São Paulo Research Foundation (FAPESP).

References

1. Abdi, A.H., Kasaei, S., Mehdizadeh, M.: Automatic segmentation of mandible in panoramic x-ray. J. Med. Imaging **2**(4), 044003–044003 (2015)
2. Al-Sarem, M., Al-Asali, M., Alqutaibi, A.Y., Saeed, F.: Enhanced tooth region detection using pretrained deep learning models. Int. J. Environ. Res. Public Health **19**(22), 15414 (2022)
3. Alam, M.K., et al.: Teeth segmentation by optical radiographic images using VGG-16 deep learning convolution architecture with R-CNN network approach for biomedical sensing applications. Opt. Quant. Electron. **55**(9), 808 (2023)
4. Almalki, A., Latecki, L.J.: Self-supervised learning with masked image modeling for teeth numbering, detection of dental restorations, and instance segmentation in dental panoramic radiographs. In: Proceedings of the IEEE/CVF Winter Conference on Applications of Computer Vision, pp. 5594–5603 (2023)
5. Astuti, E.R., et al.: The sensitivity and specificity of YOLO v4 for tooth detection on panoramic radiographs. J. Int. Dent. Med. Res. **16**(1), 442–446 (2023)
6. Bekiroglu, N., Mete, S., Ozbay, G., Yalcinkaya, S., Kargul, B.: Evaluation of panoramic radiographs taken from 1,056 Turkish children. Niger. J. Clin. Pract. **18**(1), 8–12 (2015)
7. Bisong, E., Bisong, E.: Google Colaboratory. Building Machine Learning and Deep Learning Models on Google Cloud Platform: A Comprehensive Guide for Beginners, pp. 59–64 (2019)
8. Dargan, S., Kumar, M., Ayyagari, M.R., Kumar, G.: A survey of deep learning and its applications: a new paradigm to machine learning. Arch. Comput. Methods Eng. **27**, 1071–1092 (2020)
9. Fabrice, N., Lee, J.J., et al.: SMD detection and classification using YOLO network based on robust data preprocessing and augmentation techniques. J. Multimedia Inf. Syst. **8**(4), 211–220 (2021)
10. Görürgöz, C., et al.: Performance of a convolutional neural network algorithm for tooth detection and numbering on periapical radiographs. Dentomaxillofacial Radiol. **51**(3), 20210246 (2022)
11. Hussain, M.: YOLO-v1 to YOLO-v8, the rise of YOLO and its complementary nature toward digital manufacturing and industrial defect detection. Machines **11**(7), 677 (2023)
12. Izzetti, R., Nisi, M., Aringhieri, G., Crocetti, L., Graziani, F., Nardi, C.: Basic knowledge and new advances in panoramic radiography imaging techniques: a narrative review on what dentists and radiologists should know. Appl. Sci. **11**(17), 7858 (2021)
13. Jocher, G., Chaurasia, A., Qiu, J.: YOLO by Ultralytics (2023). https://github.com/ultralytics/ultralytics
14. Koh, K., Tan, J., Nambiar, P., Ibrahim, N., Mutalik, S., Asif, M.K.: Age estimation from structural changes of teeth and buccal alveolar bone level. J. Forensic Leg. Med. **48**, 15–21 (2017)
15. Li, X., et al.: Generalized focal loss: learning qualified and distributed bounding boxes for dense object detection. In: Advances in Neural Information Processing Systems, vol. 33, pp. 21002–21012 (2020)
16. Lin, P., Huang, P., Huang, P., Hsu, H., Chen, C.: Teeth segmentation of dental periapical radiographs based on local singularity analysis. Comput. Methods Programs Biomed. **113**(2), 433–445 (2014)

17. Mourão, J., Sousa, J.: Lesão dentária na anestesiologia. Revista Brasileira de Anestesiologia **28** (2014). https://doi.org/10.1016/j.bjan.2013.04.009
18. Muresan, M.P., Barbura, A.R., Nedevschi, S.: Teeth detection and dental problem classification in panoramic X-ray images using deep learning and image processing techniques. In: 2020 IEEE 16th International Conference on Intelligent Computer Communication and Processing (ICCP), pp. 457–463. IEEE (2020)
19. Peck, S., Peck, L.: Tooth numbering progress. Angle Orthod. **66**(2), 83–84 (1996)
20. Putra, R.H., et al.: Automated permanent tooth detection and numbering on panoramic radiograph using deep learning approach. Oral Surg Oral Med Oral Pathol Oral Radiol **137**, 537–544 (2023)
21. Redmon, J., Divvala, S., Girshick, R., Farhadi, A.: You only look once: unified, real-time object detection. In: Proceedings of the IEEE Conference on Computer Vision and Pattern Recognition, pp. 779–788 (2016)
22. Rezatofighi, H., Tsoi, N., Gwak, J., Sadeghian, A., Reid, I., Savarese, S.: Generalized intersection over union: a metric and a loss for bounding box regression. In: Proceedings of the IEEE/CVF Conference on Computer Vision and Pattern Recognition, pp. 658–666 (2019)
23. on Scientific Affairs, A.D.A.C., et al.: The use of dental radiographs: update and recommendations. J. Am. Dent. Assoc. **137**(9), 1304–1312 (2006)
24. Skalski, P.: Make sense (2019). https://github.com/SkalskiP/make-sense/
25. Strong, A.: Applications of artificial intelligence & associated technologies. Science [ETEBMS-2016] **5**(6) (2016)
26. Sun, W., Xia, K., Tang, L., Liu, C., Zou, L., Liu, J.: Accuracy of panoramic radiography in diagnosing maxillary sinus-root relationship: a systematic review and meta-analysis. Angle Orthod. **88**(6), 819–829 (2018)
27. Terven, J., Cordova-Esparza, D.: A comprehensive review of YOLO: from YOLOv1 to YOLOv8 and beyond. arXiv preprint: arXiv:2304.00501 (2023)
28. Türp, J.C., Alt, K.W.: Designating teeth: the advantages of the FDI's two-digit system. Quintessence Int. **26**(7) (1995)
29. Tuzoff, D.V., et al.: Tooth detection and numbering in panoramic radiographs using convolutional neural networks. Dentomaxillofacial Radiol. **48**(4), 20180051 (2019)
30. Umer, F., Habib, S., Adnan, N.: Application of deep learning in teeth identification tasks on panoramic radiographs. Dentomaxillofacial Radiol. **51**(5), 20210504 (2022)
31. Zhang, S., Liu, J., Zhang, X.: Adaptive compressive sensing: an optimization method for pipeline magnetic flux leakage detection. Sustainability **15**(19), 14591 (2023)
32. Zhang, Z., He, T., Zhang, H., Zhang, Z., Xie, J., Li, M.: Bag of freebies for training object detection neural networks. arXiv preprint: arXiv:1902.04103 (2019)
33. Zheng, Z., Wang, P., Liu, W., Li, J., Ye, R., Ren, D.: Distance-IoU loss: faster and better learning for bounding box regression. In: Proceedings of the AAAI Conference on Artificial Intelligence, vol. 34, pp. 12993–13000 (2020)

Automatic Detection of Polyps Using Deep Learning

Francisco Oliveira[1], Dalila Barbosa[1,2(✉)], Ishak Paçal[3], Danilo Leite[1],
and António Cunha[1,2]

[1] UTAD—University of Trás-os-Montes and Alto Douro, 5001-801 Vila Real, Portugal
`a167530@alunos.utad.pt`, `dalila.i.barbosa@inesctec.pt`, {`danilol`,
`acunha`}`@utad.pt`
[2] INESC TEC—Institute for Systems and Computer Engineering, Technology and Science,
4200-465 Porto, Portugal
[3] Igdir University, Iğdir, Turkey
`ishak.pacal@igdir.edu.tr`

Abstract. Colorectal cancer is a leading health concern worldwide, with late
detection being a primary challenge due to its often-asymptomatic nature. Routine examinations like colonoscopies play a pivotal role in early detection. This
study harnesses the potential of Deep Learning, specifically convolutional neural
networks, in enhancing the accuracy of polyp detection from medical images.
Three distinct models, YOLOv5, YOLOv7, and YOLOv8, were trained on the
PICCOLO dataset, a comprehensive collection of polyp images. The comparative
analysis revealed YOLOv5's submodel S as the most efficient, achieving an accuracy of 92.2%, a sensitivity of 69%, an F1 score of 74% and a mAP of 76.8%,
emphasizing the effectiveness of these networks in polyp detection.

Keywords: Machine learning · polyp detection · colonoscopy · YOLO

1 Introduction

According to GLOBOCAN2020, colorectal cancer is the third most common cancer
worldwide, accounting for approximately 10% of all cases. This malignancy often originates from cells within the intestinal lining, which, over time, may increase into a benign
tumor or polyp. As these polyps grow, they possess an increased risk of malignancy, a
process often influenced by hereditary or spontaneous gene mutations governing cellular
regulation [1].

The presence of such polyps in the colon is a significant public health concern
due to their potential as colorectal cancer precursors. Consequently, the emphasis on
early detection methods, such as colonoscopy, becomes paramount in identifying and
addressing these polyps before their malignant transformation. Effective detection and
prevention strategies are essential for mitigating the incidence of colorectal cancer and
enhancing public health outcomes [2].

A. Cunha et al. (Eds.): MobiHealth 2023, LNICST 578, pp. 254–263, 2024.
https://doi.org/10.1007/978-3-031-60665-6_19

Polyp detection is primarily through colonoscopy, an invasive imaging procedure for the large intestine [3]. However, given its reliance on human interpretation, its effectiveness can vary. Deep learning has emerged as a tool that promises enhanced accuracy in polyp identification.

Deep learning's application in medical imaging is intriguing yet demanding. Legal considerations, especially concerning patient data rights and healthcare providers responsibilities, pose challenges [4]. Additionally, the success of deep learning often hinges on vast data sets, making data scarcity a hurdle to optimize its potential. These challenges, while formidable, invigorate researchers. The allure lies in optimizing medical practices ensuring timely and effective patient care.

This work aims to delve into deep learning models for polyp detection in colonoscopy images and juxtapose their efficacies. It entails exploring deep learning techniques for object detection, sourcing and curating public polyp databases, and training and assessing detection models.

Our research group has been involved in the development of projects using Deep Learning and Convolutional Neural Networks. In [5] is developed an unsupervised method for homography estimation in video capsule endoscopy frames, to be later applied in capsule localization systems. The pipeline is built on an unsupervised convolutional neural network, utilizing a VGG Net architecture, that estimates the homography between two images.

In [6] a variety of CNN models, such as, AlexNet, VGG16, and ResNet, were evaluated, using a transfer learning approach to maximize their efficacy, achieving a precision of 94,0% in lesion detection.

In [7] was explored abnormality classification within an unbalanced dataset of images from capsule endoscopy, using vector features extracted from the pre-trained CNNs to assess the impact of transfer learning with limited samples.

Within this paper, we have structured our content into three primary sections. Section 2 delves into an extensive literature review. Section 3 delineates the research methodology, encapsulating database preparation, training processes, polyp detection techniques, and culminating in model evaluation. Section 4 articulates the findings derived from this research.

2   Related Works

Recent advancements in deep learning techniques have substantially improved pattern recognition capabilities within medical imaging, particularly concerning polyp detection in colonoscopy videos. It follows a brief review of the principal methodologies published for automatic polyp detection in colonoscopy examinations.

A study in [8] revamped the YOLOv4 algorithm for real-time polyp detection using CSPNet and swapped activation and loss functions. Their method achieved 91.6% accuracy on the ETIS-LARIB dataset and 96.0% on the CVC-ColonDB dataset.

In [9], the YOLOv3 and YOLOv4 algorithms use data augmentation and transfer learning. By adjusting activation and loss functions, they achieved an accuracy of 97,0% on the SUN polyp dataset and 92.6% on PICCOLO.

Zhang et al. introduced a two-part CNN pipeline for polyp detection in colonoscopies [10]. Using the ResYOLO detection algorithm refined with colonoscopic images and the Effective Convolution Operators tracker, their method achieved an accuracy of 88.6% and a speed of 6.5 FPS.

Ma et al. [11] highlighted the variance in colonoscopy accuracy due to doctors' expertise and fatigue. They proposed a model based on the SSD_Inception_v2 network, achieving 94.9% accuracy and 93.7% sensitivity in polyp detection.

Nogueira-Rodríguez et al. [12] developed a YOLOv3-based deep learning model for real-time polyp detection, enhanced with object tracking. Trained on 28,576 images, it attained an F1 score of 88,0% for single images and 72.6% sensitivity for videos. The tracking addition improved the model's specificity for CAD system integration. They utilized six diverse datasets, including ImageNet and colonoscopy images. Despite its performance, the model's F1 score dropped by 13.7% on the PICCOLO and SUN datasets.

Qadir et al. [13] devised a polyp detection system using F-RNC, incorporating 2D Gaussian masks for improved polyp segmentation. This method demonstrated 86.6% sensitivity on the ETIS-LARIB dataset and 91,0% sensitivity on the CVC-ColonDB dataset. Another unnamed study using YOLOv3 achieved a 72.6% sensitivity rate.

Wan et al. [14] employed YOLOv5 for polyp detection using the Kvasir-SEG dataset and a local collection named WCY. Their results showed over 90% accuracy for both datasets. Meanwhile, Karaman et al. [15] optimized YOLOv4 with the artificial bee colony algorithm, achieving around 80,0% accuracy on the SUN and PICCOLO polyp datasets.

Gao et al. [16] presented the YOLOv5x-CG model for colorectal lesion detection using an expanded 4949-image dataset from Shanghai Sixth People's Hospital. The model employed image enhancement, k-means clustering for lesion localization, and integrated the Coordinated Attention (CA) and "Ghost" modules. It achieved accuracies of 92,3%, 95,5%, and 87,0% for polyps, adenomas, and cancer, respectively.

In a related study by Gan et al. [17], the YOLOv5x6 model was employed on the EndoCVC dataset of 2910 images, incorporating strategies like data mosaicking and Test Time Augmentation. The model achieved detection scores of 79,5% and 88,2% in two test rounds, indicating its robust performance.

3 Methodology

The methodology used in this work is outlined in the pipeline, shown in Fig. 1.

3.1 Database

The database selected was PICCOLO. It was decided on this type of dataset because it can be considered as an intermediate-level set. It does not suffer from a lack of data, but it will not give us the results that a more extensive database would provide. This dataset provided 3433 images.

The PICCOLO database presents injuries recorded between October 2017 and December 2019 at Basurto University Hospital (Bilbao, Spain). In total, the PICCOLO

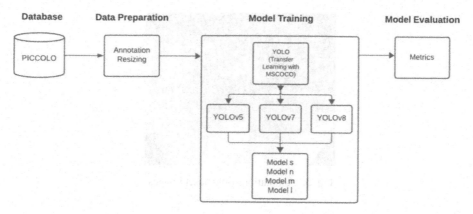

Fig. 1. Methodology pipeline

dataset included 76 lesions from 48 patients. 62 of these 76 lesions have image frames from white light (WI) and narrow-band imaging (NBI). The remaining 14 lesions were recorded using LB only (Fig. 2).

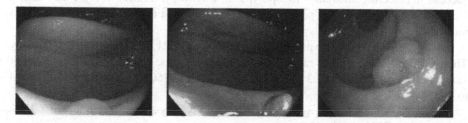

Fig. 2. Sample images from the PICCOLO database.

3.2 Data Preparation

In this study, we divided the images from the PICCOLO dataset in three sets, where 333 images were used in the test set, 2203 in the training set, and 897 in the validation set. Multiple YOLO models were utilized, necessitating the resizing of annotations to the prescribed format. This adaptation was required for the effective functioning of YOLO v5, v7, and v8. Roboflow, a dedicated tool, was used to facilitate these modifications and ensure the annotations were in the correct format. An example of these annotations is illustrated in Fig. 3.

3.3 Model Training

Transfer learning was utilized on YOLO detection models with the MSCOCO dataset, a comprehensive resource with 80 object categories and 330,000 images. This technique

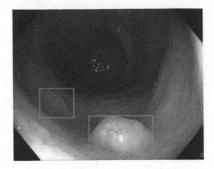

Fig. 3. Annotations on dataset images.

leveraged the MSCOCO-trained network parameters as an initial set for further training on our target datasets.

CNN models were selected for polyp detection, with a focus on the YOLO algorithm because of its speed, accuracy in crowded images, and real-time multi-class detection capabilities. This has made it a favorite in many computer vision tasks. The newer YOLO versions were specifically evaluated, including YOLOv7, v8, and v5, due to its proven success in detecting anomalies like polyps. In this study, models 'n', 's', 'm', and 'l' were tested to compare their performances, from the least to the most computationally intensive.

Models n, s, m, and l have parameters of 1.9M, 7.2M, 21.2M, and 7.2M, respectively. Their GPU processing times range from 45 ms to 224 ms, and they achieve mAP@50 values between 45.7% and 67.3%. Additionally, their mAP50-95 values vary from 28,0% to 49,0%.

YOLOv7, which shares a dataset with YOLOv5, boasts an accuracy of 69.7%, operating at a GPU speed of 3.2 ms.

Meanwhile, the latest YOLOv8 offers five pre-trained models like YOLOv5. These models, n through l, possess parameters ranging from 3.2M to 25.9M. They achieve mAP50-95 values up to 52.9%, and their GPU speeds vary between 0.99 ms and 2.39 ms.

3.4   Model Evaluation

The accuracy of a machine learning model, often defined as the ratio of correctly classified samples, is a commonly used metric for evaluation.

Standard metrics derived from the confusion matrix include sensitivity, specificity, positive predictive value (PPV), negative predictive value (NPV), F1 score, accuracy, and precision.

Considering the True Positives (TP), False Positives (FP), True Negatives (TN) and False Negatives (FN) results obtained by each model in the test set, the following metrics were calculated to evaluate their performance (Table 1).

Mean average precision (mAP) is a key metric for evaluating object detection, like polyp detection. It calculates the average precision per class considering prediction confidence.

Table 1. Metrics and their algebraic expressions.

Metrics	Expression
Precision	$P = \frac{TP}{TP+FP}$
Sensitivity	$P = \frac{TP}{TP+FN}$
F1 Score	$\frac{2 \times TP}{2 \times TP+FN+FP}$

The precision-recall curve shows how well a model classifies in binary tasks, with its shape influenced by classification thresholds. The Area Under the Curve (AUC) is a widely used metric that captures the overall performance of the model across these thresholds.

4 Results and Discussion

The result from this experiment is shown in Table 2, where it is showcased, the results obtained from state-of-the-art methodologies alongside the results from this study. This arrangement offers a comprehensive perspective, allowing for a direct comparison between the current benchmarks in the field and our contributions. The metrics used for the evaluations were accuracy, precision, sensitivity, F1-score, and mAP.

In Fig. 4 we can see the detection made by the models, in YOLOv5, where there are bounding boxes, red and green, that represent the detection made by each model, and the ground truth, respectively.

To perform a comprehensive assessment and identify the YOLO model with the best results a comparative approach was taken. Figure 5 shows the recall-precision curve of each model and reveals YOLOv5 as our dataset's top-performing model for polyp detection despite its training on smaller image sizes.

Table 2. Comparison with the state-of-the-art.

		Results			
Reference	RNC (Recurrent Neural Network)	Precision	Sensibility	F1-Score	mAP
Wan et al. [14]	YOLOv	91,3%	92,1%	91,7%	–
Pacal & Karaboga [8]	YOLOv5	96,0%	96,7%	96.4%	–
Pacal et al. [9]	YOLOv3	92,6%	79,9%	85,8%	97,0%
Karaman et al.[18]	YOLOv5x+ABC	93,3%	77,4%	–	84,5%
YOLOv5	Modelo n	98,0%	70,0%	70,0%	71,1%

(*continued*)

Table 2. (*continued*)

Reference	RNC (Recurrent Neural Network)	Results			
		Precision	Sensibility	F1-Score	mAP
YOLOv5	Modelo s	92,2%	69,0%	74,0%	**76,8%**
YOLOv5	Modelo m	98,9%	67,0%	72,0%	74,6%
YOLOv5	Modelo l	92,8%	58,0%	65,0%	70,4%
YOLOv7	-	97,5%	**75,0%**	**77,0%**	71,3%
YOLOv8	Modelo n	**99,9%**	6,0%	73,0%	71,9%
YOLOv8	Modelo s	**99,9%**	68,0%	73,0%	75,8%
YOLOv8	Modelo m	98,7%	67,0%	69,0%	66,7%
YOLOv8	Modelo l	99,6%	63,0%	70,0%	70,0%

It suggests that reducing image resolution can simplify the network's learning process for specific tasks, enhancing model speed and results. YOLO versions 7 and 8 were trained at a 640 × 640 resolution and showed a slight performance decline of 5.5% and 1%, respectively.

In general, the results were promising when it came to detecting polyps, but the best models were the YOLOv5s, with 76.8% AP, and the YOLOv8s with 75.8% mAP. This can be explained by the size of the data set used, i.e., for model n, if our set were smaller, it would possibly have better results compared to the others. For models larger than models, however, the lack of sufficient data can cause a drop in performance.

One possible reason to the version 5 of YOLO has outperformed more advanced architectures is because the dataset used in the study is not very large, and simpler models, such as YOLOv5, may do better because they have a lower risk of overfitting. More recent versions of YOLO, such as v7 and v8, can be more complex and therefore require larger datasets for effective training.

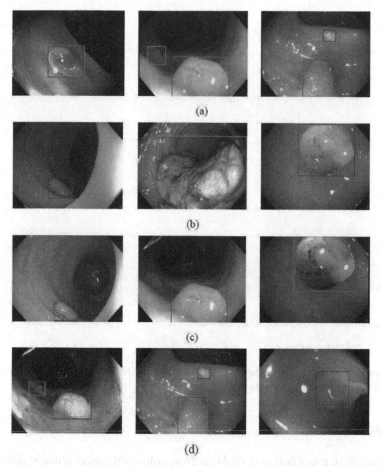

(a)

(b)

(c)

(d)

Fig. 4. Polyp Detection by YOLOv5. a) model l; b) model m; c) model s; d) model n; Red box – Prediction by the model; Green box – Ground Truth (Color figure online)

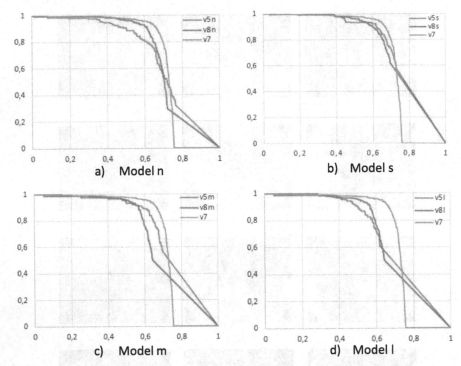

Fig. 5. Comparison of detection models. grey line – YOLOv7; orange line – YOLOv8; blue line – YOLOv5. (Color figure online)

5 Conclusions

Early detection of colon polyps is vital to prevent colorectal cancer, a major global cause of cancer deaths. Recent advances in artificial intelligence, especially convolutional neural networks, have enhanced automated polyp detection in medical imaging. This study is aimed to apply and compare deep learning methods for the identification of colon polyps. Following a brief literature survey, we selected YOLO architectures (YOLOv5, YOLOv7, and YOLOv8) for evaluation, utilizing the Piccolo dataset. Evaluations across the three YOLO iterations identified YOLOv5s as the most proficient, registering a precision of 92.2%, sensitivity of 69,0%, F1 score of 74,0%, and an AP of 76.8%. The scarcity of literature assessing YOLOv7 and YOLOv8 in polyp detection is worth noting, but our findings underscore their prospective utility.

Future research should emphasize training on dedicated colonoscopy datasets, refining pre-trained models for this niche, and leveraging strategies such as K-Fold for optimal parameter tuning.

Acknowledgements. National Funds finance this work through the Portuguese funding agency, FCT - Fundação para a Ciência e a Tecnologia, within project LA/P/0063/2020.

References

1. Henriksen, F.L.: Polyp detection using neural networks-data enhancement and training optimization. MS thesis (2017)
2. Ladabaum, U., et al.: Strategies for colorectal cancer screening. Gastroenterology **158**(2), 418–432 (2020)
3. Sakdyyah, A., Bestari, M.B., Suryanti, S.: Description of colonoscopy and histopathology of chronic diarrhea causes in non-neoplasm: literature review. Indones. J. Gastroenterol. Hepatol. Dig. Endosc. **22**(1), 52–59 (2021)
4. Castiglioni, I., et al.: AI applications to medical images: from machine learning to deep learning. Physica Med. **83**, 9–24 (2021)
5. Gomes, S., et al.: Unsupervised neural network for homography estimation in capsule endoscopy frames. Proc. Comput. Sci. **164**, 602–609 (2019)
6. Ribeiro, J., Nóbrega, S., Cunha, A.: Polyps detection in colonoscopies. Proc. Comput. Sci. **196**, 477–484 (2022)
7. Fonseca, F., et al.: Abnormality classification in small datasets of capsule endoscopy images. Proc. Comput. Sci. **196**, 469–476 (2022)
8. Pacal, I., Karaboga, D.: A robust real-time deep learning based automatic polyp detection system. Comput. Biol. Med. **134**, 104519 (2021)
9. Pacal, I., et al.: An efficient real-time colonic polyp detection with YOLO algorithms trained by using negative samples and large datasets. Comput. Biol. Med. **141**, 105031 (2022)
10. Zhang, R., Poon, C.C.Y.: Regression-based convolutional neural network with a tracker. Comput.-Aided Anal. Gastrointest. Videos 133–139 (2021). https://doi.org/10.1007/978-3-030-64340-9_16
11. Ma, Y., et al.: Polyp location in colonoscopy based on deep learning. In: 2019 8th International Symposium on Next-Generation Electronics (ISNE). IEEE (2019)
12. Nogueira-Rodríguez, A., et al.: Real-time polyp detection model using convolutional neural networks. Neural Comput. Appl. **34**(13), 10375–10396 (2022)
13. Qadir, H.A., et al.: Toward real-time polyp detection using fully CNNs for 2D Gaussian shapes prediction. Med. Image Anal. **68**, 101897 (2021)
14. Wan, J., Chen, B., Yu, Y.: Polyp detection from colorectum images by using attentive YOLOv5. Diagnostics **11**(12), 2264 (2021)
15. Karaman, A., et al.: Hyper-parameter optimization of deep learning architectures using artificial bee colony (ABC) algorithm for high performance real-time automatic colorectal cancer (CRC) polyp detection. Appl. Intell. **53**(12), 15603–15620 (2023)
16. Gao, J., et al.: White-light endoscopic colorectal lesion detection based on improved YOLOv5. Comput. Math. Methods Med. **2022** (2022)
17. Gan, T., et al.: Detection of polyps during colonoscopy procedure using YOLOv5 network. In: EndoCV@ ISBI (2021)
18. Karaman, A., et al.: Robust real-time polyp detection system design based on YOLO algorithms by optimizing activation functions and hyper-parameters with artificial bee colony (ABC). Expert Syst. Appl. **221**, 119741 (2023)

Detection of Landmarks in X-Ray Images Through Deep Learning

Mauro Fernandes[1], Vitor Filipe[1,2], António Sousa[1,2], and Lio Gonçalves[1,2(✉)]

[1] School of Science and Technology University of Trás-os-Montes and Alto Douro
(UTAD), Vila Real 5000-811, Portugal
`al31090@utad.eu`, {`vfilipe,amrs,lgoncalv`}`@utad.pt`
[2] INESC Technology and Science (INESC TEC), Porto 4200-465, Portugal

Abstract. This paper presents a study on the automated detection of landmarks in medical x-ray images using deep learning techniques. In this work we developed two neural networks based on semantic segmentation to automatically detect landmarks in x-ray images, using a dataset of 200 encephalogram images: the UNet architecture and the FPN architecture. The UNet and FPN architectures are compared and it can be concluded that the FPN model, with IoU=0.91, is more robust and accurate in predicting landmarks. The study also had the goal of direct application in a medical context of diagnosing the models and their predictions. Our research team also developed a metric analysis, based on the encephalograms in the dataset, on the type of Mandibular Occlusion of the patients, thus allowing a fast and accurate response in the identification and classification of a diagnosis. The paper highlights the potential of deep learning for automating the detection of anatomical landmarks in medical imaging, which can save time, improve diagnostic accuracy, and facilitate treatment planning. We hope to develop a universal model in the future, capable of evaluating any type of metric using image segmentation.

Keywords: Automated Landmark Detection · Deep Learning · UNet Architecture · FPN Architecture

1 Introduction

The automatic detection of reference points in medical x-ray images has assumed, in the recent past, an increasing importance at the diagnostic level, being considered as essential in a fast, accurate and effective diagnosis so that the treatment of a patient, human or non-human, is done in time in order to increase the success rate of the same.

The fact that it is an automatic but reliable detection increases the accuracy and effectiveness of the diagnosis - it reduces the time needed to analyze the images, so that each specialist can have his or her own opinion on a given image, and minimizing any potential human error. Furthermore, being accurate

A. Cunha et al. (Eds.): MobiHealth 2023, LNICST 578, pp. 264–279, 2024.
https://doi.org/10.1007/978-3-031-60665-6_20

and done automatically, it allows accurate and quantitative measurements to be made, providing highly objective information as an aid to diagnosis. These metrics can include measurements of distance, angles, and even proportions, greatly facilitating timely treatment.

In addition, the automatic detection of landmarks is also especially important in situations where the progression of diseases is being followed and monitored, and the effectiveness of treatments is being assessed. The primary benefit of this diagnostic technique is undoubtedly the standardization of medical image analysis. It ensures that within the medical community, where different specialists may typically provide varying interpretations of images and their conditions, consistent results are obtained. This standardization enhances the reliability and uniformity of the analysis, leading to more accurate diagnosis. By doing this, the ability of artificial intelligence and machine learning to train increasingly better models to detect these points of interest is also increased, thus boosting the automation of clinical processes and improving patient care by allowing the time needed for the interpretation of exams to be reduced and thus allowing health professionals to focus on more complex tasks and direct interaction with patients.

This project will apply the trained models to a specific case - the Mandibular Occlusion, which relates the upper tooth structure to the lower tooth structure. This, as we will refer to later, has three types of classification - Class I (Normal), II (Prominent Maxilla) and III (Protruding Mandible), which is obtained by analyzing the YEN angle, which is the angle formed by the Sella point, the midpoint of the anterior maxilla and the center of a circumference inside the Gnatio.

Throughout this paper we will talk a little about the state of the art in this area, then explain how we carried out our work and end with a presentation of the results and their discussion, along with the conclusions we were able to draw.

2 Related Work

The identification of landmarks in X-ray images through Deep Learning has been an essential task for several clinical procedures, such as alignment analysis, distance measurement and surgery planning. In recent years, the use of Deep Learning techniques has driven significant advances in this area, providing accurate and automated results.

However, and according to [1], the exclusive use of Deep Learning for automatic landmark detection in medical radiography images, despite having a relatively high accuracy also has a rather high risk of bias. It is therefore necessary to increase robustness and to develop new techniques that use Deep Learning as a basis to increase the reliability of studies involving this method.

One of the notable advances in this field is related to the detection of anatomical points in dental radiographs [2]. Using convolutional neural networks (CNNs), it has been possible to train models capable of accurately identifying landmarks such as the root apex, cusps, and reference lines. These automated models have shown results comparable and, in some cases, even superior to traditional methods, saving time and resources for dental professionals. Another approach to the problem proposed the use of convolutional neural networks combined with recurrent neural networks (RNNs) to identify specific anatomical landmarks, such as the tooth root and periodontal structures. This approach showed promising results, outperforming traditional manual identification methods, and providing a detailed analysis of tooth morphology.

Another proposal presents a novel learning framework for detecting anatomical landmarks in medical images, including panoramic radiographs [8]. This work uses deep learning and reinforcement learning to optimize the target accuracy in detecting multiple landmarks. The proposed method is evaluated on two datasets, one of prenatal ultrasound and another of cephalometric x-rays, demonstrating improved training stability and enhanced localization accuracy. The promising results of this study suggest that the framework can be effectively applied to landmark detection in panoramic radiographs, providing a valuable tool for health professionals in diagnosing and planning dental treatments.

In another study, an attention mechanism that incorporates multidimensional information and separates spatial dimensions is proposed [7]. This novel method is evaluated on a dataset of pelvic radiographs and demonstrates excellent performance compared to other landmark detection models. The results obtained indicate the effectiveness of this attention mechanism in accurately identifying anatomical landmarks in the pelvic region, providing a valuable tool for healthcare professionals in this field, making this automated approach one that promises to facilitate and expedite diagnosis and treatment planning, improving the efficiency and quality of patient care.

Another notable advance is focused on X-ray imaging of the spine, in which a new specialized landmark detection network is presented [6]. The proposed network consists of two stages and uses techniques such as random spinal slice augmentation and CoordConv to improve detection accuracy. These techniques allow to identify the centers of lumbar vertebrae and corners of vertebrae more accurately in X-ray images. The results obtained demonstrate high accuracy in detecting these landmarks, which can assist radiologists in analyzing lumbar x-ray images, providing important information for diagnosis and treatment planning related to spinal conditions.

Also, in the realm of spine evaluation, another study argued that the balance of the human spine depends on the accurate measurement of sagittal radiographic parameters [3]. In this study, deep learning models capable of automatically locating anatomical landmarks and generating radiographic parameters from lateral radiographs of the spine were developed. Based on a large number of annotated images, the models achieved high accuracy in locating landmarks in different areas of the spine. Moreover, the radiographic parameters predicted by the models showed a significant correlation with the actual values. Comparing the performance of the models with human intelligence, it was deduced that the deep learning model achieved results comparable to those of physicians on several parameters. This automated approach provides an accurate analysis of spinal alignment, assisting medical professionals in the diagnosis and treatment of spinal diseases.

Another application demonstrates that the use of deep learning on chest X-Ray has shown promising results on several tasks [4]. Image-level classification and regression enable the detection and diagnosis of lung diseases, such as pneumonia and lung cancer, with increasing accuracy. Segmentation aids in the precise delineation of anatomical structures, enabling the identification and measurement of lesions with greater accuracy. In addition, landmark localization and synthetic image generation contribute to the improvement of surgical planning techniques and procedure simulation. Domain adaptation enables knowledge transfer between different datasets, extending the practical applications of deep learning models. However, it is important to note that the use of public datasets has limitations, as they do not always reflect the diversity of clinical cases encountered in practice. Therefore, future research is needed to fill existing gaps and develop clinically useful systems that can handle the complexity and variability of chest radiography.

A different but interesting approach was debated in [5], where they aimed to develop an automated calibration system to make linear measurements in lateral cephalometric radiographs more efficient. The system was based on deep learning algorithms and previous medical knowledge of a stable structure, the anterior cranial base (Sella-Nasion). A two-step cascaded convolutional neural network was constructed based on 2860 cephalograms to locate the Sella, Nasion and 2 ruler points in regions of interest. The accuracy of automated landmark localization, ruler length prediction, and linear measurement based on automated calibration was evaluated with statistical analysis, with this high accuracy attributed to the inclusion of diverse training data and the application of prior medical knowledge of anatomically stable structures.

In summary, the use of deep learning techniques has revolutionized landmark identification in radiographies. Automated anatomical landmark detection in various radiographic modalities, such as dental, panoramic, cephalometric, thoracic, and orthopedic, has shown accurate and efficient results. These automated approaches can save time, improve diagnostic accuracy, and facilitate treatment planning, benefiting both healthcare professionals and patients.

3   Development

The main goal of this study was to develop a neural network that could automatically detect landmarks in X-ray images through Deep Learning. Two approaches were then developed in order to create two models capable of successfully predicting landmarks in a new untrained X-ray image.

3.1   Dataset

Our dataset consisted of 200 completely random encephalogram images from a pack of 400 images available on Kaggle, with all of them being right lateral x-ray images of the skull of different people with different anatomies, as depicted in Fig. 1. The aim of our work, by using only half of the available dataset, was

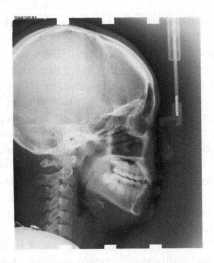

Fig. 1. Encephalogram.

to try to develop a model that would achieve reliable results even in a context where there wasn't a very large dataset for training. The original images were all 1935×2400 in size and .jpg format. They were divided, for training, validation and testing purposes, into a $60/20/20\%$ ratio (120 images for training, 40 images for validation and 40 images for testing).

Before starting the pre-processing of the 200 images, we marked 6 landmarks on all of the images as shown in Fig. 2. The points in question were the S point (Sella), M point (Midpoint of the Anterior Maxilla), the G point (Center of a circle inside the Gnatio point), the N point (Tip of the Nose), SL (Superior Lip) and IL (Inferior Lip). The choice of some of these points was not random, but rather to later calculate the YEN angle to determine the type of mandibular occlusion present in each encephalogram, as we will discuss in the results section. The resulting files, in .json format, were used to collect the coordinates of each of the points in a .csv file, using a script that performs the extraction of the points' coordinates in each of the images.

3.2   Pre-Processing

After extracting the coordinates and grouping them into .csv files for training, validation and testing purposes, a preprocessing is performed on the images in order to facilitate the further processing of the model.

Firstly the original images are loaded and transformed to grayscale and pixels are normalized. The coordinates of the landmarks are used to define rectangular regions in the mask, with dimension 20×20, defining the pixels corresponding to that region as having the value "1". After creating the masks, we resized images and masks to the model's input size, 256×256.

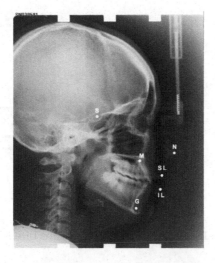

Fig. 2. Marking Landmarks in LabelMe.

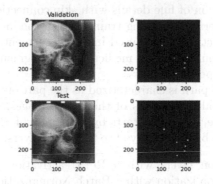

Fig. 3. Verification of the Pre-Processing.

Finally, vertical stacking of the training and validation images and masks is performed in order to create appropriate input matrices for the models.

To verify if the pre-processing was done well, the first validation image and mask is previewed, as well as the first image and mask from the testing set, to ensure that it conforms to the processing done to the image and mask sets, as represented in Fig. 3.

3.3 UNet Architecture

The first architecture we developed throughout this project was an architecture called "UNet" - a U-shaped architecture with a downsampling path and an upsampling path, with skip connections between the encoding and decoding paths to allow for fine detail reconstruction, as Fig. 4. This architecture presents fundamental characteristics for a project with the dimension of this study, due

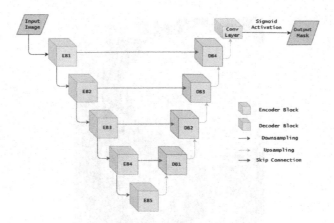

Fig. 4. Proposed UNet architecture.

to its ease of training models with small datasets. In addition, and as mentioned above, the reconstruction of fine details with skip connections and also the possibility of reducing overfitting during training with the introduction of dropout layers. It is an architecture widely used in image segmentation tasks and, with special relevance for our study, in medical image segmentation, thanks to its proven flexibility and performance.

The downsampling path is characterized as the part of the model responsible for reducing the spatial dimensions of the input images, as well as extracting fine details. In our case, this path starts by defining a block (which we will refer to as Block 1). In this block, we have the following layers:

– Two 2D convolution layers with a ReLU activation function and a "he-normal" weight initialization with a Batch Normalization layer in between.
– A dropout layer.
– A Max Pooling layer

Blocks 2,3,4 and 5 follow, with the structure very similar to Block 1. However, the number of filters doubles with each new block in order to capture more complex features as the network goes deeper.

However, there are some differences in certain blocks, relative to Block 1, that are important to note:

– In block 4 there is no dropout layer added, in order to extract features critical to the network's ability to train and learn.
– Blocks 4 and 5 do not have the Max Pooling layer.

The output of each of the blocks is fed to the input of the next block, and each of these outputs is also characterized by having a skip connection to the upsampling path.

The upsampling path is characterized by being the part of the model responsible for reconstructing the spatial resolution of the images from the features obtained in the downsampling path - features obtained by passing between the different blocks and by skip connections.

In our case, the upsampling path starts with a block, which we will call block 6:

- A transposed convolution layer.
- This is followed by a concatenation with the output of a coding block that received the information from the skip connections, allowing the fusion of low resolution information with fine details.
- Two 2D convolution layers with a ReLU activation function and a "he-normal" weight initialization with a Batch Normalization layer in between.

Blocks 7, 8 and 9 are exactly the same as block 6, with a difference in that each layer of transposed convolution and concatenation is followed by convolution followed by BatchNormalization. In the specific case of block 9, a flag is set in order to control whether there is an additional layer of convolution and Batch-Normalization - the variable "output" is optional, and if it is "True", we have 3 layers followed by convolution interleaved with BatchNormalization, and if it is "False", this additional layer is not included. This last step assumes special relevance because it is a step that can affect the performance and generalization ability of the model, being possible to adjust, by experimentation, according to the objective of the work.

At the end of all this process, we then have the addition of a final convolution layer with a sigmoidal activation (this choice falls on the fact that it is a classification function that returns a probability of each pixel belonging, or not, to the class of interest).

3.4   FPN Architecture

The second architecture developed throughout this project was an architecture called FPN - Feature Pyramid Network, chosen because it is an architecture widely used for semantic image segmentation, mainly thanks to its ability to handle objects at different scales. As with UNet, this type of architecture also has an encoding path, but then builds a FPN on the decoder path, as Fig. 5 shows.

This architecture is based on the same block system used in UNet. The encoding blocks all have the same type and the same number of layers and are called "ConvBlock". These blocks have the same type and the same number of layers:

- Two 2D convolution layers with a ReLU activation function.
- In between the convolution layers we have two BatchNormalization layers.

The encoder is the part of the model responsible for extracting high quality features at different scales from the input image. The main part of the encoding path is composed of 4 blocks (Block 1, 2, 3 and 4) with an increasing number

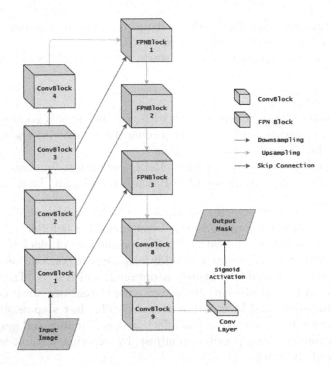

Fig. 5. Proposed FPN architecture.

of filters, where in each block a MaxPooling layer is added in order to halve the spatial dimension of the features.

After Block 4, the FPN is then built on the decoding path, responsible for refining the segmentation with the features obtained during the encoding process, while reconstructing the spatial resolution of the segmented image. The FPN has 3 blocks, with each of them being organized as follows and nominated "FPNBlock":

- An initial layer with a 2×2 stride transposed convolution, called the "up" layer.
- A "skip connection" is added between the initial layer of each block and a convolutional layer of the higher spatial resolution encoder, and a 1×1 filter and ReLU activation function is applied to this layer to combine the high-level information from the "up" layer with the information from the layer that has the higher spatial resolution.
- The outputs from the "up" layer and the "skip connection" layer are added element by element in order to combine the information from the two layers and thus allow the network to use both the high-level and lower-level features together.
- Finally, the result of this addition goes through the "ConvBlock" block, thus refining the combined features, capturing more details and improving the quality of the segmentation.

As mencioned before, this operation is performed three times (on Blocks 5,6 and 7), until two additional "ConvBlock" are added to the decoder in order to further refine the features and obtain finer details (Blocks 8 and 9). The output layer is then created with a 1×1 convolution in order to generate a segmentation map, where sigmoidal activation was used in order to produce a classification function that returns the probability of a pixel belonging, or not, to the class of interest, as happened in the UNet architecture.

3.5 Compiling and Training the Models

Before proceeding to the explanation of model compilation and training, it is first necessary to talk about the Dice Coefficient. This metric is usually used to evaluate the degree of overlap (or similarity) between two binary masks - in this specific case, between the segmentation masks generated by the model and the reference masks (generated by the true labels resulting from marking the coordinates of the points and, later, the development of a region around it in the pre-processing of the images). The Dice Coefficient measures the similarity between the predicted segmentarion region and its corresponding ground truth, with its formula described in (1), where we have set the epsilon value to be $1 * 10^{-7}$.

$$\text{Dice Coeff} = \frac{2 * \sum (y_{\text{true}} * y_{\text{pred}}) + \varepsilon}{\sum y_{\text{true}} + \sum y_{\text{pred}} + \varepsilon} \tag{1}$$

For training purposes, we will use the complementary function of the Dice Coefficient, called Dice Loss, as described in (2), where we calculate the difference between the perfect overlap, 1, and the evaluation given by the Dice Coefficient.

$$\text{Dice Loss} = 1 - DiceCoeff \tag{2}$$

Another metric we used in order to better evaluate the robustness and effectiveness of our model was the Root Mean Squared Error (RMSE). This metric is usually used to evaluate the difference between predicted values by a model (on our study case, the landmarks location) and the true values (those marked in LabelMe). It is calculated as the formula bellow shows (3), and it measures the average magnitude of the prediction errors. In terms of results - a value as close to zero indicates that there is almost no error between true labels and predicted labels, while a big value indicates that there is a discrepancy between the true and predicted labels. In the formula (3), the "n" value stands for the number of samples, while the ytrue and ypred are, respectively, the real labels and the predicted ones.

$$RMSE = \sqrt{\frac{\sum (y_{\text{pred}} - y_{\text{true}})^2}{n}} \tag{3}$$

The models were compiled taking into account the same parameters for the purpose of getting a better and trustful comparison between them:

- Adam optimizer with a learning rate of 0.001 was used.
- The loss function, as mentioned earlier, was set to be the complementary function of the Dice Coefficient.
- As metrics for the evaluation of the model both the Dice Coefficient and the RMSE were used.

The training of both models was then performed, via Google Collaboration, using their T4 GPU, 12GB RAM and 78GB disk configuration. As a definition of the training, we have the following:

- The vertically stacked matrices of the training images and training masks are used as training data.
- The batch size during training was set to be 32.
- The number of training epochs was set to be 200.
- An additional parameter, consisting of the vertically stacked matrices of validation images and validation masks, is added in order to check the performance of the model against this validation set during training.
- A callback function called "ReduceLROnPlateau" is defined, in order to dynamically adjust the learning rate during training. It was established that the variable in question would be the Dice Loss of the validation set, with a "patience" parameter of 10 and a "factor" parameter of 0.5 - after 10 consecutive epochs with no improvement in the validation Dice Loss, the learning rate is halved.

In terms of training time, Unet's architecture took 38 min to train the model, while FPN took only 28 min to complete the training.

To avoid future repetitions of the training, both models were saved at the end of the training, thus allowing them to be used in a much faster way in the future.

4   Results and Discussion

4.1   Training Metrics

$$IoU = \frac{\text{Intersection}}{\text{Union}} \tag{4}$$

After the training process of both models is done, we can then compare the results of the metrics defined as the evaluators of the training - the Dice Coefficient and the RMSE. Throughout the 200 training epochs, the Dice Coefficient and RMSE values were recorded, as documented in Table 1. We then made a measurement to find out how the model performed in the testing set using the Intersection over Union (IoU) metric, as shown in the formula (4). This is a metric that can also be known as Jaccard Index and represents the overlap between two sets - in this specific case it was calculated taking into account the overlap between the true mask and the predicted mask by each of the models, and the results are as recorded in the Table 2.

Table 1. Evaluation of Training Metrics

Model	Dice Coefficient		RMSE		Training Time
	Training	Validation	Training	Validation	(min.)
UNet	0.8426	0.7054	0.0233	0.0409	38
FPN	0.8900	0.7021	0.0198	0.0338	28

Table 2. Evaluation of Testing Set Metrics

Model	IoU
UNet	0.8342
FPN	0.9117

By analysing all the data collected, it is pretty much clear that these metrics indicate that the FPN model is more robust than the UNet model.

4.2 Predictions

The final tests were then done to see if the models could accurately detect landmarks on images that had not been trained - the images belonging to our testing set, with 40 images that were completely random and different from the training and validation sets.

To do this testing we ran the images one by one, trying to have the model of each architecture predict where the landmarks would be, thus creating a mask with those landmarks. Then we manipulated the dimensions of the test images, using the "squeeze" function to remove any unitary dimensions, doing the same with the mask generated by the models. Next, we made a figure with 4 subplots - the original test image, the actual mask created by marking the points in LabelMe, the original test image with the predicted mask applied, and finally the predicted mask, as shown in Figs. 6 and 7, both being representatives of the same test image for comparison reasons. As can be seen here, both models are extremely accurate in terms of mask definition.

4.3 Application in YEN Angle Calculation

As mentioned before, our study was not only about the automatic identification of landmarks on x-rays using Deep Learning but also about trying to use precise metrics that would allow for a quick and effective diagnostic situation. In our project, we chose to mark 6 points in each image, but will only use 3 for the calculations needed for the next step - the S point (Sella), the M point (Midpoint of the Anterior Maxilla) and the G point (Center of a circle inside the Gnatio point). These three points, when connected by vectors, form an angle between them called the YEN angle.

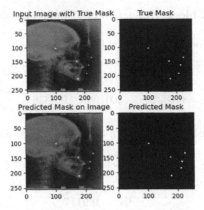

Fig. 6. Prediction made by the UNet Model.

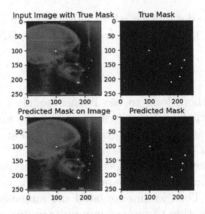

Fig. 7. Prediction made by the FPN Model.

This YEN angle is a direct metric in the evaluation of a patient's Mandibular Occlusion. It is a metric characterized by having 3 different classifications, which will now be explained:

- A YEN angle with amplitude between 117 and 123° demonstrates a Class I type of occlusion, which is the so-called normal/ideal occlusion.
- A YEN angle with amplitude below 117° is representative of a Class II type of Occlusion, which indicates a protruding maxilla.
- A YEN angle with amplitude above 123° points to a Class III type of Occlusion, which indicates that the patient has a prominent mandible.

Since our code created an ROI around the pointed landmark and the predicted mask returns small ROIs around each landmark, we calculate the centroid of each of these ROIs in order to do the YEN angle calculation. To do this step, we first converted the predicted binary mask into a label image. Next, we extracted the properties of the regions present in the label image using the

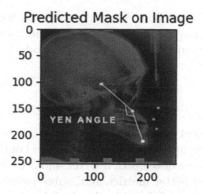

Fig. 8. YEN Angle on Predicted Mask.

"skimage" module, thus removing the information of interest for our problem - the centroid coordinates. To conclude this step, and in preparation for the next step, these centroids are converted into numpy arrays.

To calculate the angle YEN, we defined a function responsible for calculating the vectors of the segments "S-M" and "G-M" by subtracting the coordinates. Then we normalized each of these vectors by dividing them by their length, and finally used the mathematical expression in (5) in order to calculate the angle.

$$YEN = \cos^{-1}\left(\frac{v_{SM}.v_{GM}}{\|v_{SM}\| * \|v_{GM}\|}\right), \tag{5}$$

with $v_{SM} = (x_{SM}, y_{SM})$ and $v_{GM} = (x_{GM}, y_{GM})$.

By placing the 3 points (defined as S, M and G) we were then able to immediately get the value of the YEN angle of the person in question. In the test image of the FPN model, 8, the feedback was that the patient had a YEN angle of 150°. As mentioned earlier, it was then clear that the patient had prominent mandible.

4.4   Results Discussion

By analysing all the data we collected in our study, it is clear now that our FPN architecture produces a better and more robust model, capable of accurately predicting landmarks in medical images. The capability of this architecture to handle objects at different scales, alongside with feature sharing between different resolutions, makes the FPN model a success. However, slightly less robust but equally efficient, our UNet model proved itself to be capable of acurately predicting landmarks in medical images as well.

However, an issue arose throughout the process in which we developed our project - the issue of marking the landmarks. The fact that this marking is done by non-health professionals can lead to erroneous markings that will affect the training of the model and, consequently, the diagnosis.

We are left with the firm belief that with a professionally prepared dataset and prepared in such a way that the clinical case under study is well represented proportionally (i.e. without class imbalance) the model can take on even greater robustness.

5   Conclusion

The purpose of this project was to develop an architecture, based on Deep Learning, that would allow the automatic identification of landmarks in X-ray images.

Two architectures were developed, a UNet and a FPN, where it was verified that the FPN presented better metrics and, subsequently, more reliable results for the medical application of the work developed.

It was noted that the FPN model is faster in terms of training, without its speed disallowing the return of accurate landmarks, where it shone as extremely accurate and efficient. The UNet model, on the other hand, trained slowly, but still managed to detect the landmarks with high accuracy. These informations lead us to conclude that the FPN model, being faster and more accurate, is the better of the two models, showing a very high robustness.

This study also had as an additional goal the direct application in a medical context of diagnosing the models and their predictions. It was possible to develop a metric analysis, based on the encephalograms in the dataset, on the type of Mandibular Occlusion of the patients, thus allowing a fast and accurate response in the identification and classification of a diagnosis.

It is clear that these types of models are of particular clinical importance. Fast, accurate, and objective analysis of metrics can greatly facilitate the diagnostic process, enabling faster access to care/treatment, more personalized care for each patient, and allowing health professionals to have more time for even greater care for their patients.

The accuracy that has been obtained, in a diagnostic context, shows that a model with this architecture can easily calculate any type of metric that is based on landmarks - from hip dysplasia to scoliosis to osteoarthritis, various diseases can have their treatment and diagnosis made easier using tools of this type.

We hope that with the development of this project and study, we have a solid foundation to develop a universal model in the future, capable of evaluating any type of metric using image segmentation, something as simple as taking an x-ray and inserting the image for the model to predict the necessary landmarks, thus facilitating the entire process of diagnosis and subsequent treatment/follow-up.

References

1. Schwendicke, F., et al.: Deep learning for cephalometric landmark detection: systematic review and meta-analysis. Clin. Oral Invest. **25**, 4299–4309 (2021)
2. Reddy, P., Kanakatte, A., Gubbi, J., Poduval, M., Ghose, A., Purushothaman, B.: Anatomical landmark detection using deep appearance-context network. In: 2021 43rd Annual International Conference Of The IEEE Engineering In Medicine & Biology Society (EMBC), pp. 3569–3572 (2021)

3. Yeh, Y., Weng, C., Huang, Y., Fu, C., Tsai, T., Yeh, C.: Deep learning approach for automatic landmark detection and alignment analysis in whole-spine lateral radiographs. Sci. Rep. **11**, 7618 (2021)
4. Çallı, E., Sogancioglu, E., Ginneken, B., Leeuwen, K., Murphy, K.: Deep learning for chest X-ray analysis: a survey. Med. Image Anal. **72**, 102125 (2021)
5. Jiang, F., et al.: Automated calibration system for length measurement of lateral cephalometry based on deep learning. Phys. Med. Biol. **67**, 225016 (2022)
6. An, C., Lee, J., Jang, J., Choi, H.: Part affinity fields and CoordConv for detecting landmarks of lumbar vertebrae and sacrum in X-ray images. Sensors. **22**, 8628 (2022)
7. Pei, Y., et al.: Learning-based landmark detection in pelvis x-rays with attention mechanism: data from the osteoarthritis initiative. Biomed. Phys. Eng. Express **9**, 025001 (2023)
8. Zhou, G., et al.: Learn fine-grained adaptive loss for multiple anatomical landmark detection in medical images. IEEE J. Biomed. Health Inform. **25**, 3854–3864 (2021)

Performance Analysis of CNN Models in the Detection and Classification of Diabetic Retinopathy

Francisca Lúcio[1], Vitor Filipe[1,2], and Lio Gonçalves[1,2(✉)]

[1] School of Science and Technology University of Trás-os-Montes e Alto Douro (UTAD), 5000-811 Vila Real, Portugal
al74596@alunos.utad.pt, {vfilipe,lgoncalv}@utad.pt
[2] INESC Technology and Science (INESC TEC), 4200-465 Porto, Portugal

Abstract. This study focuses on investigating different CNN architectures and assessing their effectiveness in classifying Diabetic Retinopathy, a diabetes-associated disease that ranks among the primary causes of adult blindness. However, early detection can significantly prevent its debilitating consequences. While regular screening is advised for diabetic patients, limited access to specialized medical professionals can hinder its implementation. To address this challenge, deep learning techniques provide promising solutions, primarily through their application in the analysis of fundus retina images for diagnosis.

Several CNN architectures, including MobileNetV2, VGG16, VGG19, InceptionV3, InceptionResNetV2, Xception, DenseNet121, ResNet50, ResNet50V2, and EfficientNet (ranging from EfficientNetB0 to EfficientNetB6), were implemented to assess and analyze their performance in classifying Diabetic Retinopathy. The dataset comprised 3662 Fundus retina images. Prior to training, the networks underwent pre-training using the ImageNet database, with a Gaussian filter applied to the images as a preprocessing step. As a result, the Efficient-Net stands out for achieving the best performance results with a good balance between model size and computational efficiency. By utilizing the EfficientNetB2 network, a model was trained with an accuracy of 85% and a screening capability of 98% for Diabetic Retinopathy. This model holds the potential to be implemented during the screening stages of Diabetic Retinopathy, aiding in the early identification of individuals at risk.

Keywords: Diabetic retinopathy · Deep Learning · Classification · Detection · Convolutional neural network (CNN)

A. Cunha et al. (Eds.): MobiHealth 2023, LNICST 578, pp. 280–294, 2024.
https://doi.org/10.1007/978-3-031-60665-6_21

1   Introduction

Diabetic retinopathy (DR) is caused by the long-term effects of diabetes. This is a common disease that was estimated, in 2020, to affect 103.12 million people worldwide, and by 2045 this number is projected to increase to 160.50 million [1].

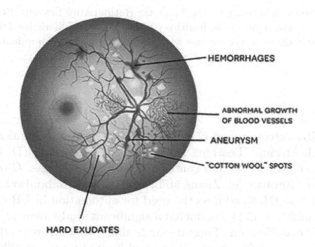

Fig. 1. Diabetic Retinopathy diagram. Image source: [24]

Diabetic retinopathy is characterized by high levels of glucose in the bloodstream causing the vascular formation of retinal microaneurysms and hemorrhages (Fig. 1), complications that may lead to cotton wool spots, hard exudates and tractional retinal detachment [25]. It is a serious public health problem being the leading cause of blindness. However, it is possible to prevent vision loss, with timely interventions and early detections, achieved by performing regular eye screenings.

The diagnosis is typically conducted by an ophthalmologist who classifies its severity into five stages (Fig. 2), according to the Diabetic Retinopathy Severity Scale [2]. DR screening is performed through fundus photography that captures the images of the retina, optic nerve head, macula, retinal blood vessels, choroid, and the vitreous [26]. Although fundus cameras have become more accessible in primary hospitals, a shortage of experienced ophthalmologists capable of conducting regular screenings, as recommended (at least annually) [3], remains a challenge. Consequently, there is a growing need for automated techniques, such as Deep Learning, to assist in DR diagnosis. The development of Deep Learning applications, in a variety of clinical settings, plays a critical role for accurate DR detection and classification. It can assist DR referrals and slow down the disease progression of patients in remote or poor areas. It can also assist clinicians in confirming their diagnosis [12].

This study aims to compare the performance of Deep Learning models for diabetic retinopathy detection and classification.

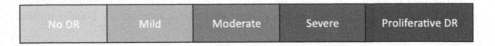

Fig. 2. Five classes according to the Diabetic Retinopathy Severity Scale. The first stage (No DR) corresponds to a healthy patient while Proliferative DR is the end-stage of advanced diabetic eye disease with vision-threatening complications.

1.1   Literature Review

The field of DR detection and classification has witnessed significant advancements through Machine Learning (ML) and Deep Learning (DL) techniques, with several noteworthy studies contributing to this progress. Giroti et al. [8], Dutta et al. [5], Revathy [6], Zhang and Nabil [9] and Alabdulwahhab et al. [4] harnessed ML and DL to address the need for automation in DR diagnosis.

Alabdulwahhab et al. [4] conducted a significant study focusing on ML techniques for DR classification. Their research aimed to address challenges in DR screening, including high patient volume and limited resources. They employed various ML algorithms, achieving 86% accuracy with the ranger random forest classifier.

In a parallel effort, Revathy [6] utilized a machine learning approach, emphasizing crucial feature extraction. Their dataset of 1000 Kaggle-sourced images underwent preprocessing, including color space conversion and filtering. For classification, they employed a hybrid approach that integrated Support Vector Machine (SVM), K Nearest Neighbors (KNN), Random Forest, Logistic Regression, and Multilayer Perceptron Network, achieving a testing accuracy of 82%. This approach demonstrates ML and image processing potential in enhancing DR detection.

Dutta et al. [5] proposed an automated knowledge model that leveraged a range of deep learning models, encompassing backpropagation Neural Networks (NN), Deep Neural Networks (DNN), and Convolutional Neural Networks (CNN). Significantly, their deep learning models outperformed the conventional NN model, underscoring the importance of intricate neural architectures for feature quantification. Furthermore, Dutta et al. [5] highlighted the significance of image preprocessing, including grayscale conversion and noise reduction through filters, which notably improved their results.

Similarly, Giroti et al. [8] conducted thorough data preprocessing, involving resizing, cropping, noise reduction, and feature detection, to enhance image quality and emphasize critical features. Their approach incorporated the EfficientNet model, aiming for an ambitious accuracy range of 87-95%. This research holds pivotal significance as it addresses the imperative need for automation in DR

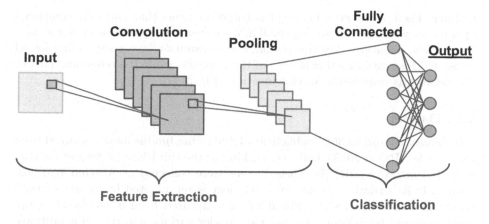

Fig. 3. Convolutional Neural Networks Diagram.

diagnosis, given the expected surge in data volume and limited availability of highly skilled professionals.

Additionally, Zhang and Nabil [9] introduced two distinct solutions to the challenge of Diabetic Retinopathy (DR) classification. In their initial approach, they introduced a shallow neural network architecture, which performed admirably in classifying the most frequent classes but faced challenges with less frequent ones. In their second approach, they leveraged a transfer learning-based method, employing the Efficientnet-B3 architecture, which significantly outperformed their shallow neural network architecture, particularly in classifying less frequent DR categories. This research underscores the superiority of transfer learning and the significance of utilizing pre-trained models on extensive datasets. It offers compelling advantages in improving DR classification accuracy, even for classes with limited representation in the dataset.

Of particular interest is the EfficientNet model, which has emerged as a standout performer in this field. EfficientNet not only achieves remarkable accuracy but also operates with exceptional efficiency, surpassing the capabilities of traditional Convolutional Neural Network (CNN) architectures [8,9,20]. This demonstrates its capacity to address the intricate challenges associated with DR diagnosis.

2   Methods

For the performance analysis of using Deep Learning in the detection and classification of diabetic retinopathy, there were trained and tested 16 Convolutional Neural Networks (CNN) models.

The CNN architectures are specifically designed to process and analyze visual data, such as images. This is possible due to their ability to accept 2D arrays as input. Their inspiration came from the human visual system [7]. Similarly, to the human visual system, CNNs are designed by multiple layers in a hierarchical manner. Their architectural concept is based on layers that apply convolutional operations, which involve sliding small filters across the input data to extract and learn relevant features. For this reason, the convolution layers are often referred to as "the feature extraction layers" of the network, while the remaining part of the network is responsible for classification (Fig. 3) [7].

2.1   Dataset

The dataset comprises 3662 publicly available retina fundus images sourced from the Kaggle APTOS 2019 Challenge, ranking as the third-largest dataset for Diabetic Retinopathy (DR) [7]. These images were collected at Aravind Eye hospital in India's rural areas and every subject is represented by images of both their right and left eyes [8]. The data was captured from a variety of equipment operated by different professionals, under various non-typical conditions. Consequently, the dataset exhibits variability in terms of image size, brightness, and, occasionally, focus. All these factors contribute to noise which causes difficulties for the algorithms to accurately classify DR. Precisely to reduce the noise from the dataset, and to achieve better color constancy, a Gaussian filter was systematically applied to all images [9]. The images were also resized into 224×224 pixels so that they can be readily used with pre-trained deep-learning models. Samples of the outcome of the pre-processing procedure are depicted in Fig. 4. Nevertheless, considering the presence of low-quality images that accurately represent the actual data, the algorithm can be effective in practical clinical applications [10].

Every image is annotated and sorted according to the stages of DR (Fig. 5). One limitation of this dataset is the large class imbalance, especially between the "No DR" and all the other classes (Fig. 6). This will heavily influence the capacity of the model to correctly classify the stages of diabetic retinopathy. The dataset was partitioned into three distinct subsets, training, validation, and testing, in order to facilitate the respective stages of model development and evaluation, as seen in Fig. 7. This procedural step has significant importance as it ensures impartial evaluation and mitigates the risk of overfitting.

2.2   CNN Architectures

In this study, a total of 16 Convolutional Neural Network (CNN) models were trained and evaluated, each employing a distinct architecture. The applied architectures were the following:

MobileNetV2. Is a network with the aim to optimize CNN architecture for mobile and embedded devices by creating a compact, power-efficient design that maintains high performance [13]. This was achieved by implementing 'depthwise separable convolution,' which decomposes the standard convolution into two distinct layers: depthwise convolution and pointwise convolution. The primary objective of testing this network was to assess whether a "lightweight" network could achieve satisfactory results in the classification of diabetic retinopathy.

VGG16 and VGG19. Are CNN models comprising 16 and 19 layers, respectively, which consist of repeated sequences of 3×3 convolutional and 2×2 pooling layers. Their uniform structure simplifies model comprehension and implementation, making them widely used choices for image classification and feature extraction [10, 14].

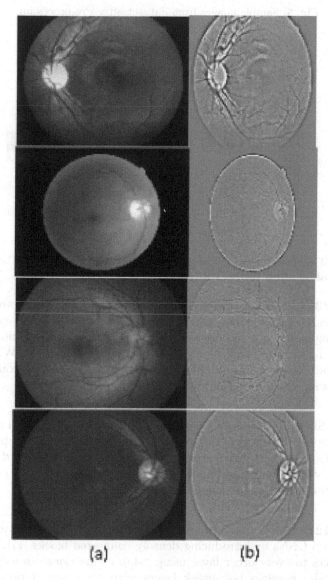

(a)   (b)

Fig. 4. (a) Sample of fundus image from APTOS 2019; (b) Corresponding sample, processed with a Gaussian filter and resized to dimensions of 254×254 pixels.

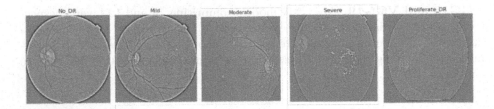

Fig. 5. Sample images from dataset after Pre-processing

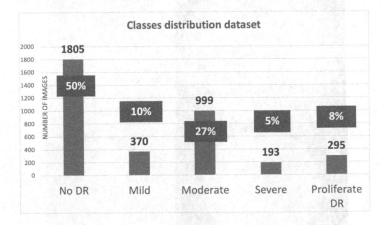

Fig. 6. Visual representation of classes distribution of the dataset; There are 3662 images in total, in which the No DR represents close to 50%.

InceptionV3 and InceptionResNetV2. Both architectures are based on inception modules, comprising parallel convolutional layers with various filter sizes, enabling multi-scale and multi-level feature extraction. InceptionResNetV2 goes a step further by incorporating residual connections [15]. While achieving strong performance, InceptionResNetV2 can demand more computational resources compared to InceptionV3 [11].

Xception. Short for "Extreme Inception", enhances the Inception architecture by employing depthwise separable convolution. This innovative approach separates spatial and channel-wise features [16], reducing parameters and operations, leading to faster training and inference. It enables the network to capture fine-grained spatial details while maintaining expressive power.

DenseNet121. Was developed to enhance information flow and parameter efficiency in deep CNNs by introducing densely connected blocks [17], where each layer connects to every other layer using "skip connections" in a feed-forward manner. It also employs bottleneck layers with 1×1 convolutions to reduce model complexity, achieving a balanced trade-off between complexity and performance.

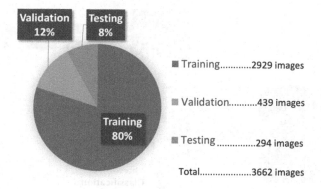

Fig. 7. Visual representation of the percentage of data splitting of the dataset.

ResNet50 and ResNet50V2. ResNet50 was developed to address the problem of vanishing gradients in deep neural networks by introducing skip connections. These connections facilitate gradient flow throughout the network, enabling the model to learn meaningful representations and enhance performance [18].

ResNet50V2, an improved iteration of ResNet50, incorporates enhancements like the pre-activation variant of residual blocks, adjusted layer ordering, and diverse weight initialization schemes for improved performance [19].

EfficientNet: EfficientNetBO to EfficientNetB6. EfficientNet was designed to improve accuracy and efficiency in image classification by employing compound scaling, which uniformly scales network width, depth, and resolution. This approach acknowledges that larger input images necessitate increased depth for capturing broader spatial information and increased width for finer pattern details [20].

In this study, seven variants of EfficientNet, ranging from EfficientNetB0 to EfficientNetB6, were trained and tested, differing primarily in network scale. EfficientNetB0 is the smallest with fewer parameters, while EfficientNetB6 is the largest variant with the most parameters. Scaling from B0 to B6 increases depth, width, and resolution, enhancing model expressiveness. However, this larger scale also demands higher computational resources.

Overall, EfficientNet has revolutionized the design of convolutional neural networks, providing a scalable and efficient solution for image classification tasks. Its wide adoption and impressive performance have solidified its position as a main choice for researchers and practitioners in the field of deep learning [21–23].

2.3 Model Training

Transfer Learning. In this study, to overcome the challenge posed by limited data, resulting in class imbalance, it is employed a technique known as transfer learning [9]. Transfer learning is a technique that enables the transfer of knowledge acquired from one task to improve learning in another task, even if the

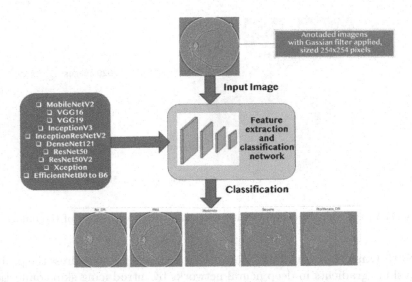

Fig. 8. Diabetic Retinopathy classification model.

domains differ [7]. In this approach, a pre-trained model, originally trained on the diverse ImageNet dataset, was fine-tuned for the task of diabetic retinopathy classification from fundus images, leveraging its high-level representations and feature extraction capabilities.

Fine-Tuning. For the performance analysis and comparison of CNN architectures in the classification of diabetic retinopathy, the model involved inputting already pre-processed data (Fig. 5, fundus images with a Gaussian filter applied and resized to 254 × 254 pixels) into a pre-trained feature extraction and classification network (Fig. 8). The model has trained with 80% of the dataset, validated with 12%, and tested with 8% (Fig. 7). For training the model, the batch size was set to 32 and was set for 40 epochs, however, the training would stop if there was no notable improvement after making three adjustments to the learning rate.

Evaluation Metrics. To evaluate the performance of the model, several metrics were utilized, including the calculation of the confusion matrix, accuracy, and F1-score. The confusion matrix provides insights into the classification results, showcasing the number of true positives, true negatives, false positives, and false negatives. Accuracy measures the overall correctness of the model's predictions, while the F1-score assesses the model's balance between precision and recall. These metrics collectively provide a comprehensive assessment of the model's performance in classifying diabetic retinopathy (DR).

3   Results and Analysis

In this study, were trained multiple CNN models to identify the most accurate architecture classifier for diabetic retinopathy. To determine the model that achieves the highest classification performance in DR classification, were employed a range of evaluation metrics, including accuracy, to assess the performance of each model.

Accuracy. In the context of this research, accuracy measures the ability of the trained models to correctly classify diabetic retinopathy cases compared to the ground truth labels. A higher accuracy value would indicate, in general, a more reliable classification performance.

The Table 1 presents the accuracy results obtained for each model, as well as the number of parameters. The experimental results confirm that, similar to the state-of-the-art studies discussed earlier, the EfficientNet networks consistently achieve the highest accuracy scores among the models tested [8,9]. EfficientNetB5 and EfficientNetB2 emerge as the top performers, achieving accuracy rates of 85.37% and 84.69%, respectively. It is worth noting that EfficientNetB2 achieves accuracy close to EfficientNetB5, with 3,6 times fewer parameters. As expected, MobileNetV2 performs poorly with only 56% accuracy.

In the performance graph (Fig. 9), it is visually evident that the EfficientNet networks achieve better accuracy results while utilizing fewer parameters. The densenet121 network also stands out, as it achieves a considerable accuracy value while using a low number of parameters, although it never surpasses the efficiency of the EfficientNet.

From the 294 images of the testing set, 50% of the images belong to the "no DR" class, with only 5% and 10% belonging to the "Severe" and "Proliferate DR", respectively (Fig. 10). Due to the highly imbalanced nature of class distribution on the dataset, evaluating performance with accuracy alone will not provide much information about the individual class-wise performance of the model in diabetic retinopathy classification. Therefore, confusion matrices were generated to gain insights into the model's performance for each specific class.

Confusion Matrix. In the context of this study, the confusion matrix will help understand how well the model is able to correctly identify different levels of retinopathy severity because it allows analyzing the distribution of correct and incorrect predictions across the classes.

By examining the confusion matrix (Fig. 11), it becomes apparent that the models are accurately classifying the most prevalent class, "No DR". However, they fall short of achieving comparable results for the less frequent classes such as "Severe", "Mild" and "Proliferate DR".

F1-Score. To assess the overall effectiveness of the models in accurately classifying diabetic retinopathy, it was analyzed the f1-score of each individual class.

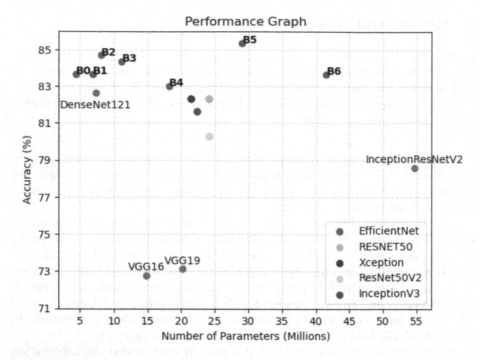

Fig. 9. Model size vs Accuracy; EfficientNet stands out as the best performance overall

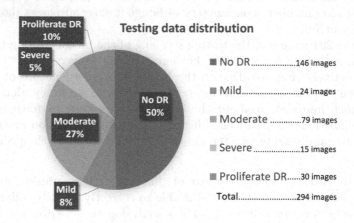

Fig. 10. Visual representation of classes distribution of the testing dataset; There are 294 images in total, in which the No DR represents 50%.

Table 2 displays the f1-score values for each class obtained by the different models. It confirms the observations made in the confusion matrices, where the models performed well in classifying the most represented class, "No DR", with the EfficientNetB6 model achieving an f1-score of 0.99. For the least represented

Table 1. Performance of the classification models: Accuracy and Number of Parameters

Architecture	Accuracy(%)	Number of Parameters(Millions)
EfficientNetB5	85,37	29,05
EfficientNetB2	84,69	8,14
EfficientNetB3	84,35	11,18
EfficientNetB0	83,67	4,38
EfficientNetB1	83,67	6,91
EfficientNetB6	83,67	41,56
EfficientNetB4	82,99	18,14
DenseNet121	82,65	7,31
RESNET50	82,31	24,12
Xception	82,31	21,49
InceptionV3	81,63	22,34
ResNet50V2	80,27	24,10
InceptionResNetV2	78,57	54,74
VGG19	73,63	20,16
VGG16	72,79	14,85
MobileNetV2	56,12	2,59

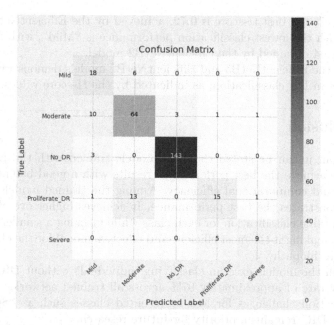

Fig. 11. Confusion Matrix of the model EfficientNetB2; The diagonal line indicates that its prediction is the same as the true value, and the more accurate the predictions are, the darker the color.

Table 2. F1-score values for each class obtained by the models

Architecture	No DR	Mild	Moderate	Severe	Proliferate DR
EfficientNetB5	0,98	0,62	0,82	0,43	0,68
EfficientNetB2	0,98	0,64	0,79	0,69	0,59
EfficientNetB3	0,98	0,60	0,78	0,55	0,65
EfficientNetB0	0,98	0,63	0,78	0,72	0,47
EfficientNetB1	0,98	0,62	0,77	0,64	0,60
EfficientNetB6	0,99	0,61	0,77	0,48	0,61
EfficientNetB4	0,98	0,62	0,77	0,45	0,57
DenseNet121	0,98	0,58	0,78	0,48	0,49
RESNET50	0,97	0,60	0,77	0,57	0,47
Xception	0,97	0,59	0,78	0,61	0,45
InceptionV3	0,98	0,53	0,76	0,57	0,42
ResNet50V2	0,96	0,54	0,75	0,59	0,39
InceptionResNetV2	0,96	0,52	0,52	0,55	0,21
VGG19	0,96	0,08	0,66	0,00	0,00
VGG16	0,95	0,31	0,65	0,00	0,00
MobileNetV2	0,81	0,31	0,20	0,00	0,14

class, "severe", the best f1-score is 0.72, achieved by the EfficientNetB0 model. The class with the lowest classification performance is "Mild", with the highest f1-score of 0.64 obtained by the EfficientNetB2 model.

Overall, the EfficientNetB5 and EfficientNetB2 models demonstrate superior performance in DR classification, as indicated by the f1-score values.

4   Conclusion

In conclusion, it can be stated that the models trained with the EfficientNet architecture achieve the best performance results with a good balance between model size and computational efficiency. Among the trained models, EfficientNetB2 demonstrates the best performance. It achieves higher overall accuracy and more specific classification for each class while utilizing a smaller number of parameters, making it the most efficient and effective model for the classification of diabetic retinopathy.

Although the models excel in classifying individuals without DR, achieving an accuracy rate of approximately 97% across all trained networks, addressing the classification challenges for less represented classes such as "Severe" and "Proliferate DR" remains a priority for future research.

Furthermore, to ensure the practical applicability of these models in clinical settings, collaboration with healthcare professionals is essential. Integrating these AI-driven solutions into clinical workflows offers a valuable solution for accurate early disease screening, particularly in cases of a deficiency of specialized doctors. Such collaborations can significantly contribute to preventing visual impairment in diabetic individuals, as DR remains one of the leading causes of blindness in adults.

References

1. Teo, Z.L., et al. Global prevalence of diabetic retinopathy and projection of burden through 2045: systematic review and meta-analysis. Ophthalmology **128**(11), 1580–1591 (2021). Elsevier
2. Zhang, J., Strauss, E. C. Sensitive detection of therapeutic efficacy with the ETDRS diabetic retinopathy severity scale. Clin. Ophthalmol., 4385–4393 (2020). Taylor & Francis
3. He, J., et al.: Artificial intelligence-based screening for diabetic retinopathy at community hospital. Eye **34**(3), 572–576 (2020). Nature Publishing Group, UK, London
4. Alabdulwahhab, K.M., Sami, W., Mehmood, T., Meo, S.A., Alasbali, T.A., Alwadani, F.A.: Automated detection of diabetic retinopathy using machine learning classifiers. Eur. Rev. Med. Pharmacol. Sci. **25**(2), 583–590 (2021)
5. Dutta, S., Manideep, B.C., Basha, S.M., Caytiles, R.D., Iyengar, N.C.S.N.: Classification of diabetic retinopathy images by using deep learning models. Int. J. Grid Distrib. Comput. **11**(1), 89–106 (2018)
6. Revathy, R.: Diabetic retinopathy detection using machine learning. Int. J. Eng. Res. **9** (2020)
7. Tsiknakis, N., et al.: Deep learning for diabetic retinopathy detection and classification based on fundus images: a review. Comput. Biol. Med. **135**, 104599 (2021)
8. Giroti, I., Das, J.K.A., Harshith, N.M., Thahniyath, G.: Diabetic retinopathy detection & classification using efficient net model. In: 2023 International Conference on Artificial Intelligence and Applications (ICAIA) Alliance Technology Conference (ATCON-1), Bangalore, India, pp. 1-6 (2023). https://doi.org/10.1109/ICAIA57370.2023.10169756
9. Hangwei, Z., Nabil, E.: Classification of diabetic retinopathy via fundus photography: utilization of deep learning approaches to speed up disease detection. arXiv preprint arXiv:2007.09478 (2020)
10. Li, T., Gao, Y., Wang, K., Guo, S., Liu, H., Kang, H.: Diagnostic assessment of deep learning algorithms for diabetic retinopathy screening. Inf. Sci. **501**, 511–522 (2019)
11. Zhang, W., et al.: Automated identification and grading system of diabetic retinopathy using deep neural networks. Knowl.-Based Syst. **175**, 12–25 (2019)
12. Ardiyanto, I., Nugroho, H.A., Buana, R.L.B.: Deep learning-based diabetic retinopathy assessment on embedded system. In: 2017 39th Annual International Conference of the IEEE Engineering in Medicine and Biology Society (EMBC), 1760–1763 (2017)
13. Sandler, M., Howard, A., Zhu, M., Zhmoginov, A., Chen, L.C.: Mobilenetv2: inverted residuals and linear bottlenecks. In: Proceedings of the IEEE Conference on Computer Vision and Pattern Recognition, pp. 4510–4520 (2018)
14. Zhao, Z., et al.: BiRA-Net: bilinear attention net for diabetic retinopathy grading. In: 2019 IEEE International Conference on Image Processing (ICIP), 1385–1389 (2019). https://doi.org/10.1109/ICIP.2019.8803074

15. Szegedy, C., Ioffe, S., Vanhoucke, V., Alemi, A.: Inception-v4, inception-ResNet and the impact of residual connections on learning. In: Proceedings of the AAAI Conference on Artificial Intelligence, vol. 31(1) (2017)
16. Chollet, F.: Xception: Deep learning with depthwise separable convolutions. In: Proceedings of the IEEE Conference on Computer Vision and Pattern Recognition, pp. 1251–1258 (2017)
17. Huang, G., Liu, Z., Van Der Maaten, L., Weinberger, K.Q.: Densely connected convolutional networks. In: Proceedings of the IEEE Conference on Computer Vision and Pattern Recognition, pp. 4700–4708 (2017)
18. He, K., Zhang, X., Ren, S., Sun, J.: Deep residual learning for image recognition. In: Proceedings of the IEEE Conference on Computer Vision and Pattern Recognition, pp. 770–778 (2016)
19. Zhang, X., Li, Z., Change Loy, C., Lin, D.: PolyNet: a pursuit of structural diversity in very deep networks. In: Proceedings of the IEEE Conference on Computer Vision and Pattern Recognition, pp. 718–726 (2017)
20. Tan, M., Le, Q.: EfficientNet: rethinking model scaling for convolutional neural networks. In: International Conference on Machine Learning, pp. 6105–6114 (2019)
21. Chetoui, M., Akhloufi, M.A.: Explainable diabetic retinopathy using Efficient-NET. In: 2020 42nd Annual International Conference of the IEEE Engineering in Medicine & Biology Society (EMBC), pp. 1966–1969 (2020). https://doi.org/10.1109/EMBC44109.2020.9175664
22. Karki, S.S., Kulkarni, P.: Diabetic retinopathy classification using a combination of EfficientNets. In: 2021 International Conference on Emerging Smart Computing and Informatics (ESCI), pp. 68–72 (2021). https://doi.org/10.1109/ESCI50559.2021.9397035
23. Lazuardi, R.N., Abiwinanda, N., Suryawan, T.H., Hanif, M., Handayani, A.: Automatic diabetic retinopathy classification with EfficientNet. In: 2020 IEEE Region 10 Conference (TENCON), pp. 756–760 (2020). https://doi.org/10.1109/TENCON50793.2020.9293941
24. Nneji, G.U., Cai, J., Deng, J., Monday, H.N., Hossin, M.A., Nahar, S.: Identification of diabetic retinopathy using weighted fusion deep learning based on dual-channel fundus scans. Diagnostics 12(2), 540 (2022). https://doi.org/10.3390/diagnostics12020540
25. Shukla, U.V., Tripathy, K.: Diabetic Retinopathy @StatPearls (2023). https://www.ncbi.nlm.nih.gov/books/NBK560805/
26. Mishra, C., Tripathy, K.: Fundus Camera @StatPearls (2023). https://www.ncbi.nlm.nih.gov/books/NBK585111/

Deep Learning Model Evaluation and Insights in Inherited Retinal Disease Detection

Hélder Ferreira[1]([✉]), Ana Marta[2,3], Inês Couto[2], José Câmara[1],
João Melo Beirão[2,3], and António Cunha[1,4]

[1] University of Trás-os-Montes and Alto Douro, 5000-801 Vila Real, Portugal
helder2003ferreira123@gmail.com
[2] Department of Ophthalmology, Centro Hospitalar Universitário de Santo António,
EPE (CHUdSA), Porto, Portugal
[3] Instituto de Ciências Biomédicas Abel Salazar (ICBAS), Porto, Portugal
[4] INESC TEC - INESC Technology and Science, FEUP Campus, Porto, Portugal

Abstract. Inherited retinal diseases such as Retinitis Pigmentosa and Stargardt's disease are genetic conditions that cause the photoreceptors in the retina to deteriorate over time. This can lead to vision symptoms such as tubular vision, loss of central vision, and nyctalopia (difficulty seeing in low light) or photophobia (high light). Timely healthcare intervention is critical, as most forms of these conditions are currently untreatable and usually focused on minimizing further vision loss.

Machine learning (ML) algorithms can play a crucial role in the detection of retinal diseases, especially considering the recent advancements in retinal imaging devices and the limited availability of public datasets on these diseases. These algorithms have the potential to help researchers gain new insights into disease progression from previous classified eye scans and genetic profiles of patients.

In this work, multi-class identification between the retinal diseases Retinitis Pigmentosa, Stargardt Disease, and Cone-Rod Dystrophy was performed using three pretrained models, ResNet101, ResNet50, and VGG19 as baseline models, after shown to be effective in our computer vision task. These models were trained and validated on two datasets of autofluorescent retinal images, the first containing raw data, and the second dataset was improved with cropping to obtain better results. The best results were achieved using the ResNet101 model on the improved dataset with an Accuracy (Acc) of 0.903, an Area under the ROC Curve (AUC) of 0.976, an F1-Score of 0.897, a Recall (REC) of 0.903, and a Precision (PRE) of 0.910.

To further assess the reliability of these models for future data, an Explainable AI (XAI) analysis was conducted, employing Grad-Cam. Overall, the study showed promising capabilities of Deep Learning for the diagnosis of retinal diseases using medical imaging.

© ICST Institute for Computer Sciences, Social Informatics and Telecommunications Engineering 2024
Published by Springer Nature Switzerland AG 2024. All Rights Reserved
A. Cunha et al. (Eds.): MobiHealth 2023, LNICST 578, pp. 295–306, 2024.
https://doi.org/10.1007/978-3-031-60665-6_22

1   Introduction

Inherited retinal diseases (IRDs) are genetic diseases that affect the normal function of light-sensitive cells (photoreceptors) and the cell layer that supports them (retinal pigment epithelium). They are the most common cause of blindness in the working-age population in some developed countries, to some degree [1].

The most common IRD, Retinitis Pigmentosa, manifests through fundoscopy, revealing characteristics like bony spicule-like pigmentations in the retina, narrowed arterioles, optic disc pallor, cataracts, and vitreous cell presence [2]. Stargardt Disease presents hiperfluorescent pisciform lesions, macular atrophy, and choriocapillaris silence due to lipofuscin accumulation. Cone-rod Dystrophy predominantly impacts the macula, causing central vision difficulties, color vision impairment, and macular atrophy.

IRDs often have unique phenotypic features that medical professionals can identify using advanced retinal imaging technology [3]. This technology allows for the rapid and non-invasive acquisition of high-resolution retinal images, requiring sometimes just a dilated pupil and causing no discomfort to the patient. Various imaging modalities, including fundus autofluorescence (FAF) and spectral-domain optical coherence tomography (SD-OCT), can be used to perform these scans [4].

For example, FAF images are critical in identifying patterns indicative of photoreceptor dysfunction and apoptosis. This is done by detecting lipofuscin and related compounds by exploiting their auto-fluorescent properties. Lipofuscin accumulates primarily in the retinal pigment epithelium (RPE) due to oxidative stress. By visualising lipofuscin distribution, FAF images provide valuable insight into the extent and location of oxidative stress-induced damage in the retina [5].

The availability of high-resolution, detailed multimodal information allows ophthalmologists to identify patterns associated with specific diseases. However, due to the rarity of these diseases, accurate clinical diagnoses require specialised expertise and experience that is limited to a small number of specialists and hospitals.

State-of-the-art machine learning models can recognise disease-specific patterns from retinal images and be used to extend the reach of accurate diagnoses to a broader population [6].

These models' importance is increased when considering the scarcity of available public data about these diseases and the existence of different modalities of retinal imaging that go from fundus photography with 30° of field of view up to Optos Ultra-Widefield with 200° [7,8].

A substantial amount of data about IRDs is generally hard to get or have access to. However, for this study, a public Portuguese hospital provided us with a private dataset involving autofluorescence retinal images, which will be used.

In this paper, standard state-of-the-art Deep Learning models were applied and evaluated to automatically classify retinal images on three inherited retinal diseases: Retinitis Pigmentosa, Stargardt Disease, and Cone-Rod Dystrophy. Additionally, Grad-CAM maps were used to identify potential biases and improve models.

2   Methodology

The methodology adopted in this study follows the standard machine learning steps. It is divided into two procedures (P1 and P2), illustrated in Fig. 1.

First, the set of retinal images, raw data (RD), underwent a preprocessing stage, where it was cleaned, restructured with proper labels and split into 2 datasets (DS1 and DS2) for model training. Then, models were chosen and trained (T1 and T2). Finally, the models are evaluated using standard classification metrics (E1 and E2) and accessed with Grad-CAM maps.

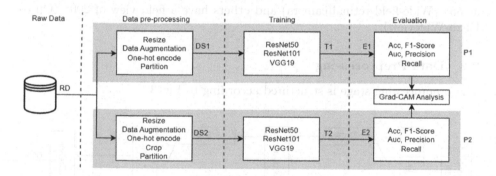

Fig. 1. Methodology pipeline

2.1   Raw Data

A collection of 491 autofluorescence retinal images was made available by a public hospital in Portugal. The images were labelled by clinical experts, with 326 identified as Retinitis Pigmentosa (RP), 81 as Cone-rod Dystrophy (CR), and the remaining 84 as indicative of Stargardt Disease (STG), as can be seen in Fig. 2.

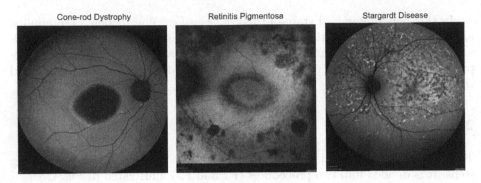

Fig. 2. Examples of images from each class

The set included images from each patient's eyes with multiple imaging modalities to capture the retinal images, adding diversity to our dataset. Some images have a field view of 30° (fundus photography), others a field of view at 55° (Wide-field retinal camera) and others have a field view of 200° (Optos Ultra-Wideview).

2.2 Data Preprocessing

The preprocessing stage is structured according to Fig. 3.

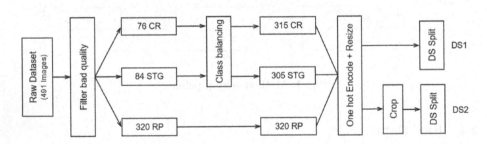

Fig. 3. Data Preprocessing Diagram

During this step, 11 images were removed for having poor quality, i.e., low resolution and too dark (unreadable), where 5 belonged to the CR category and 6 to the RP category.

To maintain data symmetry and ensure balanced class representation, we applied data augmentation techniques involving horizontal flips and image rotations within the range of -10º to 10º specifically for the Cone-rod and Stargardt classes, illustrated in Fig. 4, as those techniques allowed the increase of data while improving the efficiency of the models. This approach resulted in a balanced dataset, comprising 315 images for CR, 320 for RP, and 305 for STG. Then, all images were resized to a standard dimension of 224 × 224 pixels and transformed categorical class data into numerical attributes using one-hot encoding allowing a faster model training. Finally, both datasets were partitioned into training, validation, and testing sets, with ratios of 64:16:20, respectively.

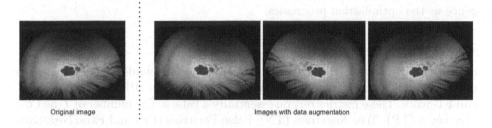

Original image   Images with data augmentation

Fig. 4. Original image (on the left) and images with data augmentation (on the right)

The diagram illustrated in Fig. 3, shows all steps taken during the preprocessing of data, including removal of unreadable images, application of data augmentation on CR and STG classes, one hot encoding and resize, crop in DS2 and finally partition on both sets.

Apart from the cropping variation between DS1 and DS2, our strategies for image preprocessing remained consistent.

In the first approach, we also identified that some of the images contained bottom text, on the RP and STG classes which could lead to model memorization during training, since it's not present in the CR class. Considering this possibility, we made a strategic decision to divide our data into two distinct datasets. One dataset (DS1) contained the raw images with bottom text, while the other dataset (DS2) was edited to remove this text by cropping 15% of the image's height. This allowed us to later determine potential model bias and ensure it focuses on the right features.

2.3   Model Training

The VGG (Visual Geometry Group) and ResNet (Residual Networks) models were selected since they are state-of-the-art classifiers with exceptional performance for medical analysis tasks. Additionally, these models are suited for problems with small datasets, just like the one we're dealing with, since they have trained weight for Transfer learning, e.g., from the ImageNet [9]. ResNet101, ResNet50, and VGG19 model versions were selected for the project.

The models went through a two-step training process for P1 and P2, utilizing DS1 for both training and validation of P1, and DS2 for both training and validation of P2, respectively.

The training was conducted using 15 epochs, which proved to be sufficient to achieve convergence in terms of performance for all models.

Transfer learning was executed by loading the state-of-the-art models, freezing all layers, and appending a final dense layer for classification with 3 neurons matching our number of classes. The training optimiser employed was the Adam Optimization Algorithm, alongside the utilization of a learning rate scheduler callback to lower the learning rate over epochs to achieve a more stable convergence as the optimisation progresses.

2.4   Model Evaluation

Standard classification metrics were used to evaluate models, including Area under the ROC Curve (AUC), Accuracy (Acc), Precision (PRE), Recall (REC), and F1-Score. These metrics rely on essentially 4 values: The number of True Positive cases (TP), True Negatives (TN), False Positives (FP) and False Negatives (FN) identified by the model. AUC metric was particularly useful in assessing the performance of our model in distinguishing between positive and negative cases.

It is essential to note, however, that while the Acc metric is the most commonly employed, it may not consistently provide the most representative evaluation, particularly when data exhibits class imbalances. For that reason, other metrics such as AUC or F1-Score can be better options [10].

The Acc, PRE, REC and F1-Score metrics are calculated according to their equations:

$$Acc = \frac{TP + TN}{TP + TN + FP + FN} \qquad F_1 = 2 \cdot \frac{TP + TN}{TP + TN + FP + FN}$$

$$Pre = \frac{TP}{TP + FP} \qquad Rec = \frac{TP}{TP + FN}$$

All models underwent a final evaluation using a dedicated test set comprising 20% of the dataset employed during training, which involved DS1 for P1 and DS2 for P2. The dataset split was performed as part of the initial data preprocessing stage.

3   Results and Discussion

This section provides an overview of the setup used for training the models and presents the results, starting with P1 with the use of DS1, then P2 with DS2, and finally a discussion between them.

3.1   Setup

When fitting the model, we used data in batches of 16 for both training and validation, for 15 epochs, while using the learning rate callback with the formula, learning rate * exp (-0.05). This formula exponentially decreases the learning rate during each epoch.

The machine learning models were trained on a PC with an Intel Core i5-7400 CPU, NVIDIA GeForce RTX 3060 GPU, and 12 GB of RAM. The system ran on Windows 10 and utilised the TensorFlow framework for training and evaluating the model.

3.2 P1 Results

The results for the initial procedure (P1) are presented in Fig. 5 and include metrics results and the confusion matrix, which provides details on how many test set images were correctly classified by each model (the values on the diagonal) and how many were misclassified (all other values).

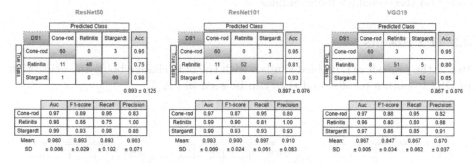

Fig. 5. ResNet101, ResNet50 and VGG19 models - Confusion matrices and metrics results when performed on DS1 with their Standard Deviation (SD)

All 3 models showed positive results in terms of mean Acc ranging from 86 to 90%. When looking at each class individually, on the Cone-rod dystrophy all models achieved an Acc of 0.95, Retinitis Pigmentosa had Accs of 0.75, 0.81 and 0.80 for ResNet50, ResNet101 and VGG19 respectively, and on Stargardt Disease these models got Accs of 0.98, 0.93 and 0.85 in the same order.

As for the other metrics, ResNet50 achieved a mean AUC of 0.980, with an F1-Score of 0.893, REC of 0.893, and PRE of 0.903. Similarly, ResNet101 obtained scores of 0.983, 0.900, 0.897, and 0.910, for mean AUC, F1-Score, REC, and PRE, respectively. On the other hand, VGG19's results were slightly lower, with values of 0.967 for mean AUC, 0.847 for F1-Score, 0.867 for REC, and 0.870 for PRE.

In addition to obtaining these results, the visualization of images for which the models made incorrect predictions is always beneficial for evaluating the justification of these errors. Some of these examples can be found in Fig. 6.

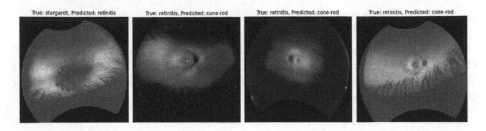

Fig. 6. Examples of images that all 3 models predicted wrong

After examining the images, it appeared they weren't that easy to predict and it's reasonable to confuse the models. It's important to remember that the dataset we used was relatively small, so we shouldn't discredit the models based solely on these challenging examples.

3.3   P2 Results

In P2, the procedure remained similar, with the only change being the utilization of DS2 to obtain results, and they can be seen in Fig. 7.

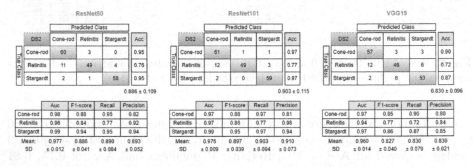

Fig. 7. ResNet101, ResNet50 and VGG19 models - Confusion matrices and metrics results when performed on DS2

P2 results were not very far apart from the P1 seen previously, this time the mean ACC ranged from 83 to 90%. On the Cone-rod dystrophy class, ResNet50, ResNet101 and VGG19 achieved an Acc of 0.95, 0.97 and 0.90 respectively. On the same order of models, Retinitis Pigmentosa had an Acc of 0.76, 0.77 and 0.72. Lastly, on Stargardt Disease these models got Accs of 0.95, 0.97 and 0.87.

In the other metrics, ResNet50 achieved a mean AUC of 0.977, with an F1-Score of 0.886, REC of 0.890, and PRE of 0.893. Similarly, ResNet101 obtained scores of 0.976, 0.897, 0.903, and 0.910, for mean AUC, F1-Score, REC, and PRE, respectively. VGG19 results were once again lower, with values of 0.960 for mean AUC, 0.827 for F1-Score, 0.830 for both REC and PRE.

The same idea of visualising images in which the models made incorrect predictions was conducted, and examples can be seen in Fig. 8.

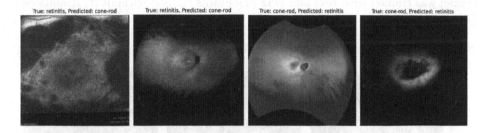

True: retinitis, Predicted: cone-rod   True: retinitis, Predicted: cone-rod   True: cone-rod, Predicted: retinitis   True: cone-rod, Predicted: retinitis

Fig. 8. Examples of images that all 3 models predicted wrong

Similarly to what happened in P1, when analysing the models' incorrect predictions, most of the images are susceptible to confusion and do not disregard the models' capabilities

3.4   Discussion and Explainability Analysis

While the results from DS1 and DS2 may not be very far off each other, their preprocessing strategies were different with the removal of extraneous text on DS2 that was present on the bottom part of images and could lead to memorization during model training, consequently affecting its generalisation. This was a real concern especially considering the text was present on the RP and STG images categories but not on the CR, so the models could use that for advantage if untreated.

To visualise if text memorization had happened in the first case (DS1), we utilised the Grad-CAM as a final analysis technique. Grad-CAM is a state-of-the-art visualization method commonly used in computer vision tasks, specifically in convolutional neural networks (CNN) for image classification [11].

By generating a heatmap, Grad-CAM allows us to identify the regions in an image that had the most impact on the network's final prediction. Unlike previous approaches, which focused solely on the last layer's feature maps, Grad-CAM analyses the gradients flowing into the final convolutional layer. This enables us to pinpoint the specific areas of the image that the model paid attention to while making its decision [11].

When visualizing these attention maps, we gain valuable insights into the decision-making process of the model. We can determine whether the model focuses on relevant image features or relies on irrelevant cues such as text, thereby validating our hypothesis about text memorization. This technique has immense potential in uncovering the inner workings of deep learning models and understanding their strengths and limitations in diverse applications, including medical image analysis.

For this evaluation, we will only be considering the DS1 and DS2 models with best results, which both correspond to ResNet101 and apply Grad-CAM on images of every category containing the bottom text, taking into account DS1 model was trained with text and DS2 model was trained without it. Results can be seen in Fig. 9.

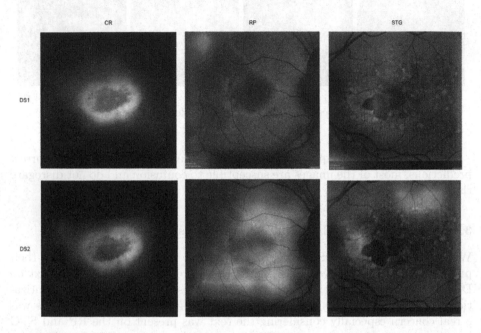

Fig. 9. Examples of Grad-CAM applications on images from each category (Cone-rod on left, Retinitis Pigmentosa on middle and Stargardt on the right) using the ResNet101 model trained with DS1 (top images) and ResNet101 trained with DS2 (lower images)

In the case of the DS1 train set, the Grad-CAM image reveals that the model seems to be memorizing irrelevant text information present in images from both RP and STG. This suggests that the model is giving excessive importance to text that may not be directly related to the task at hand and that is problematic as it may lead to overfitting and the model's inability to generalize well on unseen data.

When examining the Grad-CAM image of the DS2 train set, it is evident that the model is focusing on the important features relevant to the task. By cropping the images to only include the necessary visual elements, the model was able to disregard irrelevant information and prioritize the important aspects even when asked to make predictions on images that contain the text. This shows that the DS2 is providing more accurate and meaningful insights, allowing the model to make informed decisions.

Based on these observations, it's safe to say that the model trained with ResNet101 on DS2 is the best option for future predictions as it has good results and disregards irrelevant information allowing it to generalize well on unseen data. This highlights the importance of preprocessing and selecting relevant training data to enhance the performance and interpretability of machine learning models [12].

4 Conclusion

In our research, we have showcased the exciting potential of leveraging convolutional neural networks (CNNs) in conjunction with fundus autofluorescence (FAF) images to autonomously categorize a spectrum of inherited retinal diseases (IRDs). While it's important to acknowledge that our results may not yet attain perfection from a purely technical standpoint, they represent a significant leap forward in the realm of medical diagnostics.

As we look ahead, our research trajectory aims to explore new deep learning strategies for disease classification to improve the results. While at the same time, increasing our database with a diverse range of FAF images to enhance the robustness of our models. This expansion will undoubtedly broaden the applicability of our findings and deepen our understanding of IRDs.

Moreover, our aspiration extends beyond the confines of our work. We envision that this study will serve as a ground base for other projects with different data to enhance healthcare solutions and improve patient outcomes in the field of retinal diseases.

Acknowledgments. This work is financed by National Funds through the Portuguese funding agency, FCT - Fundação para a Ciência e a Tecnologia, within project LA/P/0063/2020.

References

1. Rachael C., et al.: Inherited retinal diseases are the most common cause of blindness in the working-age population in Australia. Ophthalmic Genet. **42**(4), 431–439 (2021)
2. Francis, P.J.: Genetics of inherited retinal disease. J. Royal Soc. Med. **99**(4), 189–191 (2006)
3. Dockery, A., Whelan, L., Humphries, P., Farrar, G.J.: Next-generation sequencing applications for inherited retinal diseases. Int. J. Mol. Sci. **22**(11), 5684 (2021)
4. Pichi, F., Abboud, E.B., Ghazi, N.G., Khan, A.O.: Fundus autofluorescence imaging in hereditary retinal diseases. Acta Ophthalmol. **96**(5), e549–e561 (2018)
5. Heiferman, M.J., Fawzi, A.A.: Discordance between blue-light autofluorescence and near-infrared autofluorescence in age-related macular degeneration. Invest. Ophthalmol. Visual Sci. **57**(12), 25–25 (2016)
6. Pontikos, N., et al.: Eye2Gene: prediction of causal inherited retinal disease gene from multimodal imaging using AI. Invest. Ophthalmol. Visual Sci. **63**(7), 1161 (2022)

7. Liesenfeld, B., et al.: A telemedical approach to the screening of diabetic retinopathy: digital fundus photography. Diab. Care **23**(3), 345–348 (2000)
8. Nagiel, A., Lalane, R.A., Sadda, S.R., Schwartz, S.D.: Ultra-widefield fundus imaging: a review of clinical applications and future trends. Retina **36**(4), 660–678 (2016)
9. Deng, J., Dong, W., Socher, R., Li, L.J., Li, K., Fei-Fei, L.: ImageNet: a large-scale hierarchical image database. In: 2009 IEEE Conference on Computer Vision and Pattern Recognition, pp. 248–255. IEEE (2009)
10. Jordaney, R., Wang, Z., Papini, D., Nouretdinov, I., Cavallaro, L.: Misleading metrics: on evaluating machine learning for malware with confidence. Technical report (2016)
11. Selvaraju, R.R., Cogswell, M., Das, A., Vedantam, R., Parikh, D., Batra, D.: Grad-CAM: visual explanations from deep networks via gradient-based localization. In: Proceedings of the IEEE International Conference on Computer Vision, pp. 618–626 (2017)
12. Famili, A., Shen, W.M., Weber, R., Simoudis, E.: Data preprocessing and intelligent data analysis. Intell. Data Anal. **1**(1), 3–23 (1997)

Informative Classification of Capsule Endoscopy Videos Using Active Learning

Filipe Fonseca[1]([⊠]) [ID], Beatriz Nunes[2] [ID], Marta Salgado[4] [ID], Augusto Silva[2] [ID], and António Cunha[1,3] [ID]

[1] Universidade de Trás-os-Montes e Alto Douro, Vila Real, Portugal
fmiguelof@gmail.com
[2] Universidade de Aveiro, Aveiro, Portugal
[3] INESC TEC, Porto, Portugal
[4] Centro Hospitalar Universitário de Santo António, Porto, Portugal

Abstract. The wireless capsule endoscopy is a non-invasive imaging method that allows observation of the inner lumen of the small intestine, but with the cost of a longer duration to process its resulting videos. Therefore, the scientific community has developed several machine learning strategies to help reduce that duration. Such strategies are typically trained and evaluated on small sets of images, ultimately not proving to be efficient when applied to full videos. Labelling full Capsule Endoscopy videos requires significant effort, leading to a lack of data on this medical area. Active learning strategies allow intelligent selection of datasets from a vast set of unlabelled data, maximizing learning and reducing annotation costs. In this experiment, we have explored active learning methods to reduce capsule endoscopy videos' annotation effort by compiling smaller datasets capable of representing their content.

Keywords: Active learning · Deep learning · Capsule endoscopy

1 Introduction

1.1 Context

The gastrointestinal tract is a carefully studied organ system since it can harbour severe conditions [1]. Several studies in the gastrointestinal tract showed that early detection of abnormalities is correlated with a significant decrease in dangerous developments and improvement in survival rates [2]. Upper and lower gastrointestinal endoscopy allow the visualisation of a substantial portion of the gastrointestinal tract, however, the small bowel was seen as the "black box" due to its hard reach for screening [3]. With the small bowel being home to multiple pathologies [3,4], there is a clear need for taking advantage of novel screening tests for the detection of small bowel diseases and its abnormalities.

A. Cunha et al. (Eds.): MobiHealth 2023, LNICST 578, pp. 307–323, 2024.
https://doi.org/10.1007/978-3-031-60665-6_23

The Wireless Capsule Endoscopy (WCE), is a pill-like, non-invasive camera that can be swallowed by the patient to be propelled through the digestive system taking advantage of its peristaltic movements, to provide an inner screening of the tract. In the course of its route, the capsule transmits images through radio frequency to a portable device attached to the patient's body [5]. The device can record for about 8 h, producing around 60 000 images. It is considered the preferred method for the diagnosis of diseases of the small bowel, given its ability to cover the whole gastrointestinal tract and its distinguished inner imaging results compared to other methods for abnormalities visualisation [6]. Despite this, the manual analysis of the resulting eight-hour-long recorded video by an expert is very time-consuming and susceptible to human error, since identifying lesions in this type of image is a very challenging task because the quality of the acquired images is not always the best, which can imply the loss of important information. Besides this, different types of lesions can be very similar, and the same type of lesion can present different colouration and shape, which makes the process of discriminating the lesions very demanding [5].

With this in mind, computer-aided diagnosis tools have been developed for automatic lesion detection in WCE imaging. However, these attempts do not perform well enough to be used in a clinical environment and have focused much more on vascular lesions than others. Therefore, there is a clear need to develop more robust approaches for the automatic analysis of Capsule Endoscopy Videos (CEV). The automatic detection of lesions on frames can drastically reduce the number of images that a physician has to analyse, allowing him to focus his attention on the relevant data only.

1.2   Motivation

The early detection of abnormalities can lead to significant improvement in the patient's health condition and avoid complications [7]. Diagnosing intestinal motility disorders involves assessing instructive frames, which can range from a few to a large number of images per CEV. Uninformative frames, which are obstructed by gastrointestinal contents like partially digested meals, intestinal secretions, or gas bubbles, are crucial for reducing video analysis time and indicating intestinal dysfunctions. Identifying uninformative frames helps reduce analysis time and helps identify intestinal material in a significant proportion.

Machine learning methodologies are used to construct binary classifiers for uninformative frames search in CEV processing. These classifiers are aided by a training set that accurately represents the underlying data population. However, challenges arise due to significant variations in colour among uninformative frames across different videos [8]. The labelling process may require human annotation of up to 50 000 frames for each video, which may be considered a naive technique.

Active learning offers effective methods for interactive labelling, reducing human involvement. The algorithm can enhance accuracy by using a smaller number of labelled training samples, provided it can choose the data to learn from [9]. It can be effective in expanding a training set without human interaction.

1.3   Objectives

Due to the limited availability of datasets which cover the CEV reality and the meticulous effort required to review and annotate whole videos on a frame-by-frame basis, the primary objective of this study is to contribute to evaluating the efficacy of active learning strategies on fully unlabelled CEV. The strategies under investigation include selecting certain samples that accurately reflect the overall distribution of data in the videos. This approach aims to enhance the efficiency of classifiers by reducing the number of labelled samples required [10].

The study utilises a deep learning model that was evaluated and trained in a prior experiment [11] to establish an initial understanding of the content of CEV. After the investigation of active learning selection strategies on a set of unlabelled videos, the objective is to augment the proficiency of the trained model to classify informative and uninformative frames. This will facilitate the accomplishment of the initial phase out of three, in an ongoing work aimed at improving strategies that could be used in a clinical environment.

2   Methodology

The methodology for this experiment's Active Learning (AL) cycle is described in Fig. 1.

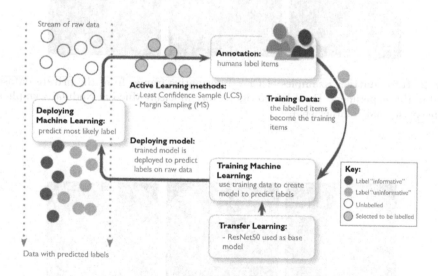

Fig. 1. The methodology used for this experiment.

Considering a base model, ResNet50, the AL cycle was initiated with the pre-trained model being introduced to new and raw data for predicting the most likely label, in our case either informative or uninformative. Then, using one AL method (either Least Confidence Sample or Margin Sample, in this experiment), a sample of predicted labels was pooled to be annotated by an oracle. Finally, the labelled items become part of the training data for the model, and the model is retrained. Then, is tested in unlabelled CEV, for performance evaluation and given the results, a new AL cycle could be initiated.

2.1 Dataset

A private dataset was used in this experiment, a CEV dataset collected from examinations at *Centro Hospitalar Universitário de Santo António*. In total, the dataset consisted of 281 videos, belonging to 238 patients, for each video was extracted the contents of the small bowel lumen, averaging 20 000 frames per video. Only 50 videos had some labelled frames. The frames were stored using the PNG format. For the experiment depicted in this paper, were randomly selected 6 unlabelled videos, hereby named V1, V2, V5, V6, V7 and V10. Figure 2 and Fig. 3 depict example frames from the private dataset for each class to classify in this experiment.

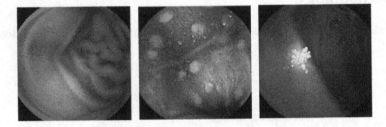

Fig. 2. Informative: Examples of CEV informative frames from the private dataset used in this experiment. From left to right: Normal Clean Mucosa; Nodular Lymphoid Hyperplasia and Xanthelasma.

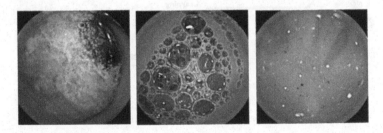

Fig. 3. Uninformative: Examples of CEV uninformative frames from the private dataset used in this experiment.

2.2   Data Preparation and Feature Engineering

To evaluate the impact of active learning strategies on classifying informative and uninformative frames of CEV from unlabelled videos, we used a private dataset. Given the dataset and the random selection of videos, we have chosen V1 to be manually annotated (following the considerations described in Sect. 2.4) in order to train the ResNet50 model. For V1, 17 137 frames were manually divided into two folders, *informative* with 6 554 frames and *uninformative* with 10 583 frames. All frames were in a dimension of 320×320 pixels.

The data of V1 was then randomly divided into 2 unbalanced sets: 70% for training and 30% for validation. The dimension of all frames was adjusted to 224×224 pixels, to meet the input conditions of the model ResNet50.

2.3   Deep and Active Learning Strategies

Deep Learning: When it comes to machine learning issues, convolutional neural network models perform exceptionally well, especially when the issues include the categorization of dataset pictures [12]. Models must be sufficiently detailed to capture similarities between image samples, such as texture, colour, and shape features. While the model's initial layers gather these high-level features, later layers collect information that links those features to the outputs, allowing the model to learn to distinguish between them. Unfortunately, there are numerous instances where there is not enough data available to use this strategy. Transfer learning addresses this issue by leveraging models that have already been trained on a sizable dataset (often trained for a different task, using the same input but providing a different output). This is accomplished by previously capturing the relationships between the data's characteristics, which may later be applied to new challenges.

Given the efficacy of transfer learning in image classification, particularly in the medical field, a methodology utilising this method was used to classify informative and uninformative frames from CEV [13]. Given that the model has already learned about data patterns in the data that was used to pre-train it, transfer learning approaches use reusable features returned by some layers as input features to enable the training of a new model that only needs to learn the relations of those features for the new problem. Transfer learning provides the benefit of improved generalisation of the models, as they underlie the phenomena more than they model the data since the model has access to many types of data, in addition to having considerably fewer parameters to train.

For this experiment, following the previous work [11] and within state-of-the-art convolutional neural networks models, we have chosen the ResNet50 architecture as the base model for transfer learning. ResNet50 is a deep convolutional neural network that has been pre-trained on a large dataset (ImageNet) and has shown excellent performance in various computer vision tasks. By using ResNet50 as the base model, we can leverage its learned features for our specific problem, which saves time and computational resources compared to training a model from scratch. The model ResNet50 was trained using two different approaches: only the last layer was updated, i.e. the pre-trained model worked as a feature extractor and only the weights of the classification layers were changed. The model was trained for 50 epochs, with a batch size of 200, and using the Adam optimisation algorithm which is an extension to the stochastic gradient descendent method that is based on adaptive estimation of the first-order and second-order moments [14]. The learning rate was set to 0.00001.

Active Learning: AL is a methodology that aims to maximize performance while minimizing the number of labelled examples required. It involves identifying the most valuable samples from unlabelled datasets and allocating them to an oracle, often a human annotator, for labelling. The goal is to minimise costs associated with labelling while maintaining performance. AL approaches can be divided into membership query synthesis, stream-based selective sampling, and pool-based AL:

- Membership query synthesis allows the learner to query the label of any unlabelled sample in the input space, even the one created by the learner [15];
- Stream-based selective sampling involves individual assessments regarding the necessity of querying the labels of unlabelled samples within the data stream, while pool-based sampling selects the optimal query sample by evaluating and ranking the entire dataset [16];
- The pool-based AL cycle involves the random selection of samples from the pool of unlabelled data, sending them to the oracle for labelling, and creating a labelled dataset. The model is trained using supervised learning techniques on the labelled dataset, and the acquired information determines the next sample to be queried. The training process is iterated until either the allocated label budget is depleted or the predetermined termination criteria are met [17].

AL differs from other approaches by using human or automated techniques to construct models with exceptional feature extraction capabilities. AL begins with datasets and designs complex query algorithms to carefully choose the most optimal samples from unlabelled datasets and request their labels. The optimisation of query criteria plays a pivotal role in determining the efficacy of AL techniques.

In this experiment, we have used two AL methods: Least Confidence Sampling and Margin Sampling, both belonging to the AL's Uncertainty Sampling technique:

- Least Confidence Sampling (LCS): This strategy selects the instances with the lowest predicted probability of belonging to the current class. It is effective when the model is uncertain about its predictions and wants to gain more confidence by labelling instances that it is least confident about.
- Margin Sampling (MS): This method is specially used when the model has some difficulties in distinguishing between multiple classes. MS is an AL

method that selects the two most confident images and calculates the uncertainty between them. Similar to LCS, these images are then presented to the oracle for annotation, added to the training set, and used to re-train the model. This approach is particularly useful when the model struggles with distinguishing between multiple classes, helping it improve its performance in such scenarios.

2.4   Annotation

In the context of CEV, the clear visualisation of internal tissue, organ lumen, or wall is sometimes hindered by the presence of intestinal juice. This fluid is often seen as a semi-opaque murky liquid, accompanied by bubbles and other artefacts related to the flux of different fluids inside the gastrointestinal tract. The presence of faecal matter, partially digested or residual foods, further complicates the problem of visibility when mixed with these secretions. Consequently, the accurate depiction of the gastrointestinal tract is impeded [18].

In this experiment, as we couldn't have an expert available to help with the annotation, it was decided that we, the technical team, would annotate the AL selected sets. This process, as well as the annotation of V1, followed the defined criteria that any frame of CEV used in this experiment would be an informative frame if it had at least 65% visible/unobstructed mucosa. A frame would be an uninformative frame if it had more than 35% of the frame obstructed.

Figure 2 and Fig. 4 depict frames from the private dataset that would be annotated as informative frames in this experiment. On the other hand, Fig. 3 and Fig. 5 depict frames that would be annotated as uninformative frames in this experiment.

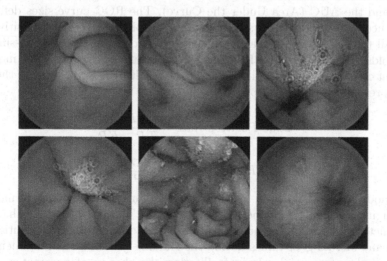

Fig. 4. Informative: Examples of CEV frames that would be annotated as informative frames from the private dataset used in this experiment.

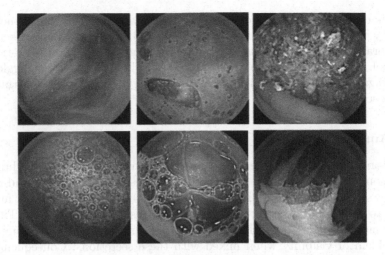

Fig. 5. Uninformative: Examples of CEV frames that would be annotated as uninformative frames from the private dataset used in this experiment.

2.5   Performance Evaluation

Considering that the efficiency was reflected in the classification distribution of true positives (TP), the correct identification of informative and uninformative frames in the set, compared with the number of false positives (FP) and false negatives (FN) classified. These values allowed the performance estimation using standard classification metrics like the Receiver Operating Characteristic (ROC) curve and the AUC (Area Under the Curve). The ROC curve sizes define the confidence of the model in its classification by plotting the true positive rate or recall (Eq. 1), versus the false positive rate (Eq. 2) at different classification thresholds. To compute the ROC, one would have to evaluate the model at different classification thresholds and plot the resulting curve. However, the AUC can express the confidence score of the model.

$$True\ Positive\ Rate = \frac{TP}{TP + FP} \tag{1}$$

$$False\ Positive\ Rate = \frac{FP}{FP + TN} \tag{2}$$

In addition, we have used loss and accuracy metrics as evaluative measures for gauging the efficacy of the ResNet50 model. The use of loss as the objective function allows for the quantification of the disparity between anticipated results and factual goal values during the training process. The aforementioned guidance plays a crucial role in facilitating the change of parameters in our model, compelling it to minimise mistakes and provide forecasts of higher accuracy. Simultaneously, Accuracy (Eq. 3) gives us a clear and simple view of how effectively our model is identifying cases, exhibiting the proportion of properly categorised data points. Nevertheless, it is important to acknowledge that when dealing with imbalanced datasets, where the distribution of classes is unequal, relying solely on high Accuracy may not be sufficient as a comprehensive measure of performance. In such cases, it becomes necessary to incorporate additional metrics such as precision, recall, and F1-score to ensure a more precise evaluation. The combination of these measures provides a comprehensive evaluation of our model's capabilities and enables us to make well-informed judgements on its suitability for the designated task.

$$Accuracy = \frac{Number\ of\ correct\ predictions}{Total\ number\ of\ predictions} \tag{3}$$

$$Precision = \frac{TP}{TP + FP} \tag{4}$$

$$Recall = \frac{TP}{TP + FN} \tag{5}$$

$$F1\text{-}score = \frac{2 \times Recall \times Precision}{Recall + Precision} \tag{6}$$

Finally, it is important to state that V10 was used to test the model throughout the steps of this experiment and served as the basis for the aforementioned metrics to be calculated. Given that the V10 had 19 097 images to be labelled, a coding strategy was implemented to randomly select 400 images to be our sample. Then those 400 images were manually labelled and became the representative sample that we used to evaluate the Accuracy of the model.

3 Results and Discussion

This section will describe the steps made throughout the experiment. The main focus of the steps was to evaluate the performance of selected AL techniques in the methodology described in Fig. 1 aimed to classify informative and uninformative frames of complete extracted videos of the small bowel lumen from full CEV.

Table 1 resumes the evolution of the model throughout the steps, as well as the impact of AL on the knowledge acquired by the model. In each step, except step 1, the model was trained and then tested in videos completely unlabelled.

The conclusions surrounding the V10 tests were drawn based on observation of the images that the model classified. The value of Accuracy will be used to prove the results that the team observed quantitatively. Given that relying solely on Accuracy may not be sufficient (as stated in Sect. 2.5), and to underline the test results, other training and validation metrics will be presented. The metrics also aim to verify that the model didn't go into overfitting and showed promising results.

Table 1. Overall view of the steps of this experiment.

# Steps	AL Methods	Data in model	Test Data	Accuracy
1	–	V1	–	–
2	–	V1	V10	0.42
3	LCS	V1, V2	V10	0.52
4	MS	V1, V2	V10	0.40
5	LCS	V1, V2, V5, V7	V10	0.54
6	LCS	V1, V2, V5, V7, V6	V10	0.41

Step 1: The model ResNet50 was trained with the V1 now labelled as stated in Sect. 2.2.

Table 2. The confusion matrix (TP, true positives; FN, false negatives; FP, false positives; TN, true negatives) and the metrics of the AUC and Loss are provided along with the Precision, Recall and F1-score for the model after Step 1.

	TP	FN	TN	FP	AUC	Loss	Precision	Recall	F1-score
Train	4717	2	7797	8	1.00	[0.0, 0.10]	1.00	1.00	1.00
Validation	1389	446	2774	4	0.98	[0.0, 0.70]	1.00	0.76	0.86

Through the analysis of the different metrics shown in Table 2 we can observe that the model already had very good results with the task in hand, which meant that no changes to the initial model were necessary. At this point, we were ready to test the model with V10 and see how efficient the model was at classifying frames into informative and uninformative, without applying any AL technique. Hence, in Step 1 there was no AL cycle.

Step 2: V10 was introduced to the model, after Step 1, to test its performance in classifying informative and uninformative frames.

It was observed, in approximately 848 images, that the model classified them inaccurately as informative frames.

Considering the method to calculate the Accuracy, 166 images were correctly predicted in the universe of 400 images, this meant an Accuracy of 0.415. With this Accuracy, we can generalise the results and conclude that the model can classify correctly approximately 42% of the images in CEV.

In Fig. 6, frames b) and c) were both considered informative and presented an equal prediction, even when we can see that frame b) is uninformative. At this point, the model hadn't yet learned that frames similar to b) weren't informative. We could see that the model, even with good results, still had room to learn.

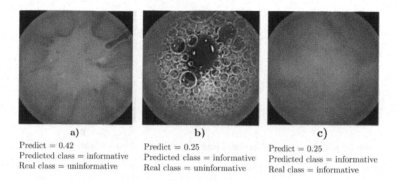

a)   b)   c)

Predict = 0.42   Predict = 0.25   Predict = 0.25
Predicted class = informative   Predicted class = informative   Predicted class = informative
Real class = uninformative   Real class = uninformative   Real class = informative

Fig. 6. Example of frames classified by the model in Step 2 as informative. The frames a) and b) were inaccurately classified as informative. The frame c) was correctly classified as informative.

Step 3: The introduction of the AL cycle to the model trained after Step 1, aimed to increase the model's knowledge with a big reduction in the effort of data annotation. The AL method chosen was Least Confidence Sampling (LCS).

V2 was the raw data for the model to predict labels and using LCS, 200 images were pooled, annotated and then inserted in the initial dataset and used to retrain the model. After re-training the model, now with the added images annotated from V2, the obtained results are stated in Table 3.

Table 3. The confusion matrix and the metrics of the AUC and Loss are provided along with the Precision, Recall and F1-score for the model in Step 3.

	TP	FN	TN	FP	AUC	Loss	Precision	Recall	F1-score
Train	4725	0	7758	241	1.00	[0.0, 0.10]	0.95	1.00	0.98
Validation	1799	36	2716	62	0.99	[0.0, 0.50]	0.97	0.98	0.97

Compared to the results of Step 1 (see Table 2), the number of FN in training and validation decreased but the number of FP increased.

V10 was again used to test the model and around 3828 images were considered as informative. After checking them, it was verified that there is still a large number of images that were inaccurately classified.

The Accuracy at this step was 0.52.

Taking into consideration Fig. 7, we could see that images similar to a) and b) were still wrongly classified as informative. It can also be noted that frame a) presented a prediction very similar to the prediction in frame c) which is an informative frame.

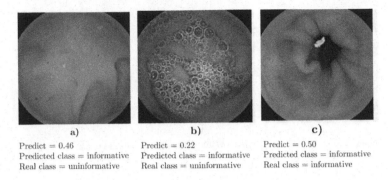

a)

Predict = 0.46
Predicted class = informative
Real class = uninformative

b)

Predict = 0.22
Predicted class = informative
Real class = uninformative

c)

Predict = 0.50
Predicted class = informative
Real class = informative

Fig. 7. Example of frames classified by the model in Step 3 as informative. The frames a) and b) were inaccurately classified as informative. The frame c) was correctly classified as informative.

Step 4: The initial conditions of Step 3 were repeated but the AL method LCS was replaced with MS, in order to assess whether another AL method was more suitable for the task that we were dealing with.

With V2 as the raw data for the model to predict labels and using MS, 200 images were pooled, annotated and then inserted in the initial dataset. After re-training the model, now with the added images annotated from V2, the obtained results are stated in Table 4.

Table 4. The confusion matrix and the metrics of the AUC and Loss are provided along with the Precision, Recall and F1-score for the model in Step 4.

	TP	FN	TN	FP	AUC	Loss	Precision	Recall	F1-score
Train	4213	513	7991	7	0.99	[0.0, 0.10]	1.00	0.89	0.94
Validation	855	980	2777	1	0.98	[0.0, 1.00]	1.00	0.47	0.64

The results obtained with MS and compared with the results from LCS, it was possible to conclude that the results with LCS presented to be better, regarding AUC, Loss and the total number of false predictions. Even with the worst results after re-training the model, we still used V10 to test the model and verified that only 319 images were classified as informative.

The model, using MS, had an Accuracy of 0.397.

Considering Fig. 8, as in the previous step with LCS, we could see that images similar to frames a) and b) were still wrongly classified as informative and images similar to frame a) presented predictions very similar to the prediction of frame c) which is an informative frame.

We concluded that with MS the model had an overall regression when compared to the results of Step 3 with LCS.

Given the aforementioned information, LCS was the AL method used for the following steps, until the end of the experiment.

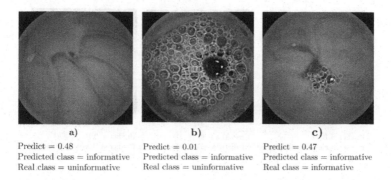

a)

b)

c)

Predict = 0.48
Predicted class = informative
Real class = uninformative

Predict = 0.01
Predicted class = informative
Real class = uninformative

Predict = 0.47
Predicted class = informative
Real class = informative

Fig. 8. Example of frames classified by the model in Step 4 as informative. The frames a) and b) were inaccurately classified as informative. The frame c) was correctly classified as informative

Step 5: The main goal of this step, was to evaluate the performance of the model's classification capability, after 3 iterations of the AL cycle.

Three iterations of the AL cycle over the trained model after Step 1, were triggered using V2, V5 and V7 as the raw data for the model to predict labels. Using LCS, in each iteration 200 images were pooled, annotated and then inserted in the initial dataset, used to train the model. After re-training the model, now with the added images annotated from V2, V5 and V7, the obtained results are stated in Table 5.

Table 5. The confusion matrix and the metrics of the AUC and Loss are provided along with the Precision, Recall and F1-score for the model in Step 5.

	TP	FN	TN	FP	AUC	Loss	Precision	Recall	F1-score
Train	4885	14	5451	2774	0.99	[0.0, 0.05]	0.64	1.00	0.78
Validation	1791	44	1822	956	0.97	[0.0, 0.20]	0.65	0.98	0.78

The results of training and validation in this step were slightly worse when compared with the results of Step 3, given that the total number of FN and FP increased.

The V10 was used to test the model and around 11 157 images were considered informative. After checking them, it was verified that there were still a large number of images that were inaccurately classified.

The Accuracy at this step was 0.54.

The Fig. 9 depicted that images similar to a) and b) continue to be difficult for the model to correctly classify, which could mean that 3 AL cycles weren't enough to testify major differences in the capability of the model to classify images of that type.

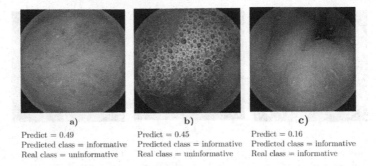

a)   b)   c)

Predict = 0.49   Predict = 0.45   Predict = 0.16
Predicted class = informative Predicted class = informative Predicted class = informative
Real class = uninformative Real class = uninformative Real class = informative

Fig. 9. Example of frames classified by the model in Step 5 as informative. The frames a) and b) were inaccurately classified as informative. he frame c) was correctly classified as informative.

Step 6: We came across V6 and verified that this video had unusual content and for that reason, we took an extra step to evaluate how the model would react to this type of content (Fig. 10).

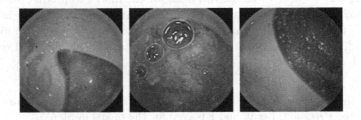

Fig. 10. V6 had an unusual amount of frames similar to images shown in this figure.

Taking the resulting model from Step 5, V6 was the raw data for the model to predict labels and using LCS, 200 images were pooled, annotated and then inserted in the initial dataset. After re-training the model, now with images from V1, V2, V5, V6 and V7, the obtained results are stated in Table 6.

Table 6. The confusion matrix and the metrics of the AUC and Loss are provided along with the Precision, Recall and F1-score for the model in Step 6.

	TP	FN	TN	FP	AUC	Loss	Precision	Recall	F1-score
Train	4770	140	8384	30	0.99	[0.0, 0.05]	0.99	0.97	0.98
Validation	1093	742	2741	37	0.96	[0.0, 0.40]	0.97	0.60	0.74

When V10 was used to test the model, it was verified that only 1314 images were classified as informative and a large percentage of those images were in reality uninformative. The Accuracy indicated that approximately 40% of the images were correctly classified.

After checking some examples of images classified as informative by the model and considering Fig. 11, we noticed that images similar to frame a) in Fig. 9 were no longer abundant, which could mean that the model had an increased capacity to deal with those images. However, it can be seen that there is still a large number of images of type b) that are wrongly classified. This could mean that the model hasn't yet learned enough to be able to correctly classify images of this type.

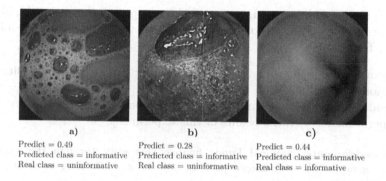

a)
Predict = 0.49
Predicted class = informative
Real class = uninformative

b)
Predict = 0.28
Predicted class = informative
Real class = uninformative

c)
Predict = 0.44
Predicted class = informative
Real class = informative

Fig. 11. Example of frames classified by the model in Step 6 as informative. The frames a) and b) were inaccurately classified as informative. The frame c) was correctly classified as informative.

4 Conclusions and Future Work

With this experiment and each of its steps, we arrived at the following conclusions:

- Introducing an AL cycle to a trained model, for classifying informative and uninformative frames of full CEV, had significant gains in reducing the time and the amount of data to be labelled, without a significant impact on the quality of the results (by comparing the results of Step 2 with Step 3);
- It was possible to observe that between LCS and MS (AL methods) the first method produced better results, given that the number of images correctly predicted is higher in the case of MS (by comparing the results of Step 3 with Step 4);
- The more iterations a model had with the AL cycle it was possible to observe that there was an increase (little one, but still an increase) in the number of correct predictions of classification (by comparing the results of Step 5 with Step 3);

– In the early stages, introducing the AL cycle to a CEV with unusual content could impact the performance of the model (by comparing the results of Step 6 with Step 5);
– Even after several iterations the model had difficulties distinguishing images with bubbles, mainly, but also with other artefacts related to the flux of different fluids inside the gastrointestinal tract from images with clear mucosa. This fact could be an indication of some ambiguity in the oracle annotation that impacted the model performance and/or the model needs more data and iterations with AL cycle to be more capable of distinguishing those types of images.

The outcome of this experiment verified the approach that using AL in classification tasks for CEV had room to grow and gave valuable cues for the following tasks as future work:

– Improving the quality of a reference dataset for tasks like abnormality classification using full CEV;
– Introducing deep active learning in classification tasks for CEV by evaluating its performance with the results of this experiment.

Acknowledgements. National Funds finance this work through the Portuguese funding agency, *FCT - Fundação para a Ciência e a Tecnologia*, within project LA/P/0063/2020.

References

1. Rawla, P., Sunkara, T., Barsouk, A.: Epidemiology of colorectal cancer: incidence, mortality, survival, and risk factors. Gastroenterol. Rev. **14**, 89–103 (2019)
2. Simadibrata, M., Adiwinata, R.: Precancerous lesions in gastrointestinal tract. Indon. J. Gastroenterol. Hepatol. Digest. Endosc. **18**, 112–117 (2017)
3. Flemming, J., Cameron, S.: Small bowel capsule endoscopy: indications, results, and clinical benefit in a university environment. Medicine **97**, e0148 (2018)
4. Spada, C., et al.: Performance measures for small-bowel endoscopy: a European society of gastrointestinal endoscopy (ESGE) quality improvement initiative. United Eur. Gastroenterol. J. **7**(5), 614–641 (2019). https://onlinelibrary.wiley.com/doi/abs/10.1177/2050640619850365
5. Lee, N.M., Eisen, G.M.: 10 years of capsule endoscopy: an update. Expert Rev. Gastroenterol. Hepatol. 4(4), 503–512 (2010)
6. Muñoz-Navas, M.: Capsule endoscopy. World J. Gastroenterol. WJG **15**(13), 1584 (2009)
7. Gueye, L., Yildirim-Yayilgan, S., Cheikh, F.A., Balasingham, I.: Automatic detection of colonoscopic anomalies using capsule endoscopy. In: 2015 IEEE International Conference on Image Processing (ICIP), pp. 1061–1064. IEEE (2015)
8. Dray, X.: Artificial intelligence in small bowel capsule endoscopy-current status, challenges and future promise. J. Gastroenterol. Hepatol. **36**(1), 12–19 (2021)
9. Radeva, P., et al.: Active labeling: application to wireless endoscopy analysis, pp. 174–181 (2012)

10. Folmsbee, J., Liu, X., Brandwein-Weber, M., Doyle, S.: Active deep learning: improved training efficiency of convolutional neural networks for tissue classification in oral cavity cancer. In: 2018 IEEE 15th International Symposium on Biomedical Imaging (ISBI 2018), pp. 770–773. IEEE (2018)

11. Fonseca, F., Nunes, B., Salgado, M., Cunha, A.: Abnormality classification in small datasets of capsule endoscopy images. Procedia Comput. Sci. **196**, 469–476 (2022)

12. Shin, H.C., et al.: Deep convolutional neural networks for computer-aided detection: CNN architectures, dataset characteristics and transfer learning. IEEE Trans. Med. Imaging **35**(5), 1285–1298 (2016)

13. Kim, H.E., Cosa-Linan, A., Santhanam, N., Jannesari, M., Maros, M.E., Ganslandt, T.: Transfer learning for medical image classification: a literature review. BMC Med. Imaging **22**(1), 69 (2022)

14. Kingma, D.P., Ba, J.: Adam: a method for stochastic optimization. arXiv preprint arXiv:1412.6980 (2014)

15. Angluin, D.: Queries and concept learning. Mach. Learn. **2**, 319–342 (1988)

16. Dagan, I., Engelson, S.P.: Committee-based sampling for training probabilistic classifiers. In: Machine Learning Proceedings 1995, pp. 150–157. Elsevier (1995)

17. Settles, B.: Active learning literature survey (2009)

18. Malagelada, C., et al.: New insight into intestinal motor function via noninvasive endoluminal image analysis. Gastroenterology **135**(4), 1155–1162 (2008)

Indoor Air Quality in a Residential Building – A Health Issue

Sandra Pereira[1,2](✉) , Andrea Santiago[1], Cristina Reis[1] , Jorge Pinto[1,2] ,
and Isabel Bentes[1,2]

[1] UTAD, Quinta de Prados, 5000 Vila Real, Portugal
spereira@utad.pt
[2] C-MADE/UTAD, Quinta de Prados, 5000 Vila Real, Portugal

Abstract. This study addresses the often-overlooked issue of indoor air quality, emphasizing its significance for the health and well-being of individuals spending a majority of their time indoors. Factors such as building occupancy, construction materials, and ventilation systems contribute to indoor air quality. Recognizing it as a critical environmental risk factor, this research focuses on assessing air quality in The Castle House, Lamego, through the measurement of PM10 and PM2.5 particles, temperature, barometric pressure, relative humidity, and carbon dioxide. The paper provides context, presents the study case, analyzes results, and concludes with implications for future research.

Keywords: indoor air quality · health and well-being · automatic monitoring

1 Introduction

When we talk about air quality, concerns usually refer to atmospheric pollution just outside buildings. However, people currently spend most of their time indoors, whether in their homes, workplaces or commercial and leisure areas, so ensuring good indoor air quality is essential for the health and well-being of these spaces' users. Indoor air quality is influenced by several factors, such as the occupancy of the building, the construction materials, the purpose for which it is intended, the activities carried out there, the building maintenance actions, and the type of ventilation and cleaning ventilation systems. Indoor air quality is an environmental risk factor of particular interest, as it can affect human health and cognitive functions and the productivity of those who spend a large part of their time in closed spaces.

The main objective of this work is to analyse the air quality in a column built to ventilate and illuminate the south facade of Casa do Castelo, which is partially buried. The Castle House is a small building located in the historic area of Lamego Castle, which was completely rebuilt to function as local accommodation. This reconstruction was carried out in accordance with the specific regulations of this historic area, in order to fully preserve the visual aspect of the heritage built inside the walls. It is a simple and poor building, with no relevant architectural value, but which is part of the set of buildings that

A. Cunha et al. (Eds.): MobiHealth 2023, LNICST 578, pp. 324–337, 2024.
https://doi.org/10.1007/978-3-031-60665-6_24

identify this classified historic area. In this building, as in most of the others that belong this complex, due to the topography and also for economic reasons, one of the facades is the wall itself or the rocky mass of the area, with the houses being partially buried, with lighting problems, ventilation and humidity. In this context, and taking into account the fact that the exterior appearance of the building had to be maintained (architecture and materials), an architectural solution was studied which consisted of maintaining the existing façades but moving the house away from the rock mass on the inside, creating a column that goes from the ground floor to the 2nd floor for ventilation and lighting through a skylight placed on the roof, but away from it to allow air circulation. After the building started operating, especially in the summer, it was found that the ground floor smelled of mould, which indicated that there was no air circulation. Thus, we analyzed the air quality in The Castle House in Lamego by measuring PM10 and PM2.5 particles, temperature, barometric pressure, relative humidity and carbon dioxide. These parameters, especially the thermal gradient, also allow us to infer whether or not there is air circulation in that column.

This paper is structured as follows. After this introduction, the main topics considered in this paper are put into context. Then, the study case is presented, and the results are analysed. Finally, the main conclusions and future works are offered.

2 Indoor Air Quality

The quality of the indoor environment is a concern that has been with man for many centuries. It is always desirable that the air is fresh and pleasant. That is, it does not harm health. There is increasing evidence that the indoor environment's quality can profoundly affect home occupants' health [1, 2]. The concept of indoor environmental quality is quite complex and comprehensive, depending on many factors, such as temperature, relative humidity, air speed, the existence of odours, the concentration of microorganisms or dust in air suspension, noise level, and lighting, among others. These factors can be grouped into four major areas: air quality, hygrothermal quality, acoustic quality and lighting quality [3]. Good air quality is of paramount importance. A high degree of air purity, large air flows and efficient air filtration are necessary to obtain a good indoor environment. Air quality depends on the degree to which the air is free of pollutants that may irritate or harm occupants. The interior environment of buildings is contaminated by various substances that result from the current use of spaces and materials used in construction. These substances can have effects on the well-being of the occupants. The design and implementation of ventilation systems must consider the sources of pollution to evacuate these polluting substances to the outside, thus avoiding contamination of the indoor air. One of the methods used to assess the quality of indoor air in buildings, to reduce the risk to the health of occupants consists of determining the production rate of existing pollutants. It is not known how all polluting substances affect indoor air quality, so they are generally considered separately. Air quality also depends directly on the volume of the compartments. For this reason, in addition to ergonomic reasons, it is recommended that no ceiling heights be lower than the minimum recommended values. Some health problems caused by poor air quality are similar to the symptoms that affect us when we have the flu, so they are difficult to associate with the workplace. The indoor environment is rarely suspected of being the cause of symptoms.

Contaminants can also originate outside the building and pass through external air inlets or, in cases where the air extracted from the building by the air conditioning system is greater than the amount of air introduced, flowing inside the building through any crack available.

2.1 Indoor Air Quality in Residential Buildings

In residential buildings, indoor air quality is ensured by natural, mechanical or mixed ventilation systems. These systems are intended to supply fresh air to the occupants of these buildings, to the combustion appliances and to ensure the extraction of combustion products. This ventilation must be provided in comfortable and safe conditions, minimising energy consumption [4].

The high rate of pollutants inside buildings originates from occupancy density, equipment, and synthetic covering materials. Poor air quality can cause immediate, short-term, and even medium and long-term effects. It is essential to take care of indoor air quality, particularly in the building's design, installation and operation. Both the activities inside buildings and the materials integrated into the construction can produce or release undesirable substances into the indoor environment. Next, the pollutants described in Portuguese regulations in air quality are analysed.

The activities inside residential buildings and the materials integrated into the construction can produce or release undesirable substances into the indoor environment. The relative humidity of indoor air can directly and indirectly influence the occupants' activity. Low relative humidity values can cause sensations of dryness, skin and mucous membrane irritation, respiratory tract infections or discomfort in contact with some materials due to the generation of static electricity. High relative humidity values can also cause discomfort, inhibiting perspiration through the skin and the development of mould and mites that cause allergies, irritations and, in more severe cases, asthma. Relative humidity values, considered adequate, must be between 30 and 70%. The occupants' metabolism and activity produce carbon dioxide (CO_2) and water vapour. Gas combustion also releases carbon dioxide and produces water vapour. Some consider that this gas is not toxic but a simple asphyxiant [5]. It is harmless at low concentrations of carbon dioxide, typically occurring inside buildings. But if the concentrations are high, it can cause drowsiness, breathing problems, headaches, fatigue, nausea, difficulty concentrating, etc.

Regarding limit values, the World Health Organization (WHO) [6] does not define a limit value for the concentration of this gas inside non-industrial buildings. However, prolonged exposure alters the body's acid-base balance, causing calcium loss in the bones. The main sources of CO_2 production are human metabolism and all combustion sources in a home. Carbon monoxide (CO) is an odourless, tasteless and colourless gas resulting from combustion, especially in environments not rich in oxygen. At extremely low concentrations, carbon monoxide causes headaches and drowsiness. As the concentration increases, symptoms begin to include problems with concentration, vision and nausea and, in extreme cases, can lead to death as blood haemoglobin reduces oxygen to insufficient levels because it has a greater affinity for carbon monoxide. Very high concentrations of this gas can cause palpitations, vomiting, and cardiovascular problems, among others. All these pollutants mentioned above cause various anomalies in buildings, which in turn harm the quality of the indoor environment.

Various polluting substances can be released inside residential buildings by construction materials. The substances that have received the most attention are volatile organic components (VOCs) and formaldehyde (HCHO) [5] due to higher values inside than outside.

Pollutants that have a source mostly outside residential buildings must also be analysed, such as radon, particles, ozone and microorganisms.

Radon is a noble gas with no smell, colour or taste, radioactive of natural origin, and present in the soil. The concentration of radon inside houses depends on the concentrations of uranium and radium in the soil and subsoil under construction, as well as the infiltration routes of that gas and the ventilation of the house. Radon usually forms in the rocky materials beneath the building's settlement and diffuses and exhales from the rocks, entering buildings through cracks, cable passages and pipes. Radon concentrations are often higher inside basements and ground floor rooms than on upper floors. Air exchange with the outside depends on the occupants' ventilation habits and the houses' natural ventilation. Building materials, as they contain varying concentrations of uranium and radium, can also be a source of radon exhaled into buildings. However, as a general rule, the main source of radon is the soil under buildings [7]. Radon, when inhaled, is a carcinogen responsible for the increase in the incidence of lung cancer in exposed populations.

Measuring radon gas in indoor spaces is the only way to determine whether radon gas concentrations exceed the national reference level. The radon concentration inside buildings is not constant, showing daily variations (generally higher at night and lower during the day), seasonal (higher in winter and lower in summer), and annual.

Particles in indoor environments can have different diameters and types and carry living organisms such as viruses, fungi and bacteria. These particles may come from tobacco smoke, combustion products or outside air. Particles can be dust, fibres, pollens, etc. Dust is fine dust particles that generally originate from outdoor dust, and when inhaled, they deposit in the respiratory system and cause rhinitis, asthma, bronchitis and respiratory allergies. The fibres originate from glass and rock fibres found in various products and irritate the eyes, skin and respiratory tract. Pollens are produced by plants outdoors, but once indoors, they persist for a long time. Their chemical composition and geometric shape vary, meaning their effects on the human body vary. However, the smaller the particles, the more adverse the effects on health, which can be associated with respiratory problems, worsening symptoms in asthma patients, reduced lung function, etc. Prolonged exposure to this type of particle can also result in chronic bronchitis.

Ozone (O3) is a compound that produces adverse effects and can seriously affect human health and well-being. Inside buildings, ozone is released, particularly by photocopiers and laser printers. Ozone can be highly oxidising and reacts with various substances outside and inside, such as perfumes, furniture, carpets, paints, varnishes, and cleaning products, generating ultrafine toxic particles. Symptoms of exposure to ozone are related, in particular, to changes in lung functions, inflammation in the airways, and the worsening of asthma problems. Other symptoms are eye irritation, headaches and accelerated heart rate.

The four most significant categories of microorganisms that occur in indoor environments are bacteria, mites, microorganisms from pets and fungi. The variety and concentration of these microorganisms increase with the number of occupants. These microorganisms can cause allergies such as rhinitis (inflammation of the nose mucosa), asthma, sneezing, tears, colds, breathing difficulties, and digestive problems.

2.2 Ventilation

Ventilation in residential buildings must be general and permanent, as renewing indoor air ensures the healthiness of spaces, thus guaranteeing better air quality.

Indoor air quality can be controlled through a control strategy or by implementing appropriate ventilation strategies. Ventilation emerges as a fundamental strategy in managing indoor air quality, with localised extraction preferred in the presence of intense and punctual emission sources, as in the kitchen. Dilution and removal should be seen as mechanisms for eliminating pollutants generated in a dispersed manner. Ventilation systems supply new air to the occupants of the dwellings, to the combustion appliances, and to ensure the extraction of combustion products. Insufficient ventilation conditions have very negative impacts on indoor air quality. Relative humidity is often the determining factor in establishing extraction flow rates in service compartments. The admissions are located in the main compartments to provide metabolic oxygen and dilute pollutants and odours from the occupants. The climate naturally influences the choice of ventilation system, ranging from fully controllable systems with low air permeability to natural ventilation systems with high permeability of the surroundings. The sizing of ventilation systems must be careful. Mechanical ventilation systems activated according to pollutant removal needs require higher flow rates. In most residential buildings, the system installed is mixed. Ventilation systems must respect pre-existing evacuation location principles and take advantage of actions promoting evacuation to allow better ventilation of the entire fire. Air permeability and ventilation flow rates must be specified, which depend on the activities carried out inside the buildings and their occupancy.

Natural ventilation is the renewal of air promoted by natural actions (thermal and wind), which ensure controlled airflow between exterior air intake openings (windows and grilles) and air extraction openings (chimneys). In Portugal, natural ventilation in residential buildings must follow the specifications of standard NP 1037-1: 2002 (Ventilation and evacuation of combustion products from rooms with gas appliances. Part I: Residential buildings) [8]. The ventilation system is intended to ensure indoor air quality, supplying "new" air to the combustion appliances and ensuring the exhaustion of combustion products, which must be provided in comfortable and safe conditions. The ventilation rates of this system depend on the size and distribution of openings in the building envelope and wind pressure. Wind pressure depends on weather conditions, and openings in the building envelope must be controlled according to the weather. The World Health Organization states that very high ventilation rates should be avoided. Natural ventilation is carefully designed and constructed to ensure adequate ventilation rates, although occupants generally have to adjust openings when necessary. Like many other systems, natural ventilation has advantages and disadvantages [8].

Mechanical ventilation is the renewal of air promoted by mechanical fans, which ensures controlled and uninterrupted air flow between external air intake openings and air extraction openings connected to ducts. There are systems with mechanical inflation and extraction and systems with extraction fans only. Mechanical ventilation is a way of ventilating spaces that allows constant airflow to be imposed, regardless of external actions and users. It can include air supply and/or extraction and also heat recovery. It ensures the necessary flow to be inflated in spaces with an adequate interior temperature and allows humidity control, avoiding building pathologies. Collective systems installed in multi-family buildings must operate 24 h a day. Double-flow systems can be adopted to improve efficiency in colder areas, with heat recovery, which allows the new air to be pre-heated by crossing it with the extracted air. When a mechanical source provides ventilation, the building envelope can be closed. The air supplied for ventilation can be clean, that is, without pollutants from outside air. Furthermore, heating and cooling can be easily combined with mechanical ventilation systems. These systems can also control pressure differences over the building envelope and prevent damage, such as moisture, in the building structures.

Mixed ventilation occurs when there is natural and mechanical ventilation. New air enters through openings in the surroundings and is extracted through exhaust fans and extractors. It is possible to improve the resolution of the natural ventilation system by introducing mechanical support. Mixed ventilation often uses a low-energy auxiliary extraction fan in a natural ventilation duct. The fan is operated when forces are low or reverse flow is to be avoided. Its efficiency can be improved by zoning the building so that some parts operate under natural conditions while others are under mechanical ventilation. A mixed system may include a natural ventilation system combined with mechanical ventilation utterly independent of the system. Thus, natural ventilation is used for as long as possible, and the mechanical ventilation system takes over when this no longer occurs.

The following table presents a comparative analysis of the main advantages and disadvantages of natural, mechanical, and mixed ventilation systems.

3 Legislation

The national indoor air quality policy emerged following the transposition into domestic law of European Directive 2002/91/EC [10].

In existing buildings, the indoor air quality index for each pollutant was calculated based on the arithmetic mean of the maximum mean concentration values of the pollutant measured in each area of the home. The Indoor Air Quality Index (IQAI) of a building will be defined based on the pollutant with the worst classification [11].

With the publication of Directive 2010/31/EU [12], relating to the energy performance of buildings, the regime established by Directive 2002/91/EC was reformulated, reinforcing the promotion of energy performance in buildings and highlighting the goals and challenges agreed upon by the European Member States for 2020. This time, the new national regulations, Decree-Law 118/2013 [13], defined a non-mandatory indoor air quality certification, which constituted a setback. However, it considers the minimum values of fresh airflow per space and the protection thresholds for indoor air pollutant concentrations to safeguard health and well-being. It also highlights that adequate natural ventilation must be prioritised over forced ventilation from a perspective of optimising resources, energy efficiency and cost reduction. Indoor air quality audits are also eliminated. However, controlling pollution sources and adopting preventive measures are maintained, both in terms of the design of buildings and their operation, to comply with the legal requirements to reduce possible risks to public health.

In this context, to comply with the changes imposed by Decree-Law no. 118/2013, Ordinance 353-A/2013 of December 4 was published [14]. Table 1 presents the protection thresholds for radon, CO2, CH2O, CO, VOC and particulate matter (PM10 and PM2.5). Regarding indoor air quality in homes, it should be noted that there is no specific legislation, leaving it up to the occupants to ensure the air quality in their homes. However, in residential buildings, the only regulatory requirement related to indoor air quality refers to an air exchange rate of 0.6 h-1, as mentioned in the old decree-law. In the current legislation, the hourly calculation of the air exchange rate is based on the method that meets the requirements of standard EN 15242 [15] for commercial and service buildings.

Table 1. Protection threshold and tolerance margin for physical-chemical pollutants according to Ordinance No. 353-A/2013 [14]

Pollutants	Unit	Protection threshold	Tolerance margin [%]
Particulate matter (PM10 fraction)	$\mu g/m^3$	50	100
Particulate matter (PM2.5 fraction)	$\mu g/m^3$	25	100
Total Volatile Organic Compounds (VOCs)	$\mu g/m^3$	600	100
Carbon monoxide (CO)	mg/m^3	10	-
Formaldehyde (CH2O)	$\mu g/m^3$	100	-
Carbon dioxide (CO2)	mg/m^3	2250	30
Radon	Bq/m^3	400	-

- The concentrations in $\mu g/m^3$ and mg/m^3 refer to a temperature of 20 °C and a pressure of 1 atm (101.325 kPa);
- The protection thresholds indicated relate to an average of 8 h;
- The margins of tolerance shall apply to existing buildings and new buildings without mechanical ventilation systems;
- Radon analysis is mandatory in buildings built in granite areas, namely in the districts of Braga, Vila Real, Porto, Guarda, Viseu and Castelo Branco.

4 Case Study

4.1 The Castle House in Lamego

The Castle House in Lamego is a house intended for local accommodation, consisting of 3 floors and, as already stated, the south facade is partially buried. In this building, due to the topography and also for economic reasons, part of the south facades was the rocky mass of the area, causing lighting, ventilation and humidity problems. The house was completely rebuilt three years ago but taking into account the fact that the exterior appearance of the building had to be maintained (architecture and materials), an architectural solution was studied which consisted of maintaining the existing elevation but moving the house away from the rock mass on the inside, creating a column that goes from the ground floor to the 2nd floor for ventilation and lighting through a skylight placed on the roof, but away from it to allow air circulation (Fig. 1).

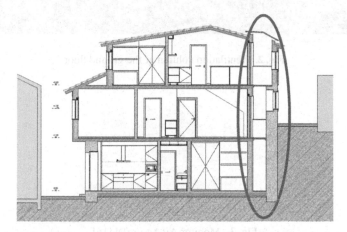

Fig. 1. Column for ventilation and lighting through a skylight placed on the roof

After it started operating, especially in the summer, it was found that the ground floor (Fig. 2) smelled of mould, which indicated that there was no air circulation and, probably poor air quality.

In this context as thought to analyse the air quality by measuring PM10 and PM2.5 particles, temperature, barometric pressure, relative humidity and carbon dioxide. The thermal gradient and the barometric pressure also allow us to infer whether or not there is air circulation in that column.

To this end, two devices, monitor AirAssure™ [16], Fig. 3, were placed inside the column, one on ground floor, "Walls", and the other on floor 2, "Tower", to collect data regarding air quality, Fig. 3 (Fig. 4).

Sixty-seven measurements were carried out on each AirAssure device/monitor between 3:27 pm on February 21, 2023, and 10:29 am on February 24 2023. The monitoring time was short because the main objective was to compare the air quality at the level of the ground floor, which is a non-ventilated area that, from time to time, smells mold, and the most ventilated area, which is the 2nd floor, next to the skylight. On the

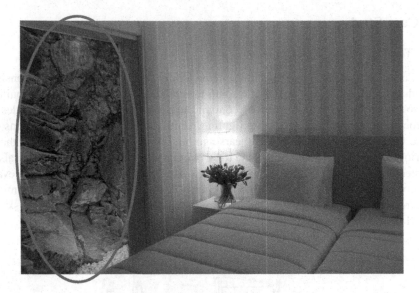

Fig. 2. Ventilation column at the ground floor

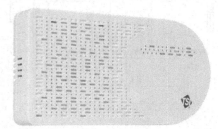

Fig. 3. Monitor AirAssure™ [16]

other hand, it was also intended to understand whether or not air was circulating in the ventilation column without mechanical ventilation.

In the Fig. 5, it can be observed all the data collected by the monitors placed, one on the "Wall" and on the "Tower" in the studied period.

Analysis of Results

Regarding PM10 and PM2.5 particles, we found a greater concentration in the Tower, because the outside air contained more particles than the indoor air and since at the level of the "Tower" (2nd floor) the space is immediately connected to the outside by the skylight, the concentration of particles is higher at that level. Nevertheless, in both, they are lower than 50 mg/m³, obtaining an AQI considered Good for health levels.

The carbon dioxide values are identical, as the average of the two measurements is very close, 421 ppm in the Wall and 416 ppm in the Tower.

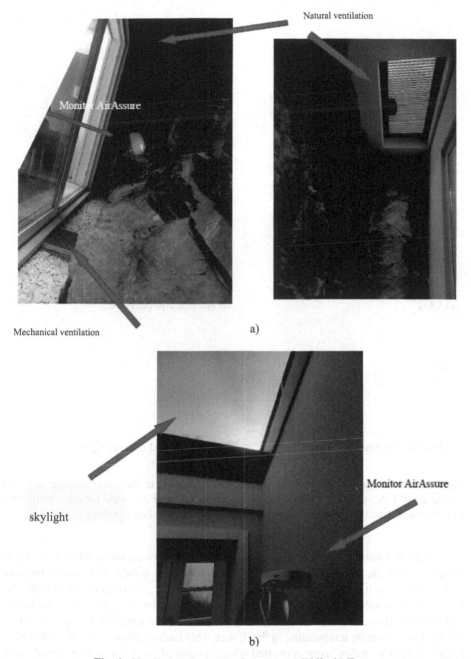

Fig. 4. Ventilation devices and sensors. a) Walls, b) Tower

We found that the barometric pressure is lower in the Tower because it is a higher floor (2nd floor) in relation to the Wall which is the ground floor but the variation between the Wall and the Tower is more or even constant.

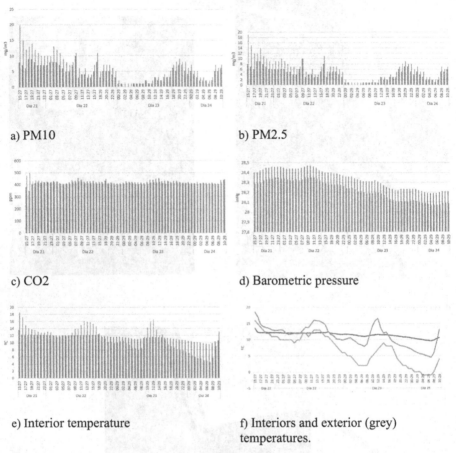

a) PM10

b) PM2.5

c) CO2

d) Barometric pressure

e) Interior temperature

f) Interiors and exterior (grey) temperatures.

Fig. 5. Datta collected by the monitors in the Wall (blue) and in the Tower (orange) between 21 and 24 of February 2023. a) PM10, b) PM2.5, c) CO2, d) Barometric pressure, e) Interior temperature, f) Interiors and exterior (grey) temperatures. (Color figure online)

The temperature in the Wall is constant because it is buried, and therefore very much protected from the action of the sun and other atmospheric agents. The same is not true in the Tower, as it is higher during the day than at night. If we compare it with the temperature outside, we see the same variation between the temperature of the Tower and outside. However, it should be noted that the outside temperature recorded was always lower than the temperature in the Tower. This finding allows us to infer that next to the skylight a "buffer" zone is created where a mass of air is hotter than outside and, as the area of connection to the outside is small, it is not enough to give the exit of this warmer air outside. The temperature in the Wall is generally lower than in the Tower and the pressure is higher, so it is difficult to circulate air from the Wall to the Tower, and it seems advisable to increase the ventilation area next to the skylight and use mechanical air circulation.

The relative humidity in the Wall is higher than in the Tower, reaching values of 80% humidity. The maximum value reaches 75% in the Tower, and the average during the period under analysis is 69% in the Wall and 63% in the Tower. We can conclude that the relative humidity in some measurements is above the recommended parameters. It is for this reason, and because there is no air circulation, that the mold smell appears.

Table 2 shows the mean values, mode and standard deviation of the readings recorded for the various parameters.

Table 2. Statistical analyses of the collected data.

Parameter		Device 1 – Walls			Device 2 - Tower		
		Mean	Mode	Standard deviation	Mean	Mode	Standard deviation
Temperature	°C	11,506	12,10	0,805	11,196	12,00	3,341
Relative humidity	%	69,269	61,00	9,033	63,090	68,00	8,350
Barometric Pressure	mmHg	28,338	28,23	0,098	28,223	28,35	0,099
CO2	ppm	421	412,00	14,85	416	408,00	16,267
PM10	mg/m^3	4,343	5,00	2,609	6,358	7,00	4,166
PM2.5	mg/m^3	4,090	5,00	2,460	5,985	7,00	3,808

5 Conclusions and Future Work

The quality of the indoor environment is a very complex, comprehensive and highly important topic. However, it depends on several factors. For good air quality inside buildings, it is always desirable that the air that circulates is fresh and pleasant and does not negatively impact the health of the occupants. But today, there is increasing evidence that the indoor environment can profoundly affect the health of building occupants. The occupancy density of buildings and installed equipment are some factors that pollute the interior. Air pollutants can originate from human activity (for example, water vapour and relative humidity), construction materials (volatile organic compounds), and other types of pollutants, such as radon. All pollutants cause poor air quality that can affect human health. Indoor air quality is a parameter that affects all types of buildings, from residential buildings, offices, schools, day-care centres and kindergartens. In these locations, this parameter is ensured by ventilation systems intended to supply new air to the combustion appliances and provide the extraction of combustion products. It must be guaranteed to be in comfortable and safe conditions. For indoor air quality to be good, it is important that the two established criteria exist and are respected, which are the determination of limit values for polluting substances depending on the length of time occupants remain in the contaminated environment and the finding of criteria related to sensory effects caused by polluting substances in humans. However, the air quality in a building is assessed to satisfy the health and comfort criteria of the inhabitants/occupants. Ventilation is essential to control indoor air quality. The most used systems in Portugal are natural, mechanical and mixed ventilation. However, the most used system is the natural ventilation system, which ensures the desired ventilation rates and has greater efficiency in extracting pollutants. When sizing a system of this type, it is mandatory to be very careful. Thermal comfort essentially depends on the temperature and relative humidity of the air. Still, it also depends on the air velocity, the asymmetry of the radiant temperature, the floor temperature and the difference in air temperatures. If the occupants feel a simple draft or a very sharp temperature difference, they will feel very uncomfortable.

Regarding the case study, it should be noted that the quality of the outdoor air influences the quality of the indoor air and the ventilation, temperature, pressure and humidity are very important parameters in the circulation of air and therefore in its quality. As future work, it is very important to repeat this procedure in the summer, when the system works worst, due to the direct action of the sun on the skylight and accumulation of hot air next to the skylight.

Acknowledgements. This work was supported by the FCT (Portuguese Foundation for Science and Technology) through the project UIDB/04082/2020 (CMADE).

References

1. Nica, R.M., Hapurne, T., Dumitrascu, A.I., Bliuc, I., Avram, C.: Proposal for a small two-story living room house based on air-quality monitoring, Proc. Manuf. **22**, 268–273 (2018). https://doi.org/10.1016/j.promfg.2018.03.041. ISSN 2351-9789
2. Figols González, M., Díaz de Garayo Balsategui, S., Aláez Sarasibar, X.: Indoor air quality monitoring as a tool for evaluating and improving the healthiness of a space. Anales de Edificación **6**(3), 13–20 (2020). https://doi.org/10.20868/ade.2020.4610. ISSN 2444-1309
3. Pinto, M., Freitas, V.P., Viegas, J.: Qualidade do Ambiente Interior em Edifícios de Habitação. Revista "engenharia&vida", ano IV, No 38, setembro 2007
4. Amaral, M.: Sistemas de Ventilação Natural e Mistos em Edifícios de Habitação. Tese de Doutoramento, Orientador: Prof. Dr. Vasco Manuel Araújo Peixoto de Freitas, Faculdade de Engenharia da Universidade do Porto, Porto, setembro 2008
5. Mascarenhas, J.: Sistemas de Construção IX - Contributos para o Cumprimento do RCCTE, Detalhes Construtivos sem Pontes Térmicas, Materiais Básicos (6ª parte): o Betão, 2ª edição, Livros Horizonte, Lisboa (2008)
6. WHO Air quality and health, Guidelines Review Committee, WHO guidelines for indoor air quality: selected pollutants. World Health Organization (2010). 454 p. ISBN 9789289002134
7. Carvalho, F.P., Reis, M.C.: Radon in Portuguese houses and workplaces. In: Oliveira Fernandes, E., Gameiro da Silva, M., Rosado Pinto, J. (eds.) Proceedings of the International Conference Healthy Buildings HB 2006, Lisbon, vol. II, pp. 507–511 (2006)
8. Instituto Português da Qualidade -IPQ [Portuguese Institute of Quality], -Ventilation and combustion products evacuation from places with gas-burning appliances, Part 1: Dwellings, Natural ventilation [in Portuguese], prNP 1037-1 (2002)
9. Gomes, R.: Estudo e conceção de sistemas de Ventilação natural em edifícios de habitação, dissertação para grau de mestre, Universidade da Madeira (2010)

10. European Union. On the Energy Performance of Buildings. Directive 2002/91/EC of the European Parliament and of the Council, Official Journal of the European Communities; Brussels (2002)
11. Pourkiaei, M., Romain, A.-C.: Scoping review of indoor air quality indexes: characterization and applications. J. Build. Eng. **75**, 106703 (2023). https://doi.org/10.1016/j.jobe.2023.106703. ISSN 2352-7102
12. European Communities: Directive 2010/31/EU of the European Parliament and of the Council of 19 May 2010 on the energy performance of buildings (recast) (2010)
13. Decree-Law No. 118/2013 of 20th August. 2013. Diário da República, 1.a série, No. 159. Ministry of Economy and Employment, Portugal
14. Ordinance 353-A/2013 of 4th December, 2013. Diário da República, 1.ª série, N.º 235. Ministry of Environment, Territory Planning, Health and Solidarity, Employment and Social Security. Lisbon, Portugal (2013)
15. EN 15242, Ventilation for buildings - Calculation methods for the determination of air flow rates in buildings including infiltration. European Committee for Standardization: Brussels, Belgium (2007)
16. Tslink: Continuous IAQ Monitoring Instruments. https://tsi.com/products/indoor-air-quality-meters-instruments/continuous-iaq-monitoring-instruments/. Accessed Nov 2023

Identification and Detection in Building Images of Biological Growths – Prevent a Health Issue

Sandra Pereira[1,2(✉)] ⓘ, António Cunha[1,3] ⓘ, and Jorge Pinto[1,2] ⓘ

[1] Quinta de Prados, UTAD, 5000 Vila Real, Portugal
spereira@utad.pt
[2] C-MADE / UTAD, Quinta de Prados, 5000 Vila Real, Portugal
[3] INESC TEC-INESC Technology and Science (Formerly INESC Porto), Porto, Portugal

Abstract. Building rehabilitation is a reality, and all phases of rehabilitation work need to be efficiently sustainable and promote healthy places to live in. Current procedures for assessing construction conditions are time-consuming, laborious and expensive and pose threats to the health and safety of engineers, especially when inspecting locations that are not easy to access. In the initial step, a survey of the condition of the building is carried out, which subsequently implies the elaboration of a report on existing pathologies, intervention solutions, and associated costs. This survey involves an inspection of the site (through photographs and videos). Also, biological growth can threaten the humans inhabiting the houses. The World Health Organization states that the most important effects are increased prevalences of respiratory symptoms, allergies and asthma, as well as perturbation of the immunological system. This work aims to alert to this fact and contribute to detecting and locating biological growth (BG) defects automatically in images of the facade of buildings. To make this possible, we need a dataset of images of building components with and without biological growths. At this moment, that database doesn't exist. So, we need to construct that dataset to use deep learning models in the future. This paper also identifies the steps to do that work and presents some real cases of building façades with BG and solutions to repair those defects. The conclusions and the future works are identified.

Keyword: Sickness prevention · Biological growths · Deep Learning

1 Introduction

Building rehabilitation is already a reality. Moreover, it is an excellent way to improve the construction sector's sustainability and indoor air quality [1–3]. International policy frameworks propose measures that include innovation, digitalisation, lower carbon emissions, and the fight against climate change as the main goals to be achieved in the search for sustainable development [3]. So, betting on solutions that facilitate all the tasks of a rehabilitation process is welcome. The traditional methods for this work commonly include engaging building surveyors to undertake a pathology report that involves a laborious site inspection. That results in a description of the physical conditions of the

A. Cunha et al. (Eds.): MobiHealth 2023, LNICST 578, pp. 338–350, 2024.
https://doi.org/10.1007/978-3-031-60665-6_25

building elements with the use of images, note-taking, drawings and information provided by the owner. The data collected is then analysed to produce a report. The report summarises the condition of the building, its elements [4], possible causes, and ways to repair the damages. This information also creates renewal, repair, and maintenance price estimates. Current assessment pathology report procedures are time-consuming and laborious and sometimes put the surveyor's health and safety at stake, particularly at height and roof levels that are usually not easy to access for those inspections [5].

Image analysis techniques for detecting defects have been proposed as an alternative to manual on-site inspection methods. In recent years, researchers have experimented with applying several soft computing and machine learning-based detection techniques to increase the automation of asset condition inspection. Whilst the latter is time-consuming and unsuitable for quantitative analysis, image analysis-based detection techniques, on the other hand, can be pretty challenging and entirely dependent on the quality of images taken under different real-world situations (e.g., light, shadow and noise) [5–13].

This paper proposes a deep learning methodology to detect and locate biological growth defects in images of facade walls of buildings. It is organised as follows: first, a brief discussion of selecting the most common defects that arise from biological growth in building façades is presented. This discussion is followed by a brief overview of deep learning methods used to solve fundamental computer vision problems. This quick overview provides the theoretical basis of the work that will be undertaken in the future. It follows the presentation of the deep learning-based detection and localisation model using transfer learning utilising the VGG-16 model for feature extraction and classification. It presents some real cases of building façades with BG and solutions to repair those defects. The images taken so far will contribute to constructing a dataset of images with and without BG to make the use of the methodology proposed possible. Finally, conclusions and future work are presented.

2 State of the Art

2.1 Biological Growths in Building Facades

Fungi, algae, mosses, and lichens are the biological agents that most affect building facades [14]. The growth of fungi and algae is usually caused by the absence of fungicidal and/or algicidal additives in the construction process. Stains resulting from biological colonisations can be caused by algae, fungi, lichens or parasitic vegetation, that is, microorganisms of animal or vegetable origin. In the presence of organic material, microorganisms of animal origin, such as fungi, grow in dark environments with little ventilation. Those of plant origin, such as algae, develop in hot environments with sun exposure in the presence of carbon dioxide [15].

Biological growths (BG) are the primary type of stone pathology that develops most quickly under usual conditions [16].

World Health Organization (WHO) concludes that the most critical effects of biological growths are increased prevalences of respiratory symptoms, allergies and asthma, and perturbation of the immunological system [3].

Humidity is a fundamental factor for biological growth. When exposed facades are at high-temperature levels, whether due to water infiltration or condensation, an environment conducive to developing fungi, algae and lichens is created. Shaded areas with little ventilation tend to retain more moisture, favouring biological growth.

Although biological growth can occur in shady areas, exposure to sunlight plays an important role. Direct sunlight and ultraviolet (UV) radiation can negatively affect biological growth, inhibiting its spread. However, areas with prolonged shade or indirect light can facilitate BG growth.

Temperature conditions also influence biological growth. Some organisms can develop in various temperatures, while others are more sensitive and prefer specific climates. Mild and humid temperatures, especially in regions with mild winters and summers, can favour biological growth on facades.

Atmospheric pollution, including gases and particles in the air, can affect biological growth on facades. Some pollutants can provide nutrients that promote BC development, while others can be toxic and inhibit their growth. Air quality can also influence the availability of nutrients and the ability of organisms to establish themselves on facade surfaces.

Some construction materials, such as bricks, concrete, stone and wood, can provide favourable substrates for biological growth. Porous, irregular surfaces or surfaces with accumulation of dust and debris are more likely to harbour organisms. Furthermore, the type of coating applied to facades can affect the surface's ability to retain moisture and, consequently, influence BG growth if the facade is exposed to high humidity conditions, whether due to humid weather conditions, lack of adequate ventilation or drainage problems, this can create a favourable environment for the growth of biological organisms. Areas of the facade that receive little direct sunlight and are in shadow for long periods are prone to biological growth. The lack of the sun reduces the rate of moisture evaporation, creating wetter conditions favourable to the development of moss, fungi and lichens.

Certain building materials, such as mortar, concrete, bricks and porous stone, can absorb and retain moisture for longer, providing an environment conducive to biological growth. These porous materials can provide enough nutrients and moisture to support the development of biological organisms.

2.1.1 Fungi

Fungi are the primary agents of degradation of facade surface coatings, considering that they are highly adaptable to environments with low humidity, sudden temperature variations and a minimum amount of nutrients for their nutrition [17, 18].

Fungi are organisms that need organic matter, dead or alive, for their development, which is why they establish themselves in places where it is deposited by other living beings or by the action of the wind [19].

According to [20], most fungi are aerobic, as they require oxygen at least in one phase of their life cycle. An optimal pH is also crucial for the metabolism of fungi. Most of them grow at optimum pH values between 4 and 6. However, many species can grow between 2 and 9 [20].

According to [21], the stains resulting from the accumulation of filamentous fungi on any substrate can be scientifically designated as mould. These microorganisms cause the appearance of dark spots with black, brown or greenish tones, which not only affect the visual quality of the facades but also gradually deteriorate the coverings and the support itself. In Figs. 1a and b, it is possible to see an example of the presence of fungi on a facade.

The consequences caused by the presence of fungi are worrying, as they feed, above all, on organic materials attached to facades, some dirt, and carbon monoxide. They can also feed on some components present in surface coating resins, such as paints and varnishes. These materials have a high concentration of organic material in their composition so that fungi can damage the paint film [14].

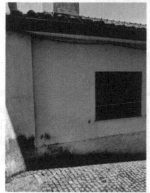 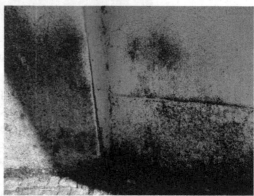

a) Façade with the presence of BG   b) Detail of fungus in the façade

Fig. 1. Presence of BG in a building façade.

Algae

According to [18] algae are photosynthetic organisms. That is, they use sunlight to produce their food. Therefore, they do not depend on the constituents of the material they adhere to develop. Like vegetables, algae need water and light, favouring their growth, especially in external environments.

Mosses

Mosses are bryophytes that preferably live in damp and shady walls, on which their reproduction depends. The humidity may be due to infiltrations or ineffective waterproofing. Figure 2 shows an example of mosses on facades.

This pathology begins from a seed, seedling or spore that reaches the facade of the building. The main ways are through the wind and bird faeces. Light, water (humidity) and nutrients are needed for germination or seedling development. The proliferation of mosses (bryophytes) in cracks or very porous concrete is mistakenly confused with fungi.

Lichens

Uemoto, K. et al. [18] clarifies that lichens are particular living organisms developed due to symbiosis (mutualistic relationship between two organisms where there are advantages

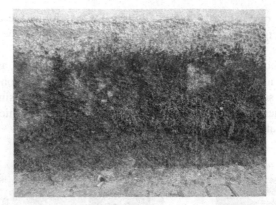

Fig. 2. Detail of a building façade with mosses.

for both individuals) between algae and fungi. Honda, N. K. et al. [22] defines lichen more precisely as a symbiotic organism composed of a fungus and one or more algae. In this symbiotic relationship, the algae produce organic food and photosynthesis. The fungus, on the other hand, guarantees protection and a suitable environment for the development of the algae. Therefore, it is concluded that for lichens to exist, fungi and algae must exist together.

Lichens are more frequent on rocky substrates Fig. 3a) and b) [20].

According to [21], like algae, lichens are photosynthetic and do not depend on the constituents of the materials to which they are attached. The damage that lichens cause to surfaces is similar to that of algae and fungi. They grow more slowly than algae and are generally not found on new surfaces until the algae and fungi have become established. They are usually found embedded in masonry, forming a thin layer firmly adhered to the substrate, or in the form of flat sheets, forming rosettes and poorly adhered to the base. In the initial stage, lichens can be easily confused with fungi and algae.

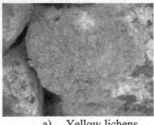
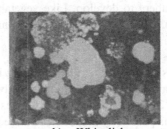

a) Yellow lichens   b) White lichens

Fig. 3. Lichen in a rocky substrat [20].

Prevention, Control and Repair Methods

Prevention and control of biological growths generally involve cleaning strategies, adequate maintenance, chemical treatments, selection of resistant materials and environmental control measures. Great care must be taken when deciding whether or not to carry out an intervention. When choosing the best method, evaluating the different aspects involved in the problem is necessary.

Initially, it is recommended that a preliminary project be carried out, defining proper procedures for greater effectiveness. On very degraded substrates, preliminary consolidation must be carried out to avoid further deterioration of the state of conservation, and the stone must be partially dried to improve the treatments' [20].

Afterwards, the most appropriate method for treatment must be chosen. The selection of the mechanical, physical or chemical treatment method depends on the type of organism present, the type of substrate to be treated, the state of conservation, and the costs involved.

Mechanical methods involve physically removing biological material with manual instruments such as scalpels, brushes, spatulas, scrapers, etc. These methods are widely used due to their simplicity and immediate results.

Physical interventions have no preventive power. They only eliminate living organisms. Examples of physical interventions include ultraviolet radiation and washing using water jets, which can also be used to remove biological growths.

In the chemical method, chemicals are responsible for eliminating macro and microorganisms, although some products also have preventive action on biological growth. The effectiveness of any chemical depends on the type of substrate, the type of organism or organisms involved, and the application method. In addition to chemicals, there are also biocides. The term biocide refers collectively to bactericides, algaecides, fungicides, and herbicides, distinguished by the specific organism to attack: bacteria, algae, fungi, lichens and plants, respectively [16].

2.2 Deep Learning Methods

Deep learning has increased in different research fields, with the potential to overcome the most challenging and laborious problems by using various layers of information processing in deep architectures for pattern recognition or classification [11, 22]. Convolutional Neural Networks (CNNs) dominate computer vision tasks and image processing, where the input data is usually 2D. CNN recognises visual patterns directly from the image using multiple-layer neurons and uses shared weights in each convolutional layer [11, 23]. CNNs are usually composed of layers organised according to their functionalities designed to learn spatial hierarchies of features automatically and adaptively, from low to high-level patterns. There are three main layers: convolutional, pooling and fully connected, where the first two perform feature extraction and the third maps the extracted features into the final output classification [23].

VGG16 is an example of a CNN model proposed by K. Simonyan and A. Zisserman from Oxford University. The model achieves 92.7% top-5 test accuracy in ImageNet, a dataset of over 14 million images belonging to 1000 classes. It improves AlexNet by replacing large kernel-sized filters with multiple 3×3 kernel-sized filters one after another [24].

Transfer learning appears to optimise and minimise the error through weight initialising the convolutional layers using pre-trained CNN weights with the same architecture to avoid training a CNN from scratch. The exception is the layer whose nodes depend on the number of classes. The early layers learn low-level features, and the late layers learn high-level features specific to the problem in the study [25, 26]. After the weight initialisation in the last fully connected layer, the network can be fine-tuned, starting with only the previous layer tuning and then the remaining layers, incrementally including more layers in the update process until the desired performance.

3 Methodology

This research aims to develop a model that detects (the presence or absence of biological growths) in the facades of buildings.

The pipeline used for the automatic detection of biological growths is described in Fig. 4.

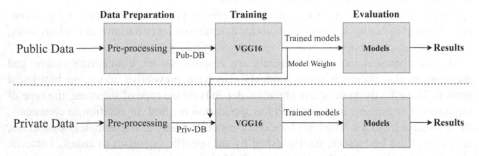

Fig. 4. Workflow of the research.

First, the data will be collected (from public and private databases) to be pre-processed and organised in datasets. The images of the private database will be collected and annotated by the authors. These datasets will train the deep learning model (VGG16) to classify images with or without biological growths. A model will be trained with public data, and then, with transfer learning methods using the weights of this model, a new one will be pre-train and fine-tuned on the private data. After the training, the models will be evaluated, and the results will be discussed in future work.

3.1 Data Preparation

A private database (Priv-DB) will be constructed. The dataset will be divided into 70% of the images for training, 15% for validation and 15% for testing the models.

3.2 Training

For the classify the images as with or without BG, a VGG16 pre-trained model will be used. The VGG16 is a state-of-the-art classification model with high-accuracy results, similar to the other available models, and for this reason, was the one chosen.

3.3 Evaluation

The standard metrics for model classification in machine learning were used for the model's evaluation. The accuracy (1) represents the fraction of predictions that the model hit.

$$Accuracy = (TP + TN)/(TP + TN + FP + FN) \qquad (1)$$

where TP is the true positive, TN is the true negative, FP is the false positive, and FN is the false negative. Sensitivity (2) measures the proportion of correctly identified positives, and specificity (3) measures the proportion of correctly identified negatives.

$$Sensitivity = TP/(TP + FN) \qquad (2)$$

$$Specificity = TN/(TN + FP) \qquad (3)$$

The area under the curve (AUC) represents the degree or measure of separability. It tells how much the model is capable of distinguishing classes. The higher the AUC, the better the model predicts the classes.

4 Results and Discussion

4.1 Vila Real Climatic Conditions

The city of Vila Real is located in the Northern Region of Portugal. Its geographical location is 41° 18' North latitude and 7° 44' West longitude, on a plateau at approximately 450 m altitude, on the promontory formed by the confluence of the Corgo and Cabril rivers, where its oldest part is located (Vila Velha).

The Serras do Marão and Alvão act as natural barriers for the region. Due to this geographical situation, it has a climate with some continentality compared to the Portuguese west coast. The climate of Vila Real is Mediterranean. The average annual relative humidity is 74%. The summer is moderately hot and dry but is already transitioning to a temperate maritime climate, given the average annual temperature of 13.3 °C and the accumulated yearly precipitation exceeding 1000 mm. Winter is relatively long, with temperatures occasionally reaching below 0 °C.

4.2 Biological Growths on Building Façades

Below are some photographs of biological growths on building facades in Vila Real, most of which are on buildings in the city's historic centre. Most of the facades where biological growth was detected are oriented to the North and West, and some are located on narrow streets that cause the main facade of the building to be shadowed for most of the day.

The biological growths found were fungi, algae, mosses, lichens and vegetation in yellow, black, white and various shades of green.

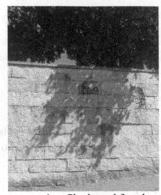
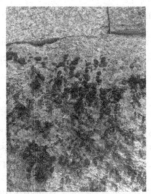

a)   Shadowed façade   b)   Details of the mosses in the façade

Fig. 5. Shadowed building façade.

In Figs. 5a) and b), on a facade facing west, it is possible to observe that the growths are located on the rough stones and have a more significant protrusion, and for part of the day, they are under the shade of tree branches.

Broken tiles and leaks from downpipes are relatively common causes of biological growth. Leaks in downpipes can be due to broken pipes or insufficient sections to dispatch the volume of water from the gutters. Figure 6 (facade facing west) is an excellent example of the two situations mentioned, where it is possible to observe the presence of algae and vegetation growth.

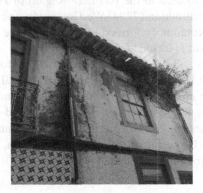

Fig. 6. Vegetation and algae in building façade.

In Fig. 7a) and b), on a facade facing west, stains associated with biological coloni-sation (moss, lichens) are visible near the base of the walls in contact with the exterior floor of the house.

The presence of these biological colonisations is associated with frequent humidi-fication of stone elements and lack of maintenance. The humidity on the facades may be due to rising dampness or rainwater that runs down, is absorbed by the facade, and accumulates at its base.

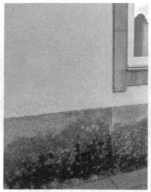
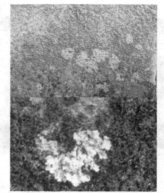

a)   Lichens and mosses in façade   b)   Detail of yellow and white lichens

Fig. 7. Building façade with lichens and mosses.

The absence of a drip tray on the top of the facade to direct water leads to a constant presence of water in the same places, providing a favourable environment for microorganisms. In Fig. 8a) and b), the façade facing south is wholly filled with mosses of different colours.

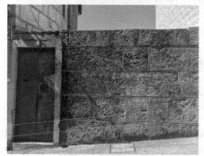
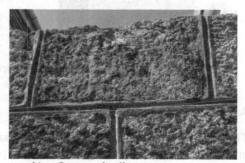

a)   Building wall with mosses   b)   Green and yellow mosses

Fig. 8. Building with a stone wall with the presence of mosses.

In the lower parts of buildings close to the pavement, it is common for rainwater to accumulate. Even if the water does not run down the facade, the rain splashes deposit residue and wet the surface of the materials. In the long term, this action provides a favourable environment for the growth of biological colonisation. Figures 9a) and b) show a facade facing North with a significant presence of mosses and fungi in the lower part.

The previously mentioned phenomenon also causes the appearance of algae, as shown in Fig. 10a) and b).

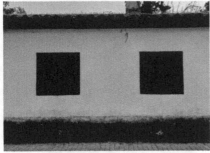
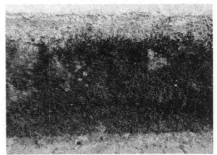

a) Building façade   b) Detail with fungus and mosses

Fig. 9. Building façade with several types of BG.

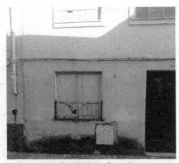
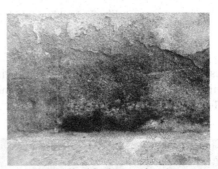

a) Building façade   b) Detail with algae and mosses

Fig. 10. Building façade with algae and mosses

4.3 Repair of Biological Growths

The first step to repairing biological growth is cleaning the facade to remove existing growth thoroughly. Depending on the type of growth (such as moss, fungi, lichens) and severity, appropriate cleaning methods may be used, such as washing with water and detergent, gentle brushing, low-pressure blasting, or using specific cleaning agents.

After cleaning, an antimicrobial treatment is recommended for the facade surface. This treatment will help prevent the future growth of biological organisms by inhibiting their proliferation.

It is necessary to check whether damage or cracks in the facade could allow moisture to enter and encourage biological growth. If present, it is crucial to carry out appropriate repairs, such as filling cracks with appropriate sealants, replacing damaged bricks or mortar, or any other action necessary to ensure the integrity of the facade.

Check that the facade has an adequate drainage system to direct water away from the surface. Excessive humidity can promote biological growth. It would help if it ensured that the gutters and drainage pipes were in good working order and the water was correctly directed away from the facade.

To prevent recurrent biological growth on the facade, a regular maintenance routine must be established. This maintenance may include periodic cleaning, visual inspections to identify problem areas, and preventive measures, such as removing leaves or debris that may accumulate moisture on the facade.

Depending on the conditions and history of biological growth on the facade, it may be helpful to consider applying specific protective coatings, such as anti-algae, anti-fungus or water-repellent coatings. These coatings help to create an additional barrier against biological growth and protect the facade.

5 Conclusions and Future Works

The appearance of biological growth is directly related to the building's solar orientation and the climatic conditions of its location, as well as shading and the rainwater drainage system from the roof, gutters, and downpipes. The most common types of CB were lichens, mosses, algae, and fungi found on facades facing north and west.

Finally, a periodic maintenance plan is essential. It must be programmed and followed, considering the growth rates of the species involved and the dynamics of recolonisation. This makes it possible to intervene in the initial phases of evolution or even prevent such a situation.

As a suggestion for future work, we intend to increase the database with the various types of biological growths in photographic records, apply deep learning models to this database, and obtain automatic detection results.

Acknowledgements. This work was supported by the FCT (Portuguese Foundation for Science and Technology) through the project UIDB/04082/2020 (CMADE).

References

1. Qualharini, E.L., Oscar, L.H.C., Da Silva, M.R.: Rehabilitation of buildings as an alternative to sustainability in Brazilian constructions. Open Eng. **9**(1), 139–143 (2019)
2. Almeida, C.P., Ramos, A.F., Silva, J.M.: Sustainability assessment of building rehabilitation actions in old urban centres. Sustain. Cities Soc. **36**, 378–385 (2018)
3. World Health Organization Regional Office for Europe: WHO guidelines for indoor air quality:dampness and mould. World Heal. Organisation, pp. 228 (2009)
4. C. W086: W086 - Building Pathology - CIB (2021)
5. Perez, H., Tah, J.H.M., Mosavi, A.: Deep learning for detecting building defects using convolutional neural networks. Sens. (Switzerland) **19**(16), 3556 (2019)
6. Cheng, H.D., Chen, J.-R., Glazier, C., Hu, Y.G.: Novel approach to pavement cracking detection based on fuzzy set theory. J. Comput. Civ. Eng. **13**(4), 270–280 (1999)
7. Słoński, M.: A comparison of deep convolutional neural networks for image-based detection of concrete surface cracks. Comput. Assist. Methods Eng. Sci. **26**(2), 105–112 (2019)
8. Cha, Y.J., Choi, W., Suh, G., Mahmoudkhani, S., Büyüköztürk, O.: Autonomous structural visual inspection using region-based deep learning for detecting multiple damage types. Comput. Civ. Infrastruct. Eng. **33**(9), 731–747 (2018)
9. Zhang, A., et al.: Automated Pixel-level pavement crack detection on 3D Asphalt surfaces using a deep-learning network. Comput. Civ. Infrastruct. Eng. **32**(10), 805–819 (2017)
10. Chaiyasarn, K., Sharma, M., Ali, L., Khan, W., Poovarodom, N.: Crack detection in historical structures based on convolutional neural network. GEOMATE J. **15**(51), 240–251 (2018)

11. Li, S., Zhao, X.: Image-based concrete crack detection using convolutional neural network and exhaustive search technique. Adv. Civ. Eng. **2019** (2019)
12. Eriksson, L.: Detection of facade cracks using deep learning (2020)
13. Dais, D., Bal, İE., Smyrou, E., Sarhosis, V.: Automatic crack classification and segmentation on masonry surfaces using convolutional neural networks and transfer learning. Autom. Constr. **125**, 103606 (2021)
14. Felipe, A., Silva, D.A.: Manifestações patológicas em fachadas com revestimentos argamassados: estudo de caso em edifícios em Florianópois (2007)
15. Rodrigues, M.P., Eusébio, M.I., Ribeiro, A.: Revestimentos por pintura. Defeitos, causas e reparação (2011)
16. Sofia, D., Fernandes Coutinho, S.: Revestimentos biológicos em pedras graníticas do património construído : ocorrência, limpeza e prevenção, September 2009
17. Allsopp, Dennis, Seal, K.J.: Introduction to Biodeterioration, Very Good, 1st edn. Liberty Book Shop (1986)
18. Uemoto, K., Agopyam, V., Brazolim, S.: Degradação de pinturas e elementos de fachada por organismos biológicos. EPUSP, São Paulo (1999)
19. Sousa, V., Pereira, F.D., de Brito, J.: Rebocos Tradicionais: Principais Causas de Degradação. Eng. Civ. (23), 5–18 (2005)
20. Ranalli, G., Sorlini, C.: Bioremediation, in plant biology for cultural heritage., Plant Biol. Cult. Herit. Biodeterior. Conserv. 340–346 (2008)
21. Shirakawa, M.A., Monteiro, M.B., Selmo, S.M.D.S., Cincotto, M.A.: Identificação de fungos em revestimentos de argamassas com bolor evidente. In: Anais. Goiania, Ufgo (1995)
22. Honda, N.K., Vilegas, W.: The chemistry of lichens. Quim. Nova **22**(1), 110–125 (1999)
23. Jia, F., Lei, Y., Lin, J., Zhou, X., Lu, N.: Deep neural networks: A promising tool for fault characteristic mining and intelligent diagnosis of rotating machinery with massive data. MSSP **72**, 303–315 (2016)
24. Yamashita, R., Nishio, M., Do, R.K.G., Togashi, K.: Convolutional neural networks: an overview and application in radiology. Insights Imaging **9**(4), 611–629 (2018)
25. Simonyan, K., Zisserman, A.: Very deep convolutional networks for large-scale image recognition. In: 3rd International Conference on Learning Representation ICLR 2015 – Conference on Track Proceedings, September 2014
26. Tajbakhsh, N., et al.: Convolutional neural networks for medical image analysis: full training or fine tuning? IEEE Trans. Med. Imaging **35**(5), 1299–1312 (2017)

Multimedia e-health Data Exchange Services. Signal/Data Processing and Computing For Health Systems

Develop Method to Efficiently Apply Image-Based Facial Emotion Classification Models to Video Data

Hee Min Yang[1], Joo Hyun Lee[1], and Yu Rang Park[1,2(✉)]

[1] Department of Biomedical Systems Informatics, Yonsei University College of Medicine, Seoul, South Korea
yurangpark@yuhs.ac
[2] Department of Artificial Intelligence, Yonsei University, 50-1 Yonsei-ro, Seodaemun-gu, Seoul 03722, South Korea

Abstract. The ability to recognize emotions through facial cues, in childhood, is helpful for social interactions. Image-based facial emotion recognition models need low computing power, but cannot accept sequential information from video data. Conversely, video-based facial emotion recognition models require high computational power, so it cannot be easily applied in a low computing environment. In this paper, we propose a method that classifies the emotion from facial expression video data by applying threshold using an image-based model. The proposed method improves the accuracy of 3.67%, 24.74%, and 15.13% for each video dataset by reducing the non-emotion in the video and responding more sensitively to the expressed emotion than other methods that simply select the most frequent emotion in the video. The results of the study showed the threshold method can improve the performance of emotion classification without modifying the facial emotion classification model.

Keywords: Facial Emotion Recognition · Deep Learning · Computer Vision · Child

1 Introduction

The ability to recognize and express one's own and others' emotions based on facial cues is directly linked to an individual's ability to interact with others. This skill is even more important in childhood, when the first social interactions occur, before speech is fully developed [1, 2]. The inability to recognize facial emotions is closely linked to child development problems [3]. It can be one of the reasons for developmental delay in basic social skills needed to adapt to social life. Low emotional knowledge in children is associated with negative outcomes, including poor social functioning, low academic achievement, and internalizing/externalizing behavior problems [1] [4, 5].

Facial emotion recognition has been reported to be helpful for children with developmental behavioral conditions that make it difficult to recognize emotions, such as

A. Cunha et al. (Eds.): MobiHealth 2023, LNICST 578, pp. 353–360, 2024.
https://doi.org/10.1007/978-3-031-60665-6_26

autism spectrum disorder (ASD) [6–8]. However, most emotion recognition studies focus on adult data, so when applied to children's faces, performance decreases. Park et al. (2022) showed that emotion classification after splitting of child and adult facial image data achieved an accuracy improvement of 22.4% compared to before splitting [9]. As a result of the emotion classification of children's facial expressions by machine learning, children tend to be highly expressive in terms of positive emotions and ambiguous in terms of negative emotions [10, 11]. For example, when children are ambiguously angry in terms of negative emotions, they sometimes show neutral expressions, making it difficult to know what emotions the child is experiencing.

Video-based facial emotion recognition models require high computational power because they use the sequential information of video data [12, 13]. Conversely, image-based models can also be implemented at low computational power [14], but have the problem of not accepting sequential information of a video data. In an environment where computational power is limited, such as mobile devices, a method is needed to efficiently apply image-based models to video data.

Therefore, we aimed to (1) develop a method based on the classification of human emotions in the video to select the representative emotion of a video using an image-based facial emotion classification model for children, and (2) evaluate the applicability and effectiveness of the developed method by applying it to a real public video dataset.

2 Materials and Methods

2.1 Dataset

We used the two child facial expression video datasets, the DuckEES databases [15] and the LIRIS Children Spontaneous Facial Expression Video [16]. The DuckEES dataset contains facial expressions of emotion created by children and teenagers between the ages of 8 and 18. The video dataset contains 251 videos with six facial expressions of emotion (happy, sad, fear, disgust, pride, embarrassment) and 'neutral', and the emotion labels were evaluated by 36 human cross-validators. We use 121 videos with an accuracy of 0.7 or higher based on cross-validation, which is the cutoff for the final dataset presented by the DuckEES researchers, excluding embarrassment and pride videos for which the image-based classification model did not learn about these labels. Of the 121 videos, there are 36 happy, 17 sad, 18 fear, 20 disgust and 30 neutral videos. The video was recorded in 25 frames. The LIRIS-CSE dataset contains 180 videos that have six facial emotion expression labels (happy, sad, angry, fear, surprise and disgust) and the participants' mean age is 7.3 years. The 180 videos include 61 happy, 26 sad, 1 angry, 32 fear, 51 surprise and 9 disgust. The video was also recorded in 25 frames. And we created the combined dataset using DuckEES and LIRIS-CSE as described above. There is no additional processing and they were simply used together. For this study, we chose the following seven labels for the two datasets: happiness, sadness, anger, fear, surprise, disgust, and neutral.

2.2 Proposed Method: Threshold

The proposed method, threshold, selects the representative emotion of a video using an image-based facial emotion classification model, which consists of two parts (Fig. 1). In part A: the part of classifying the emotion of each frame in a video by the classification model, the method used facial video data with the true label about the facial emotion, which was labeled by the labeler with cross-validation. The facial video data is divided into frames, and the frames are used as a kind of image data as input to the image-based emotion classification model. Using the frame images of the video, the facial emotion classification model predicts the emotion for each frame. This procedure generates tabular data composed of the predicted emotion results for each frame, which is used in the next part. In part B: the part of determining the representative emotion for a video, the number of emotions for each frame of the facial video is aggregated and sorted in the order of the most emotions. Threshold is the ratio of sensitivity to non-neutral emotions. When Eq. (1) is satisfied,

$$\max emotion(\text{without neutral}) \geq (threshold \times numberofframetotal) \qquad (1)$$

the representative emotion of the video becomes the emotion of the maximum number. If Eq. (1) is not satisfied, the most frequent emotion or neutral is selected as the representative emotion. The accuracy of the current threshold is calculated by comparing the selected representative emotion to the true label on each video. The architecture for this study is summarized and visualized in Fig. 1.

2.3 Evaluation Metrics

We use accuracy and F1-score as the evaluation metrics. Accuracy measures how close the predicted value is to a true or accepted value of being true. The F1-score is an integrated indicator of how accurately the model predicted and whether the model actually captured all important outcomes.

2.4 Experimental Setting

We conducted our experiments on a desktop computer equipped with an Intel Core i7–9700 CPU, 16 GB of RAM, and a 256 GB SSD. GPU processing was not used for this project, only CPU power was used.

We used the image-based model [17] pre-trained on the FER2013 dataset (Facial Expression Recognition 2013 Dataset) [18] using Mini-Xception as the model architecture, a miniature version of Xception [19]. And we set the threshold to increase from 0.05 to 1.00 in 0.05 increments to find the optimal value.

There are two settings for categorizing emotions, the broad emotion setting and the specific emotion setting. In the broad emotion setting, the emotion is categorized by three labels: negative, positive, and neutral, to clearly compare non-emotion and emotion [10, 11]. On the other hand, the specific emotion setting is for evaluating the robustness of our method in more complicated classification tasks. The emotion has seven labels: happiness, sadness, anger, fear, surprise, disgust, and neutral [20]. In each setting, we compare our threshold method to the baseline Top 1 method using evaluation metrics. Top 1 is a method that selects the most frequent emotion in each frame of a facial expression video as the representative emotion.

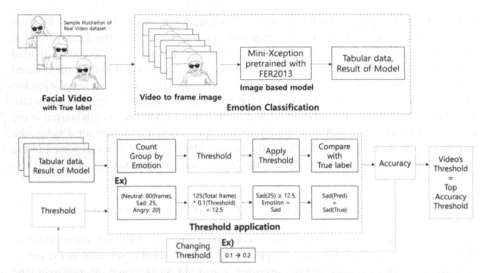

Fig. 1. The figure shows the architecture of the threshold method. The architecture has Part A, where an image-based model classifies the emotion for each frame (i.e., image) of the facial video, and Part B, where the classified emotion results are used to determine the threshold for selecting the representative emotion for that facial video.

2.5 Method Validation

We used 5-fold cross-validation to validate the proposed method. In this method, the original data is divided into 5 subsets of equal size. Then, one of these subsets is used as validation data, and the rest of the subsets are used as training data to learn the model. This process is repeated 5 times, with different subsets selected as validation data each time. As a result, we estimate the performance of the final model by averaging the model performance of 5 times.

3 Result

3.1 Broad Emotion Test (3 Label)

We expanded the range of emotions and tested three broad ranges of emotions. This is to evaluate negative emotions by uniting them. Experimental performance is measured by the average accuracy from 5-fold cross-validation. For the DuckEES data set, the optimal threshold was 0.15, 0.05 for LIRIS-CSE, and 0.05 for DuckEES+LIRIS-CSE. The accuracy of the method applying the optimal threshold to each data set is 0.8545, 0.7468, and 0.7813. Top 1 accuracies were 0.8087, 0.4944, and 0.6211. That is, the threshold showed improvements in accuracy of 0.0458, 0.2474, and 0.1602 compared to the baseline top 1. It can be seen that the threshold method outperforms top1 in DuckEES and DuckEES+LIRIS-CSE (Table 1).

We compare the threshold (with the optimal value of 0.05) and the top 1 with the combined dataset (DuckEES+LIRIS-CSE) for each emotion with the performance of

Table 1. Evaluation result of Top1 and Threshold based on 3 labels (Neutral, Positive, Negative).

Dataset	Threshold		Top 1 Accuracy	Difference*
	Accuracy	Optimal threshold		
DuckEES [15]	0.8545	0.15	0.8087	0.0458
LIRIS-CSE [16]	0.7468	0.05	0.4944	0.2474
DuckEES+LIRIS-CSE [15, 16]	0.7813	0.05	0.6211	0.1602

* Difference is the difference between the accuracy of Threshold and the accuracy of Top1.

accuracy and F1-score. As a result, the threshold has higher accuracy and F1-score values than the top 1 in all three emotions. In particular, in F1-score, the threshold is 0.1558, 0.0554, 0.0854 and 0.1598 higher in the order of negative, positive, neutral and average of three emotions (Table 2).

Table 2. Comparison results of top 1, threshold (with optimal threshold value 0.05) and threshold with median value for the combined dataset of DuckEES [15] and LIRIS-CSE [16]. The higher results are highlighted in bold.

	Emotion							
	Negative		Positive		Neutral		Average of 3 emotions	
	Threshold(0.05*)	Top 1	Threshold	Top 1	Threshold	Top 1	Threshold	Top 1
Accuracy	**0.7879**	0.6844	**0.9226**	0.8970	**0.8519**	0.6611	**0.8540**	0.7475
F1-score	**0.8000**	0.6442	**0.8878**	0.8324	**0.4054**	0.3200	**0.7811**	0.6213

* The optimal value of the threshold from the combined dataset, each threshold value is 0.05 in this table.

3.2 Specific Emotion Test (7 Label)

We experimented with seven labels from two video dataset. Experimental performance is measured by the average accuracy from 5-fold cross-validation. Threshold was tested by raising it to 0.05 units from 0.05 to 1.00 to find the optimal value. For the DuckEES data set, the optimal threshold was 0.20, LIRIS-CSE was 0.05, and DuckEES+LIRIS-CSE was 0.20. The accuracy of the method applying the optimal threshold to each data set is 0.6635, 0.4216, and 0.5153, which is higher than the top1 accuracy of 0.6440, 0.3222, and 0.4519. That is, the threshold showed accuracy improvements of 0.0195, 0.0994, and 0.0634 for the Top 1 baseline. The experimental results can be seen in Table 3.

4 Discussion

In this study, we proposed to use thresholds in an image-based classification model to select representative emotions from child facial videos. In particular, we applied the method to a real public video dataset to evaluate its feasibility and efficacy. As a result of

Table 3. Evaluation result of Top1 and Threshold based on 7 labels (Neutral, happy, sad, angry, fear, surprise and disgust).

Dataset	Threshold		Top 1 Accuracy	Difference*
	Accuracy	Optimal threshold		
DuckEES [15]	0.6635	0.30	0.6440	0.0195
LIRIS-CSE [16]	0.4216	0.05	0.3222	0.0994
DuckEES+LIRIS-CSE [15, 16]	0.5153	0.20	0.4519	0.0634

* Difference is the difference between the accuracy of Threshold and the accuracy of Top1.

the evaluation by the two datasets and the combined dataset, our method shows higher accuracy than the so-called Top 1, which is a method of selecting the most frequent value among the emotions in the video. The same image-based emotion classification model was used, but the accuracy performance of our method was outperformed.

Performance comparison between the threshold (with the optimal threshold value) and the top 1, the F1-score difference of negative emotion between the two methods is larger than that of positive emotion, which shows that when the Top 1 method selects the most frequent emotion as the representative emotion for the facial emotion video, the actual negative emotion tends to be buried in Neutral due to the many Neutral frames in the video [10, 11]. Threshold, in contrast, finds the emotions that have been buried in Neutral and also shows the result of preserving Neutral as itself in the Neutral video.

Our threshold method captures the instantly appearing facial emotions and selects them as the representative emotions of the video more accurately than before. This is because studies on human emotion recognition have shown that people recognize emotions by estimating the context of the situation [20, 21], and studies on the importance of different parts of the face for emotion recognition have found that sufficient information is needed in the important areas (the study identified the eyes and mouth) for emotion recognition [22, 23]. So, like humans, our method captures emotional expressions that have strong facial information and context (laughing, frowning, or crying) that appear for a while, rather than the basic neutral state in the video, to determine what emotion the video has. And the Threshold method improves performance by efficiently interpreting the results of the classification model without having to develop or replace additional models. So far, regardless of each facial emotion recognition model's type, the proposed method can be easily applied, and can be expected to achieve higher performance in the research results.

This proposed method has a limitation that requires a process of finding an appropriate threshold for the recording environment and the participants' faces. Therefore, prior data for the threshold search is required to be used in the actual environment. In addition, since this study used facial data from children, further research with adult data is needed to verify whether adults have the same substantial performance improvement.

5 Conclusions

The results of the threshold-based emotion classification method proposed in this study suggest that emotion classification performance can be improved without modifying the classification model itself, especially in children's data where emotion classification is difficult.

Acknowledgement. This work was supported by Institute of Information & communications Technology Planning & Evaluation (IITP 2022-0-00064) grant funded by the Korea government(MSIT).

References

1. Izard, C.E.: Emotional intelligence or adaptive emotions? Emotion **1**, 249–257 (2001)
2. Barth, J.M., Andrea, B.: A longitudinal study of emotion recognition and preschool children's social behavior. Merrill-Palmer Q. (1982), 107–128 (1997)
3. Harms, M.B., Martin, A., Wallace, G.L.: Facial emotion recognition in autism spectrum disorders: a review of behavioral and neuroimaging studies. Neuropsychol. Rev. **20**, 290–322 (2010)
4. Trentacosta, C.J., Fine, S.E.: Emotion knowledge, social competence, and behavior problems in childhood and adolescence: a meta-analytic review. Soc. Dev. **19**(1), 1–29 (2010)
5. Ensor, R., Spencer, D., Hughes, C.: You feel sad? Emotion understanding mediates effects of verbal ability and mother–child mutuality on prosocial behaviors: findings from 2 years to 4 years. Soc. Dev. **20**(1), 93–110 (2011)
6. Happé, F., Frith, U.: Annual research review: towards a developmental neuroscience of atypical social cognition. J. Child Psychol. Psychiatry **55**(6), 553–577 (2014)
7. Hobson, R.P., Ouston, J., Lee, A.: Emotion recognition in autism: coordinating faces and voices. Psychol. Med. **18**(4), 911–923 (1988)
8. Carolien, R., et al.: Emotion regulation and internalizing symptoms in children with autism spectrum disorders. Autism **15**(6), 655–670 (2011)
9. Park, H., et al.: Facial emotion recognition analysis based on age-biased data. Appl. Sci. **12**(16), 7992 (2022)
10. Washington, P., et al.: Improved digital therapy for developmental pediatrics using domain-specific artificial intelligence: machine learning study. JMIR Pediatrics Parent. **5**(2), e26760 (2022)
11. Anwar, S., Milanova, M.: Real time face expression recognition of children with autism. Int. Acad. Eng. Med. Res **1**(1), 1–8 (2016)
12. Xia, X., Zhao, Y., Jiang, D.: Multimodal interaction enhanced representation learning for video emotion recognition. Front. Neurosci. **16**, 1086380 (2022)
13. Wei, Q., Huang, X., Zhang, Y.: FV2ES: a fully End2End multimodal system for fast yet effective video emotion recognition inference. IEEE Trans. Broadcast. **69**, 10–20 (2022)
14. Pandey, S., Sonakshi, H.: Facial emotion recognition using deep learning. In: 2022 International Mobile and Embedded Technology Conference (MECON). IEEE (2022)
15. Giuliani, N.R., et al.: Presentation and validation of the DuckEES child and adolescent dynamic facial expressions stimulus set. Int. J. Methods Psychiatric Res. **26**(1), e1553 (2017)
16. Khan, Rizwan Ahmed, et al.: A novel database of children's spontaneous facial expressions (LIRIS-CSE). Image Vis. Comput. **83**, 61–69 (2019)

17. Arriaga, O., Valdenegro-Toro, M., Plöger, P.:Real-time convolutional neural networks for emotion and gender classification. arXiv preprint arXiv:1710.07557 (2017)
18. Goodfellow, I.J., et al.: Challenges in representation learning: a report on three machine learning contests. In: Neural Information Processing: 20th International Conference, ICONIP 2013, Daegu, Korea, November 3–7. Proceedings, Part III 20. Springer, Heidelberg (2013)
19. Chollet, F.: Xception: Deep learning with depthwise separable convolutions. In: Proceedings of the IEEE Conference on Computer Vision and Pattern Recognition (2017)
20. Ekman, P.: Universals and cultural differences in facial expressions of emotion. In: Nebraska Symposium on Motivation. University of Nebraska Press (1971)
21. Frijda, N.H.: Recognition of Emotion. Advances in Experimental Social Psychology, vol. 4, pp. 167–223. Academic Press (1969)
22. Birmingham, E., et al.: The moving window technique: a window into developmental changes in attention during facial emotion recognition. Child Dev. **84**(4), 1407–1424 (2013)
23. Kim, M., Cho, Y., Kim, S.-Y.: Effects of diagnostic regions on facial emotion recognition: the moving window technique. Front. Psychol. **13**, 966623 (2022)

DeepSquitoes: A Mobile System Framework for the Surveillance of Disease-Carrying Mosquitoes

Sudha Cheerkoot-Jalim[1]([✉]), Camille Simon-Chane[2], Zarine Cadersaib[1],
Leckraj Nagowah[1], Zahra Mungloo-Dilmohamud[1], Denis Sereno[3],
Kavi Kumar Khedo[1], Shakuntala Baichoo[1], Soulakshmee D. Nagowah[1],
Abha Jodheea-Jutton[4], Fadil Chady[1], and Aymeric Histace[2]

[1] Faculty of Information, Communication and Digital Technologies, University of Mauritius,
Réduit, Mauritius
s.cheerkoot@uom.ac.mu
[2] ETIS UMR 8051, CY Cergy Paris University, ENSEA, CNRS, Cergy, France
[3] Institut de Recherche Pour Le Développement, Montpellier, France
[4] Faculty of Medicine and Health Sciences, University of Mauritius, Réduit, Mauritius

Abstract. Insects that spread diseases like malaria, chikungunya and Lyme disease are found all over the world because of climate change, economic fluctuations, human migration, and international trade. In this study, we propose *DeepSquitoes*, a mobile system framework for insect identification and fast data dissemination, with the goal of improving the management of public health hazards. *DeepSquitoes* specialises in the quick identification of mosquitoes, which are common in tropical areas, and can be used to monitor insect population movements in real-time. To maximise user interaction and data accuracy, the application includes geolocation-based identification, sophisticated preprocessing, and specialised annotation. Image preprocessing techniques like Gaussian Blur and contour extraction are applied on mosquito wing images to ensure data quality. Deep learning algorithms are trained on the preprocessed images for mosquito species classification. The image recognition model performs well, with a 93% training accuracy and a 74% validation accuracy using MobileNetV2 from TensorFlow. Our local dataset, which included 154 images of eight different insect species, had a commendable recognition accuracy rate of 76%.

Keywords: Entomological Surveillance System · Deep Learning · Image Classification

1 Introduction

Bloodsucking insects are involved in the transmission of causative agents of diseases of parasitic (malaria, leishmaniasis, trypanosomiasis, filariasis), viral (chikungunya, dengue, phlebovirus, bluetongue, fever, Rift Valley, West Nile fever) or bacterial origin (bartonellosis, heartwater, Lyme disease) [1]. They are also responsible for the dissemination of pathogens by phoresy (passive transport) that cause foodborne diseases.

A. Cunha et al. (Eds.): MobiHealth 2023, LNICST 578, pp. 361–373, 2024.
https://doi.org/10.1007/978-3-031-60665-6_27

Climatic disturbances, global economic development, migration and the intensification of intercontinental trade have led to striking changes in their worldwide distribution. For instance, there has been the introduction and colonisation of new climatic areas by the tiger mosquito (Aedes Albopictus), an established vector of chikungunya and dengue viruses in several countries, including Mauritius and France [2].

Mosquitoes are vectors of various pathogens that can cause diseases such as dengue fever, malaria, chikungunya, West Nile fever, yellow fever, heartworm disease and filariasis [3]. Mosquitoes belong to the order Diptera (two-winged flies) and suborder Nematocera, which also includes many flies of economic importance like sand flies, midges, mothflies, and black flies [4]. Mosquito-borne diseases are those spread by the bite of an infected mosquito and often cause outbreaks resulting in immense suffering for humans. They have become increasingly widespread and pose a major worldwide public health problem [5]. The species mostly involved in the transmission of infections are contained in the genera Aedes, Culex, Anopheles, Ochlerotatus and Mansonia, belonging to the subfamilies Anophelinae and Culicinae [6].

In Mauritius, the most abundant species are Aedes Albopictus, Culex Quinquefasciatus and Anopheles Arabiensis[1]. Aedes Albopictus is known to transmit chikungunya and dengue, Culex Quinquefasciatus is known to transmit West Nile fever and Anopheles Arabiensis transmits Malaria and Filariasis. There are also some less common species like Anopheles Coustani and Aedes Fowleri that can transmit Rift Valley Fever Virus, and some rare ones like Anopheles Merus that can transmit malaria [6]. These diseases may cause major economic losses and affect many sectors, including the tourism industry, which is one of the major pillars of the Mauritian economy.

Mosquito-borne disease outbreaks can be foreseen by tracking the dynamics of pathogen-bearing mosquitoes in the field [7]. Through surveillance, entomologists can identify species composition, population dynamics, and the threat of dangerous mosquito-borne diseases. Decision-makers can use this information to choose the most effective management approach to control mosquitoes and protect community members in their area. One example of a mosquito surveillance system is the ArboNET[2], an arboviral surveillance system managed by the CDC (Centers for Disease Control and Prevention) and state health departments of the USA. ArboNET can create an online disease map to guide decision makers.

In low and middle-income countries (LMIC), surveying disease vectors can be quite expensive and excessively laborious for continuous and widespread monitoring. Large-scale monitoring in traditional surveillance of mosquitoes is difficult and expensive since it requires dedicated personnel to perform regular manual inspection and reporting. Novel surveillance approaches relies on smartphones and the Internet to permit people to upload pictures of mosquitoes whenever they come across them. The Mosquito Alert citizen science system[3], equipped with a specialized mobile application for the collection of geotagged photographs, serves as an illustrative example of a citizen science system [8].

---

[1] Source: Vector Biology and Control Division (VBCD) of the Ministry of Health and Wellness.

[2] https://wwwn.cdc.gov/arbonet/maps/adb_diseases_map/index.html.

[3] http://www.mosquitoalert.com/en/.

The aim of this study is to implement an entomological surveillance system usable in most parts of the world and particularly in tropical and subtropical areas. The system is composed of interconnected tools that enables the rapid, cost-effective and non-destructive identification of different species of mosquitoes. It consists of a mobile phone (device and app) and a macro low-cost camera for a fast and accurate classification of mosquitoes on the field in order to have a real-time view of their evolution in terms of population and migration. This work demonstrates the application of deep learning methods integrated in a mobile system framework, for the accurate classification of mosquito species, based on wing images. The rest of the paper is structured as follows: Sect. 2 describes the related works, while Sect. 3 details the proposed solution. The results are discussed in Sect. 4 and finally, Sect. 5 concludes the paper.

2   Related Works

This section discusses related works on automatic recognition and classification of insects along with mobile insect recognition applications.

2.1   Automatic Recognition and Classification of Insects

Mosquito-borne diseases pose a considerable threat to global health. Entomological surveys, which include the collection and identification of mosquitoes, are needed to gain a better understanding of the transmission dynamics of vectors of such diseases. These surveys are therefore of paramount importance to plan for effective control measures and to monitor their impact. Species identification is the first step in entomological studies, and misidentification negatively impacts public health. In order to make species identification more efficient for entomologists, many studies have investigated the use of mobile applications coupled with image processing and machine learning algorithms for fast and accurate species classification.

In a recent survey by Martineau et al. [9], an in-depth analysis was conducted on insect classification, with emphasis on image acquisition methods, feature extraction techniques and automated classification algorithms. The authors categorized image acquisition protocols into two main types: laboratory-based and field-based images. There is a fixed protocol to acquire laboratory-based images from the insect trapping to its placement. The insect is positioned manually based on a particular set-up and the image is captured and retained for future processing. On the other hand, field-based images are taken from cultivated fields.

Furthermore, Sereno et al. [10] patented a dataset of Wing Interference Patterns (WIPs) for experiments carried out in the fields and proposed an automatic recognition system that classifies hematophagous diptera genus. Feature extraction techniques were employed for the purpose of image classification. The authors performed feature extraction with hand-crafted features using SIFT for building global representations with VLAT [11] and used linear support vector machines (SVM) to classify these genus. An improved version of this algorithm was proposed in [12] taking benefits of a Convolutional Neural Networks (CNN) architecture (MobileNetV2).

The Automatic Insect Identification System (DAIIS) is an example of a tool, which is based on wing outlines [14]. Wing outlines, being stable and diverse in nature, are used for insect identification [15]. Users are only required to upload a minimal set of images to utilize the tool, which then performs wing outline digitisation and Elliptic Fourier transformation. It carries out classifier model training by pattern recognition of SVM and model validation. The tool makes use of 120 owlfly specimens, representing seven distinct species for training an owlfly classifier. The mean accuracy for species identification varied between 90% and 98%.

In their study, Rustom et al. [16] have proposed a system based on Machine Learning (ML) and Deep Learning (DL) for classifying two distinct mosquito genera, namely Aedes and Culex. The system employs ML as well as CNN models. Feature selection was facilitated through ROI-based image filtering and wrappers-based FFS technique. The system used images from a dataset from the IEEE data port. Among the ML algorithms tested on the dataset, Extra-Tree Classification has outperformed with an accuracy of 99.2% and VGG16 has outperformed other CNN models with an accuracy of 98.6%.

2.2 Mobile Insect Recognition Applications

Various architectures have been proposed for deployment on mobile devices for real-time applications [17]. Minakshi et al. [13] proposed a mobile phone application, which allows any user with a smartphone to take images of a still mosquito, after spraying or trapping. The species identification approach comprised several steps, including image resizing, noise removal, background segmentation, feature extraction, dimensionality reduction and finally unsupervised clustering and classification using the Support Vector Machine algorithm. The authors reported an overall accuracy of 77.5%, which could be highly improved by the use of deep learning and transfer learning algorithms.

Conversely to most applications, the model developed by Munoz et al. [18] performs image recognition of mosquito species by classifying images of mosquito larvae, pupa and eggs. For accurate classification of the genus of larvae, close-up photos of the head and tail are imperative. To achieve this, images are captured using a smartphone camera, with a 60X Clip Light-Emitting Diode (LED) microscope affixed to the device. The centrally located recognition module uses a CNN classifier to predict the possible class of the insect. The resulting data can be streamlined to a visualisation tool using Google Maps. The authors believe that the performance of their system could be improved by executing the classification algorithm on the user application.

Zhu et al. [19] investigated the use of an application embedded in smartphones and image processing approaches for the rapid and precise identification and enumeration of insects in stored grain. The objective of the work was to preprocess the acquired insect image characterized by non-uniform brightness and dark background. One sliding window-based binarization was adopted to normalize the non-uniform brightness in insect photographs captured via mobile phones. Subsequently, domain-based histogram statistics were implemented to identify and enumerate the insects in the stored grain. By adapting the sliding window size, the system was able to distinguish tiny insects. The model achieved a counting accuracy of 95%, which surpasses that of conventional methods.

He et al. [20] used an approach based on deep learning to detect oilseed rape pests. They built a dataset consisting of 3,022 images and divided them into 12 categories. The dataset consisted of images captured using both a mobile phone and a digital camera. The Single Shot Detector (SSD) was selected as the meta-architecture for the optimal detection model, owing to its multiscale capabilities and rapid high-accuracy feature. Additionally, a mobile application was also developed to enable farmers to capture the images of the pests and detect the oilseed rape pests in real time. It also provided suggestions on pest controlling.

Motta et al. [21] used a model based on a CNN, capable of recognizing adult mosquitoes from the species Aedes Aegypti, Aedes Albopictus and Culex Quinque-fasciatus. The authors trained their neural networks using a dataset comprising over 4000 mosquito images. DC light traps and suction tubes were utilised for capturing the adult insects. The collected insects were next euthanised with ethyl acetate and stored in entomological collection tubes. Their images were then taken using a digital camera or a mobile phone. Automatic taxonomic classification of the insects was performed through the image feature acquisition techniques that enabled differentiation between species. Three neural networks, including LeNet, AlexNet and GoogleNet were used for this purpose.

Chudzik et al. [22] came up with a mobile real-time grasshopper detection frame-work, MAESTRO, which employs deep learning techniques on RGB images for insect identification. The framework includes a mobile application that performs real-time detection of grasshoppers locally based on a deep learning model. The mobile applica-tion also performed data aggregation and collected ancillary information such as temper-ature, soil moisture, wind speed, and solar radiation. Upon availability of internet con-nection, the data is relayed to a cloud system for the purpose of forecasting grasshoppers movements and outbreaks.

Buschbacher et al. [23] have proposed DeepABIS, a system based on the founda-tional principles of the Automated Bee Identification System (ABIS). It is a mobile Android application capable of identifying live bees both in indoor and outdoor environ-ments. Automated feature generation using deep convolutional neural networks (CNN) was used for species identification. Additionally, it facilitates participatory sensing and the collaborative gathering of data and insights. DeepABIS adopts the MobileNetV2 architecture and utilizes two distinct datasets for its operations: the *Apoidea* dataset, comprising bee images collected from Germany, Brazil, the United States and China and *Lepidoptera* dataset featuring butterflies collected from Germany, Italy, Spain and Kaza-khstan. ABIS reports identification results with an average top-1 accuracy of 93.95% and a top-5 accuracy of 99.61% applied to data material.

Table 1 provides a comparative analysis of the related works. It can be observed that none of the studies has considered the classification of mosquito species based on wing images. The approach used in the present study for image capture and classification is based on a mobile system, which can be easily deployed in-the-field. The design and development of *DeepSquitoes* is described in detail in the following section. As articu-lated in the preceding section, the primary objective is to devise a low-cost approach for implementing an entomological surveillance system while maintaining a commendable recognition accuracy.

3 Materials and Methods

3.1 Data Acquisition

Experiments were carried out at the Vector Biology and Control Division (VBCD) laboratory of the Ministry of Health and Wellness to first build the dataset of wing images. Samples of different labelled species of mosquitoes were gathered for the project, mainly for the construction of the dataset of mosquito species. This dataset was further augmented with data images captured from the microscope and mobile device. Figure 1 shows how the microscope was set up to capture images of mosquito wings.

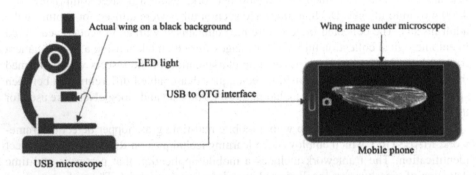

Fig. 1. Microscope and mobile device set-up

The mosquito wings were carefully dissected from their body using a precision tweezer, placed on a black background surface, and viewed under the microscope connected to the mobile device. A black background projects a better image quality in terms of colours and shape of the wing. The mobile app, MScope was used to view the digital image. To maintain consistency, the orientation of the wing was aligned as depicted in Fig. 1. The LED's light brightness was minimised to avoid any undesirable luminescence. Lastly, for each species, the picture of the wing obtained from MScope was saved to its respective folder.

3.2 Model Training

Upon completion of image capture, the dataset was ready for the preprocessing and model training phases. The wing images were preprocessed using the OpenCV package⁴. Their width, height and RGB colour channel was saved in a temporary matrix, after which, Gaussian Blur was applied to ensure a smooth background. After generating the wing outline, the image was cropped, and the canvas converted to dataURL jpeg file format.

In this work, the Tensorflow Hub MobileNetV2 model architecture was utilized, given its optimization for mobile device compatibility [24]. However, hyperparameter tuning was needed to ensure optimum performance. The input image size was changed to 116 x 256 pixels and the batch size was changed from 32 (default) to 16 since the

---

⁴ https://docs.opencv.org/4.x/.

Table 1. Comparative table of the related works

Mobile Application	Region	Type of Insect/Dataset	Image capture details (how are images taken)	Type of equipment used	Image processing details	Algorithms used	Visualisation	Challenges/Limitations
[14]	China	Owlflies	Owlfly images were captured using a digital camera	Canon 60D, 60 mm lens	Outline Digitization and Elliptic Fourier Transformation Pattern recognition of SVM machines	SVM and EF coefficients	In tool	The tool has not been tested on data other than owlflies wings
[13]	Tampa, Florida, USA	9 different vector-carrying mosquito species	Take images of still mosquito, either alive or dead, after spraying or trapping	Smartphone camera, Mosquito traps with CO_2 used as a bait to attract female mosquitoes	Reduce image size to 256×256 pixels for faster processing and run-time execution Noise removal using median filters Background segmentation Feature extraction	Unsupervised clustering and SVM for species classification	N/A	Since the dataset consisted of only 303 images, Deep Learning techniques could not be applied
[18]	New York, USA	4 possible labels for mosquito species, Images of egg, larva and pupa	Images are saved in cloud storage, together with its geolocation, Use of overlays to assist the user in taking a picture	60X Clip LED microscope that can be attached to any Android smartphone, Smartphone camera	Automatically by the CNN	Deep Learning	Google Maps	Image recognition is quite slow, since the recognition module is centrally located
[19]	China	tiny storage grain insects	Image captured using smartphone camera	Android OPPO R7 rear 13 million HD camera	Image preprocessing based on Sliding Window	Sliding window with changeable optimal threshold used for binary processing	On the mobile application	The separation of the connected domain is a key issues to improve identification accuracy
[20]	China	Oilseed rape pests (3,022 images divided into 12 categories)	Image captured using smartphone camera	HUAWEI Honor V10 mobile phone	Cuts the input image into a fixed size	SSD (single-shot multibox detector)	On the mobile application	Inappropriate detection when two pests overlap
[21]	Salvador, Bahia, Brazil	Aedes aegypti, Aedes albopictus and Culex quinquefasciatus	CDC light traps and suction tubes were used to collect adult insects Image species were then taken using a digital camera or a mobile phone	Digital camera or mobile phone. Exact model not mentioned	Automatically by the CNN	LeNet, AlexNet and GoogleNet	N/A	Dataset is limited in size and its balance between the different classes

(continued)

Table 1. (*continued*)

Mobile Application	Region	Type of Insect/Dataset	Image capture details (how are images taken)	Type of equipment used	Image processing details	Algorithms used	Visualisation	Challenges/Limitations
[22]	Inner Mongolia, China	Grasshoppers, GHCID dataset	RGB images of adult grasshoppers collected from the wild using a smartphone	Huawei P20 Pro and Nubia Z11 mini smartphones	Images are re-scaled proportionally so that their dimensions lie between 800 and 1333 pixels	Deep Learning, CNN, Multibox SSD MobileNetV2, stochastic gradient descent (SGD) training algorithm	On the mobile application	The detection performance of the stationary method and the mobile App are 78 and 49 percent respectively. The detection performance of the mobile model is low
[23]	Germany, Brazil, US, China	Live bees, butterflies	Picture of a bee's wing is captured from camera or chosen from storage		Automatically by the CNN	Deep Learning, CNN	On both the mobile and the web application	Incorporating additional information about species like their geographic distributions may result in wrong predictions
[16]	USA, Pakistan	Mosquitoes (Aedes and Culex), Dataset - IEEE data port			Uses ML and CNN for mosquito identification	Machine Learning, Deep Learning, CNN		Dataset consisted of only 1404 images

number of images was limited. Batch size is proportionate to the learning rate of training. Table 2 shows the dataset built for this project as well as the number of images in each species.

Table 2. Dataset

Species name	Family	Genus	Number of images
Albopictus	Culicidae	Aedes	23
Arabiensis	Culicidae	Anopheles	18
Fowleri	Culicidae	Aedes	23
Mascarensis	Culicidae	Anopheles	14
Arboricollis	Culicidae	Orthopodomyia	21
Quinquefasciatus	Culicidae	Culex	30
Tigripes	Culicidae	Lutzia	14
Tritaeniorhynchus	Culicidae	Culex	11

The training and validation dataset was built using the images acquired. Our dataset comprises 154 images, spanning eight distinct species. It is imperative to designate the directory where the image folders for each species are stored, with each subfolder named according to the species it represents. In our configuration, 20% of the data were allocated for validation purposes, while the remaining 80% were utilized for training. None of the images used for training were used for validation and only one image of each sample was taken. For the testing dataset, new images of pre-labelled mosquitoes were captured at the VBCD using the *DeepSquitoes* app.

3.3 *DeepSquitoes* Mobile Application

The *DeepSquitoes* mobile app, which is the main component of the *DeepSquitoes* mobile system framework, is a full REST API-based application with the front-end directly connected to the Firebase services without using a middleware. Figure 2 shows how the mobile app is connected to different Firebase services using Javascript API. Firebase authentication is used to manage the registration and login from the back-end. Firebase Storage is used to store mosquito images uploaded by registered users along with their annotations, which are saved in Firebase Firestore NoSQL database. Firebase hosting is used as the web server to publish the *DeepSquitoes* website and Firebase API is used to get all the verified data of the uploaded mosquito instances.

The *DeepSquitoes* mobile app was developed using Android Studio IDE. To get the address location of a specific mosquito, a user can either manually enter an address or use the smartphone GPS to get the exact location. Each captured image of the wing undergoes preprocessing to remove excess background before being uploaded to an online Firebase database. After the object detection and image classification, the user is redirected to a page dedicated to the identification of mosquito species. Upon successful classification,

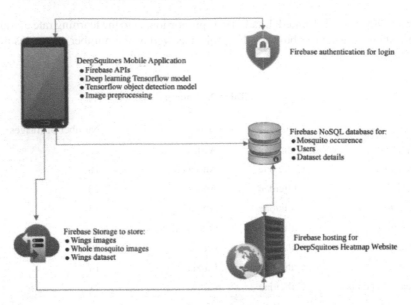

Fig. 2. Architecture Diagram

the name of the mosquito species is displayed within the mobile app. Expert users have the additional facility to annotate a mosquito species and append comments for further clarification. In addition, following the classification process, an expert user is presented with the option to review three potential matching outcomes, each accompanied with the species name and corresponding percentage match.

4   Results and Discussion

The *DeepSquitoes* mobile app enables users to upload images of insects for subsequent classification into eight different species. The images and their classification are uploaded on a cloud platform and the *DeepSquitoes* website retrieves all the insects' information and displays them on a map along with their images. The microscope was controlled directly from the mobile app due to API limitations. Native application provided by the microscope was used for taking pictures that were uploaded into the mobile application as shown in Fig. 3 and Fig. 4. For the testing phase, *DeepSquitoes* allows the user to capture multiple images of the same insect for a more accurate classification.

The mobile application has the capability to swiftly load deep learning and object detection models, thereby classifying images from mobile phones within a few seconds. Additionally, the application supports on-device image filtering by utilizing the OpenCV library. Furthermore, the architecture of the application is designed such that other deep learning models can be integrated seamlessly without requiring any modifications.

The deep learning model employed here is based on the MobileNetV2's feature extraction architecture from Tensorflow, selected for its superior performance; it is also consistent with the DL model created by Souchaud et al. [12]. The model achieved a validation accuracy of 74%. Despite the low quality of the microscope, the model attained a recognition accuracy of about 76% on our testing dataset, which is satisfactory given the low number of images in our dataset. Figure 5 shows the classification results of the mosquito species along with the percentage matched. In this figure, the identified species is *Arboricollis* and the matching percentage is 88%.

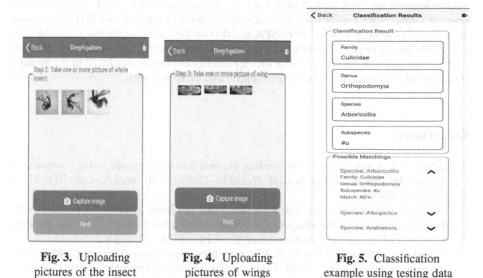

Fig. 3. Uploading pictures of the insect	**Fig. 4.** Uploading pictures of wings	**Fig. 5.** Classification example using testing data

5   Conclusion

This study presents *DeepSquitoes*, a mobile application for insect identification and fast data dissemination which has the potential to improve the management of public health hazards. The mobile application is able to identify mosquito vectors and monitor the insect population movements in real-time. *DeepSquitoes* was developed using the Ionic angular framework using Firebase as data storage. Object detection and image processing were performed using Tensorflow and OpenCV respectively. The deep learning model was developed using the Tensorflow Hub MobileNetV2 model architecture and was parameterised and adapted for the requirements of the project. The equipment set up included the mobile device, the portable microscope with LED lights and the platform to place the mosquito wings. The application is designed to be easily deployable on the iOS platform without requiring additional implementation. This system provides a viable option for monitoring the spread of various mosquito species worldwide, but limited by the quality of the citizen scientists' photos. Images submitted to the system undergo expert entomological review and labelling, serving dual purposes: informing public health agencies, and providing valuable feedback to volunteering citizens. The system is reported to be highly accurate with an area under the receiver operating characteristic curve score of 0.96. In the future, the dataset is expected to expand by increasing the number of mosquito species and the number of training images. It is also planned to host the system online to facilitate seamless updates. In addition, enhancing the microscope's capabilities for feature extraction and integrating it with an API directly into the application can significantly enhance the effectiveness of the deep learning algorithm in accurately predicting the taxonomy of a mosquito vector. Finally, techniques such as hold-out and cross-validation, although not always used in Deep Learning, can be investigated.

Acknowledgements. This study is the result of a collaborative work by the Health Informatics Research Group of the University of Mauritius, the ETIS lab of ENSEA, and IRD. It was based on the previous works performed by ENSEA and IRD on the deep learning-based classification of dipteran species using, as features, the wing interference patterns (WIPs) of insects. We wish to extend our special thanks to the Vector Biology and Control Division (VBCD) of the Ministry of Health and Wellness, Mauritius, for their support and valuable inputs.

References

1. El-Sayed, A., Kamel, M.: Climatic changes and their role in emergence and re-emergence of diseases. Environ. Sci. Pollut. Res. Int. **27**, 22336–22352 (2020). https://doi.org/10.1007/s11356-020-08896-w
2. Caminade, C., Medlock, J.M., Ducheyne, E., et al.: Suitability of European climate for the Asian tiger mosquito Aedes albopictus: recent trends and future scenarios. J. R. Soc. Interface **9**, 2708–2717 (2012). https://doi.org/10.1098/rsif.2012.0138
3. Nebbak, A., Almeras, L., Parola, P., Bitam, I.: Mosquito vectors (Diptera: Culicidae) and mosquito-borne diseases in North Africa. Insects **13** (2022). https://doi.org/10.3390/insects13100962
4. Alikhan, M., Al Ghamdi, K., Mahyoub, J.A., Alanazi, N.: Public health and veterinary important flies (order: Diptera) prevalent in Jeddah Saudi Arabia with their dominant characteristics and identification key. Saudi J. Biol. Sci. **25**, 1648–1663 (2018). https://doi.org/10.1016/j.sjbs.2016.08.014
5. Alenou, L.D., Nwane, P., Mbakop, L.R., et al.: Burden of mosquito-borne diseases across rural versus urban areas in Cameroon between 2002 and 2021: prospective for community-oriented vector management approaches. Parasites Vectors **16**, 136 (2023). https://doi.org/10.1186/s13071-023-05737-w
6. Bamou, R., Mayi, M.P.A., Djiappi-Tchamen, B., et al.: An update on the mosquito fauna and mosquito-borne diseases distribution in Cameroon. Parasites Vectors **14**, 527 (2021). https://doi.org/10.1186/s13071-021-04950-9
7. Fang, Y., Zhang, W., Xue, J.-B., Zhang, Y.: Monitoring mosquito-borne arbovirus in various insect regions in China in 2018. Front. Cell. Infect. Microbiol. **11**, 640993 (2021). https://doi.org/10.3389/fcimb.2021.640993
8. Pataki, B.A., Garriga, J., Eritja, R., et al.: Deep learning identification for citizen science surveillance of tiger mosquitoes. Sci. Rep. **11**, 4718 (2021). https://doi.org/10.1038/s41598-021-83657-4
9. Martineau, M., Conte, D., Raveaux, R., et al.: A survey on image-based insect classification. Pattern Recogn. **65**, 273–284 (2017). https://doi.org/10.1016/j.patcog.2016.12.020
10. Sereno, D., Cannet, A., Akhoundi, M., et al.: Systeme et procede d'identification automatisee de dipteres hematophages (2015)
11. Picard, D., Gosselin, P.-H.: Improving image similarity with vectors of locally aggregated tensors. In: 2011 18th IEEE International Conference on Image Processing, pp. 669–672. IEEE (2011)

12. Souchaud, M., Jacob, P., Simon-Chane, C., et al.: Mobile phones hematophagous Diptera surveillance in the field using deep learning and wing interference patterns. In: 2018 IFIP/IEEE International Conference on Very Large Scale Integration (VLSI-SoC), pp. 159–162. IEEE (2018)

13. Minakshi, M., Bharti, P., Chellappan, S.: Leveraging smart-phone cameras and image processing techniques to classify mosquito species. In: Proceedings of the 15th EAI International Conference on Mobile and Ubiquitous Systems: Computing, Networking and Services, New York, NY, USA, pp. 77–86. ACM (2018)

14. Yang, H.-P., Ma, C.-S., Wen, H., et al.: A tool for developing an automatic insect identification system based on wing outlines. Sci. Rep. **5**, 12786 (2015). https://doi.org/10.1038/srep12786

15. Zhan, Q.-B., Wang, X.-L.: Elliptic Fourier analysis of the wing outline shape of five species of antlion (Neuroptera: Myrmeleontidae: Myrmeleontini). Zool Stud. **51** (2012)

16. Rustam, F., Reshi, A.A., Aljedaani, W., et al.: Vector mosquito image classification using novel RIFS feature selection and machine learning models for disease epidemiology. Saudi J. Biol. Sci. **29**, 583–594 (2022). https://doi.org/10.1016/j.sjbs.2021.09.021

17. Guilbaud, C.S.E., Guilbaud, T.G.D.P.V.: Mosquito mapper: a phone application to map urban mosquitoes. Sci. Phone Appl. Mob. Devices **3**, 6 (2017). https://doi.org/10.1186/s41070-017-0018-9

18. Munoz, J.P., Boger, R., Dexter, S., et al.: Image recognition of disease-carrying insects: a system for combating infectious diseases using image classification techniques and citizen science. In: Proceedings of the 51st Hawaii International Conference on System Sciences. Hawaii International Conference on System Sciences (2018)

19. Zhu, C., Wang, J., Liu, H., Mi, H.: Insect identification and counting in stored grain: image processing approach and application embedded in smartphones. Mob. Inf. Syst. **2018**, 1–5 (2018). https://doi.org/10.1155/2018/5491706

20. He, Y., Zeng, H., Fan, Y., et al.: Application of deep learning in integrated pest management: a real-time system for detection and diagnosis of oilseed rape pests. Mob. Inf. Syst. **2019**, 1–14 (2019). https://doi.org/10.1155/2019/4570808

21. Motta, D., Santos, A.Á.B., Winkler, I., et al.: Application of convolutional neural networks for classification of adult mosquitoes in the field. PLoS ONE **14**, e0210829 (2019). https://doi.org/10.1371/journal.pone.0210829

22. Chudzik, P., Mitchell, A., Alkaseem, M., et al.: Mobile real-time grasshopper detection and data aggregation framework. Sci. Rep. **10**, 1150 (2020). https://doi.org/10.1038/s41598-020-57674-8

23. Buschbacher, K., Ahrens, D., Espeland, M., Steinhage, V.: Image-based species identification of wild bees using convolutional neural networks. Ecol. Inform. **55**, 101017 (2020). https://doi.org/10.1016/j.ecoinf.2019.101017

24. Sandler, M., Howard, A., Zhu, M., et al.: MobileNetV2: inverted residuals and linear bottlenecks. arXiv (2018). https://doi.org/10.48550/arxiv.1801.04381

BrainGain: A Technological Approach
for Increasing Consciousness in Coma Patients

Rita Pinto[1] and António Jorge Gouveia[1,2(✉)]

[1] School of Science and Technology, University of Trás-os-Montes and Alto Douro, Vila Real, Portugal
a173979@alunos.utad.pt, jgouveia@utad.pt
[2] C-MADE/UTAD, Quinta de Prados, 5000 Vila Real, Portugal

Abstract. Coma is a state of reduced consciousness that affects thousands of people each year. Despite advances in medicine, many patients remain in a coma for long periods of time, and many never fully recover consciousness.

This prototype is an initial version of the application, more simplified and will allow exploring and validating concepts, functionalities, and interfaces. The BrainGain application will be an innovative tool designed to help coma patients recover consciousness more quickly, through personalized stimuli and activities. The application allows the customization of the rehabilitation program for each patient, based on their needs. Patients can engage in cognitive stimulation exercises, physical activities, and therapies, all aimed at improving their quality of life. Initial results suggest that BrainGain may be a valuable tool in coma patient rehabilitation.

Keywords: awareness · coma · stimuli · activities · family · medical team

1 Introduction

Coma, or loss of consciousness, is a state of deep unconsciousness caused by various medical conditions. During a coma, the person does not respond to external stimuli and is unable to wake up or communicate consciously [1]. Treatment involves identifying and treating the underlying cause, carefully monitoring brain function, and rehabilitation. The duration of a coma can vary from a few hours to years, with varying prognosis [2–4].

Traumatic brain injury (TBI) is considered a current public health problem due to its contribution to global death and trauma-related disability [5]. Each year, 500–800 cases per 100,000 people are recorded according to multiple studies conducted in the United States and New Zealand [6]. Death occurs subsequently in 64.6% of total cases, with the most frequent cause being neurological disorders and unintentional injuries or trauma (such as falls) [7] [8] [4]. TBI is a brain injury resulting from impact or injury to the head, varying in severity and symptoms. Loss of consciousness is a frequent symptom associated with this diagnosis, which can have varying durations and result from the temporary interruption of normal brain activity due to the impact or injury. The

A. Cunha et al. (Eds.): MobiHealth 2023, LNICST 578, pp. 374–385, 2024.
https://doi.org/10.1007/978-3-031-60665-6_28

need for immediate medical attention is evidenced by the loss of consciousness, which may indicate a severe brain injury and require urgent medical treatment. Treatment can include supportive care, such as rest and pain medication, or surgical intervention to treat serious complications [9–11].

To combat this symptom, the patient should be highly stimulated to regain consciousness, both by the medical team and family. The stimuli are diverse, but can be divided into two main branches, personal and mechanical. Personal stimuli are those directed to the patient's intimate sphere, such as familiar and friendly voices, favorite music, personal tastes, familiar smells, and sensory stimuli, in short, stimuli that appeal to the use of memory. Mechanical stimuli are more general, such as following orders, repeating orders, interacting with the environment, and requested movements. The stimuli vary depending on the patient's level of consciousness.

The *BrainGain* application serves as a valuable platform that collaborates with the patient, their family, and the medical team in the process of regaining consciousness. This application offers a wide range of resources and tools, such as personalized stimuli ideas, progress tracking and reporting features, informative articles explaining the medical condition and treatment processes, as well as communication tools to foster collaboration between the medical team and families. By addressing the issue of communication gaps between these parties, the application aims to enhance the overall support system for the patient's recovery.

Utilizing software to stimulate patients who have experienced head trauma and recently emerged from a coma brings numerous significant advantages to the rehabilitation and neurological recovery process [5]. The software can be tailored to cater to the specific needs of each individual, providing exercises and interactive activities that target the impaired cognitive and motor functions resulting from the coma period. Moreover, the digital approach ensures a safe and controlled environment, allowing healthcare professionals to closely monitor the patient's progress and adapt activities according to the evolving clinical condition. The incorporation of gamification and interactivity in the software makes the rehabilitation process more engaging and motivating for patients, encouraging active participation and dedication to treatment, thereby potentially expediting the recovery process and enhancing the post-head trauma quality of life.

The personalized stimuli provided by the *BrainGain* application are particularly important, as they can help to stimulate the patient's brain activity and encourage the return of consciousness. These stimuli can include familiar voices, music, and other sensory cues that are meaningful to the patient. By providing a range of personalized stimuli options, the *BrainGain* application can help caregivers to find the most effective stimuli for each individual patient. In addition to personalized stimuli, the *BrainGain* application provides a range of other valuable features to support patients and caregivers. These include progress tracking and reporting tools, which allow caregivers to track the patient's progress over time and adjust their care plan as needed. The application is intended for those responsible for patients when they are not conscious and for the initial gain of consciousness.

This paper will present the development of the first prototype of the mobile application designed to assist coma patients in regaining consciousness.

2 Methodology

The development of the *BrainGain* mobile application prototype, aimed at assisting individuals in emerging from a comatose state, was carried out following a careful and rigorous methodological process. The work was divided into several phases, as shown in Fig. 1, allowing for a structured and efficient approach.

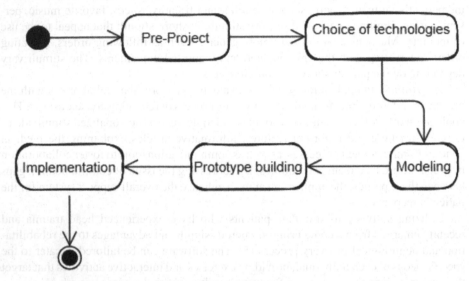

Fig. 1. Development pipeline

2.1 Pre-project

The pre-project phase is a fundamental step in the development process, whose main objectives are to deepen the understanding of the subject in question and obtain a comprehensive overview of the scope and activities that will be carried out. During this phase, we seek to collect relevant information, conduct research and analyze feasibility studies to identify needs and challenges related to the project. This preliminary exploration is crucial to defining clear goals and objectives, determining required resources, and establishing a solid strategy for project development. At the end of this phase, we are expected to be well grounded and prepared to move on to the next step in the process, with a solid understanding of what will be performed and what results to expect to achieve [12].

So, in the pre-project phase, an in-depth study of the technologies to be used was conducted. A thorough analysis of available options was performed, considering criteria such as performance, compatibility, and usability. Additionally, a detailed study of the most suitable programming language for the application development was conducted, ultimately opting for React Native and JavaScript. This choice was based on prior experience with these technologies and their ability to provide a smooth and intuitive user interface for both iOS and Android devices.

2.2 Choice of Technologies

The use of React Native presents itself as a strategic and advantageous choice in the development of mobile applications. By choosing this framework, it is possible to save time and resources, since it allows creating applications for iOS and Android from a single source code, avoiding the need to develop two different versions for each platform [13, 14]. In addition, React Native provides a fluid and fast user experience, as it can generate native interfaces, which results in performance and responsiveness similar to applications developed natively for each platform. Its wide community and the availability of pre-built components also facilitate the task of developers, accelerating the development process and allowing the creation of applications with the latest features and trends in the mobile market. One of the advantages of using JavaScript with React Native is language efficiency. JavaScript is an interpreted programming language, which means that the code is executed directly by the browser or by the interpreter, instead of being compiled before being executed. This makes the development process faster and more efficient, with less waiting time for compilation and debugging [15].

Finally, JavaScript can provide a fluid and intuitive user interface for mobile applications. React Native being component-based allows developers to build a consistent, reusable UI across their entire app, resulting in a more consistent and easier-to-use user experience [16, 17].

2.3 Modelling

The modeling phase was divided into two parts, Functional and Data modeling.

During the functional modeling phase of the project, we conducted a survey of the essential requirements and the detailed specification of the application. In this context, we thoroughly studied the specific needs of comatose patients, as well as the requirements of health professionals and families engaged in their rehabilitation process. By employing Use Case diagrams (not included in this paper), we successfully developed a robust functional model tailored to the identified needs.

Requirements Gathering – Macro Functionalities

The quality of the produced software is closely tied to requirements gathering [18].

In this subsection, we present a list that outlines the specifications for everything that must be implemented. These requirements can be classified into two categories: functional and non-functional requirements. Functional requirements pertain to the services the system should provide, while non-functional requirements are associated with specific characteristics or limitations of the system.

In this paper we will present a listing of macro functionalities instead of individual requirements. This approach is justified by the search for a more comprehensive and results-oriented view of the software development process.

Rather than focusing on detailed requirements, identifying macro functionality allows us to group the high-level functionality of the system, highlighting its main capabilities and overall goals. This approach makes it easier for stakeholders to understand the breadth and complexity of the software, allowing for better prioritization and decision-making throughout the development cycle. In addition, the list of macro functionalities promotes more efficient communication between the development team and stakeholders, facilitating the identification of critical areas and enabling a more precise allocation of resources and efforts throughout the project. In short, the macro functionality listing offers a strategic and integrated view of the software, providing a solid foundation for successful project planning and execution [19].

1. The *BrainGain* application must be able to manage several types of stimuli - visual, auditory, and tactile.
2. The *BrainGain* application must allow customizing the stimuli according to the individual characteristics of the patient.
3. The *BrainGain* application must allow the storage of monitoring and brain stimulation data - allowing the analysis of patterns and trends.
4. The *BrainGain* application must allow communication with the medical team responsible for treating the patient in a coma.
5. The *BrainGain* application must ensure safe and secure access to patient data.
6. The *BrainGain* application must allow multiple reports.
7. The *BrainGain* application should be multi-patient and multi-caregiver.

Data Modeling
Data modeling plays a crucial role in the field of data management and information systems as it serves as the basis for organizing and representing data in a structured and meaningful way. By defining the relationships between different data entities and attributes, data modeling helps to create a clear and standardized structure for databases, facilitating data integration, retrieval and analysis [20].

The Entity Relationship Diagram (ERD), as we can see in Fig. 2, enabled us to define the structure of the database required for efficiently storing and managing information essential to the recovery of comatose patients. Furthermore, we outlined the user interfaces for both the back-office and front-office through the creation of mockups. This approach ensures a cohesive and engaging user experience.

- *Patient*: represents the patient in a coma, with information such as name, age, gender, medical history and level of consciousness.
- *BrainStimuli*: represents the brain stimuli applied to the patient, including information such as type of stimulus, intensity, duration and frequency.
- *Medical_Team*: represents the medical team responsible for the patient's treatment, including information such as name, specialization and position.
- *Family*: represents the patient's relatives, with information such as name, relationship with the patient and contact data.
- *User_Account*: represents the user accounts created for each member of the family, with information such as name, email and password.
- *Reports*: represents the reports generated by the application, including information about the patient's progress, brain stimulation results and trends over time.
- *Settings*: represents application settings, including information such as personalization of brain stimuli and security and privacy settings.

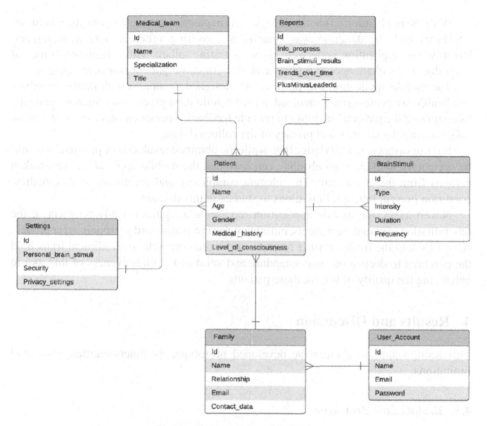

Fig. 2. Entity Relationship Diagram

3 Prototype Building and Implementation

The use of prototypes in software development offers numerous advantages that contribute significantly to the success of the project. First, a prototype allows developers and stakeholders to visualize a tangible representation of the proposed solution, facilitating communication and mutual understanding of expectations. In addition, prototypes allow for rapid iteration and validation of concepts, enabling early identification of failures and adjustment needs, which saves time and resources throughout the development cycle. Another advantage is the ability to get feedback from end users before full development, ensuring the final product best meets their needs and preferences. With the possibility of carrying out tests and simulations on prototypes, it is possible to mitigate risks and make more informed decisions, culminating in a more refined and satisfactory final delivery for all those involved in the project [21].

In the subsequent phase, focusing on prototyping, both the backend and frontend configurations of the application were meticulously developed, incorporating essential libraries to ensure smooth operation. The database's physical model was implemented using SQL light language, a crucial step that played a pivotal role in upholding the system's data integrity.

With the application's functional logic now in place, a seamless connection between interfaces and the database was established, ensuring efficient data management. Notably, the application underwent rigorous testing, albeit with a limited number of users due to the challenges in finding available comatose patients for participation.

The mobile application was purposefully designed to support both family members and healthcare professionals involved in the rehabilitation process of comatose patients. Recognizing the patients' inability to provide feedback, special emphasis was placed on safeguarding the security and privacy of the collected data.

It is important to acknowledge that, while the obtained results show promise, it would be premature to claim with absolute certainty that the mobile application can awaken patients from the coma state. The inherent complexity and variability of this medical condition present inherent limitations to studies in this domain.

Nevertheless, the mobile application represents a significant advancement in the rehabilitation of comatose patients, introducing an innovative and personalized approach. As we look to the future, further research and more comprehensive clinical trials hold the potential to deepen our understanding and validate the effectiveness of this tool in enhancing the quality of life for these patients.

4 Results and Discussion

This section aims to present the developed prototype, its functionalities, tests, and limitations.

4.1 BrainGain – Prototype

Three of the most relevant options made available by the prototype are the homepage, the menu, and the recovery diary.

The homepage (see Fig. 3, middle image) provides access to a calendar, a board with future activities, and a mood board. The main objective of this page is to customize the application according to each patient's needs. The right image in Fig. 3 represents the recovery diary, where any relevant records that contribute to the patient's improvement can be daily inserted. Over time, these records can be evaluated and included in medical records, combating forgetfulness or lack of attention during critical moments. Finally, the menu (left image in Fig. 3) presents the user with various options available in the application, including activities, stimuli, and additional information on the subject.

Figure 4's left image showcases the "Learn more about it" page, offering a vast collection of articles to enhance users' knowledge about their prognosis. Selecting an article automatically opens a complete webpage, aiming to educate individuals and raise awareness on multiple levels.

The middle image of Fig. 4 represents the stimuli section, containing a huge list of stimuli to be performed for the patient. When selecting one of these stimuli, a brief explanatory note opens (image on the right in Fig. 4).

The prototype also provides an 'Activities' section (left image of Fig. 5). This section offers a selected list of exercises and stimulating therapies for coma patients, promoting sensory, cognitive, and emotional engagement. This feature empowers caregivers and

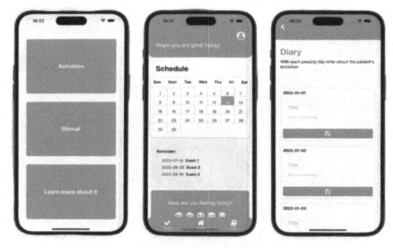

Fig. 3. Menu, homepage, and recovery diary

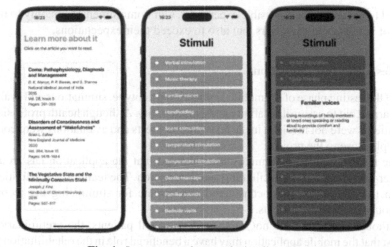

Fig. 4. Learn more about and stimuli pages.

enhances patient care, improving outcomes and aiding recovery from a coma. In the middle and right images of Fig. 5, we can see two examples of activities. The first activity consists of two circles, one green and one red, to stimulate the patient's perception and reasoning. In the second activity, we use music to stimulate the patient's auditory and emotional senses.

Thus, the prototype presented here aims to contribute significantly so that the future application represents a true advance in the field of technology, with a focus on increasing consciousness in coma patients. With an intuitive interface and innovative features, we are fully confident that it will become an indispensable tool for users and patients alike. We firmly believe that the prototype will contribute to every detail being meticulously

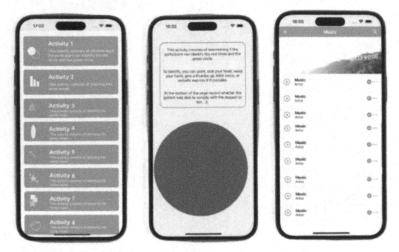

Fig. 5. Activities available example

planned to ensure the best possible experience. Our commitment is not only to meet the needs of patients and caregivers, but also to exceed their expectations.

4.2   Tests and Test Limitations

During the testing phase of the mobile application prototype, simulations and evaluations were carried out to assess its usability and functionality. Although health professionals or real patients were not involved in the tests, internal tests and evaluations were conducted by people close to the project.

The results of these preliminary tests showed that the application has an intuitive and user-friendly interface, facilitating user interaction. The features and activities available in the application were considered appropriate for stimulating the recovery of consciousness in coma patients.

Although the tests were not conducted with real patients, the preliminary results suggest that the mobile application may have a beneficial role in the rehabilitation process of coma patients. However, it is important to emphasize that further research and tests with real patients are needed to effectively validate the effectiveness and benefits of the application.

All procedures and techniques used were documented in detail to ensure reproducibility. However, given the limitations, exact replication of the tests may not be possible.

The Mobile application BrainGain project, which aims to help people recover from a coma, is a promising and important initiative in the healthcare field. By using technologies such as React Native and JavaScript, the application offers an intuitive and user-friendly interface for IOS and Android devices.

One of the main benefits of the Mobile application BrainGain is that it provides specific resources and activities to aid in the recovery of coma patients. By providing visual and auditory stimuli, the application can help awaken consciousness and improve cognition in patients.

However, it is important to note that the effectiveness of the Mobile application BrainGain has not yet been fully validated through clinical trials on real patients. While preliminary tests conducted internally suggest that the user interface is intuitive and easy to use, it is essential that the application be tested on real patients to evaluate its effectiveness in helping them recover from a coma.

Additionally, it is important that the application be used in conjunction with other treatments and therapies, such as physiotherapy and occupational therapy, to ensure that patients receive the best possible care.

The Mobile application BrainGain can be a valuable tool to complement these treatments but should not be considered a sole solution for the treatment of coma patients.

In summary, the Mobile application BrainGain is a promising and important initiative in the healthcare field, but it is essential that it be subjected to clinical trials and used in conjunction with other treatments to ensure the best possible chance of helping people recover from a coma.

5 Conclusion

This study addressed the development and evaluation of the Mobile application with the aim of helping individuals in a coma state to regain consciousness. Although we faced significant limitations, such as the lack of a real sample of comatose patients, the results obtained through the simulations carried out by some people indicate a promising potential of the application.

Users highlighted the importance of the Mobile application as an innovative and personalized tool in the field of rehabilitation of comatose patients. Through the customization of stimuli and activities, the application proved to be capable of eliciting responses and stimulating brain activity in simulated patients. These results suggest that the application can play a significant role in the rehabilitation process, providing adequate stimuli for the recovery of consciousness.

It is important to emphasize that, due to the lack of a real sample of coma patients, we cannot fully generalize the results obtained. However, the insights and feedback from experts provide a solid foundation for future investigations and larger clinical studies.

Considering the limitations inherent to this field of research, including the complexity and variability of the coma state, the Mobile application represents a significant advance in the therapeutic approach and in improving the quality of life for patients. The customization of stimuli and activities offered by the application, combined with the intuitive and fluid interface, demonstrated the potential to stimulate the recovery of consciousness.

It is recommended that future studies be conducted with a real sample of comatose patients to validate and further deepen the results found. Additionally, the incorporation of specialized health professionals and careful consideration of the ethical aspects involved are essential for the development and proper implementation of the mobile app.

Overall, the mobile application prototype proved to be a promising tool for future application development. This application could be a strong ally in the rehabilitation of comatose patients, paving the way for new therapeutic approaches and improving the understanding of this complex health condition. With the continuous advancement of technology and interdisciplinary collaboration, it is expected that the future mobile application can contribute to the recovery and quality of life of these patients, representing an important innovation in the field of medicine and intensive care.

Acknowledgements. This work was supported by the FCT (Portuguese Foundation for Science and Technology) through the project UIDB/04082/2020 (CMADE).

References

1. Bateman, D.E.: Neurological assessment of coMA. J. Neurol. Neurosurg. Psychiatry **71**(suppl. 1), i13–i17 (2001)
2. Levin, H.S., Gary, H.E., Eisenberg, H.M., Ruff, R.M., Barth, J.T., Kreutzer, J., et al.: Neurobehavioral outcome 1 year after severe head injury: experience of the Traumatic Coma Data Bank. J. Neurosurg. **73**(5), 699–709 (1990)
3. Braine, M.E., Cook, N.: The Glasgow Coma Scale and evidence-informed practice: a critical review of where we are and where we need to be. J. Clin. Nurs. **26**(1–2), 280–293 (2017)
4. Rabinstein, A.A.: Coma and Brain Death. Continuum (Minneap Minn). **24**(6), 1708–1731 (2018)
5. Christopher, E., Alsaffarini, K.W., Jamjoom, A.A.: Mobile health for traumatic brain injury: a systematic review of the literature and mobile application market. Cureus **11**(7), e5120 (2019)
6. Vadan, I.: Estimating the global incidence of TBI2019 01/06/2023. https://brain-amn.org/global-incidence-of-tbi/
7. Strauss, D.J., Shavelle, R.M., Anderson, T.W.: Long-term survival of children and adolescents after traumatic brain injury. Arch. Phys. Med. Rehabil. **79**(9), 1095–1100 (1998)
8. Colantonio, A., Escobar, M.D., Chipman, M., McLellan, B., Austin, P.C., Mirabella, G., et al.: Predictors of postacute mortality following traumatic brain injury in a seriously injured population. J. Trauma Acute Care Surg. **64**(4), 876–882 (2008)
9. Albensi, B.C., Knoblach, S.M., Chew, B.G.M., O'Reilly, M.P., Faden, A.I., Pekar, J.J.: Diffusion and high resolution MRI of traumatic brain injury in Rats: time course and correlation with histology. Exp. Neurol. **162**(1), 61–72 (2000)
10. Langlois, J.A., Rutland-Brown, W., Wald, M.M.: The epidemiology and impact of traumatic brain injury: a brief overview. J. Head Trauma Rehabil. **21**(5), 375–378 (2006)
11. Sudhakar, S.K., Sridhar, S., Char, S., Pandya, K., Mehta, K.: Prevalence of comorbidities post mild traumatic brain injuries: a traumatic brain injury model systems study. Front. Hum. Neurosci. **17**, 1158483 (2023)
12. Gibson, E., Gebken, R.: Design quality in pre-project planning: applications of the Project Definition Rating Index. Build. Res. Inf. **31**(5), 346–356 (2003)
13. Adam, B., Roy, D., Mikhail, S.: React and react native: build cross-platform JavaScript Applications with Native Power for the Web, Desktop, and Mobile, 1 p. Packt Publishing (2022)
14. Roy, D.: React Projects: Build advanced cross-platform projects with React and React Native to become a professional developer, 1 p. Packt Publishing (2022)
15. Danielsson, W.: React Native application development – a comparison between native Android and React Native: Linköpings universitet (2016)
16. Gill, O.: Using React Native for mobile software development: Metropolia University of Applied Sciences (2018)

17. Silva, D.A., Sousa, C.Fd.: Construção de Application com React Native. Revista Tecnologias em Projeção **10**(1), 1–152019
18. Ramesh, M.R.R., Reddy, C.S.: Metrics for software requirements specification quality quantification. Comput. Electr. Eng. **96**, 107445 (2021)
19. Petrov, P., Buy, U., Nord, R.L. (eds.): Enhancing the software architecture analysis and design process with inferred macro-architectural requirements. In: 2012 First IEEE International Workshop on the Twin Peaks of Requirements and Architecture (TwinPeaks), 25 September 2012
20. Meredith, M.: Data modeling: a process for pattern induction. J. Exp. Theor. Artif. Intell. **3**(1), 43–68 (1991)
21. Suranto, B. (ed): Software prototypes: Enhancing the quality of requirements engineering process. In: 2015 International Symposium on Technology Management and Emerging Technologies (ISTMET), 25–27 August 2015 (2015)

PHPlace: A New Perspective on Managing Pelvic Organ Prolapse Through Mobile Applications

Yanlin Mi[1,2]([✉]) [iD], Reut Rotem[3,4], Yair Daykan[5,6] [iD], Barry A. O'Reilly[3] [iD], and Sabin Tabirca[1,7] [iD]

[1] School of Computer Science and Information Technology, University College Cork, Cork, Ireland
y.mi@cs.ucc.ie

[2] SFI Centre for Research Training in Artificial Intelligence, University College Cork, Cork, Ireland

[3] Department of Urogynaecology, Cork University Maternity Hospital, Cork, Ireland

[4] Department of Obstetrics and Gynecology, Shaare Zedek Medical Center, Affiliated with the Hebrew University School of Medicine, Jerusalem, Israel

[5] Department of OBGYN, Meir Medical Center, Kfar Saba, Israel

[6] Sackler School of Medicine, Tel Aviv University, Tel Aviv, Israel

[7] Faculty of Mathematics and Informatics, Transylvania University of Brasov, Brasov, Romania

Abstract. In the rapidly evolving field of digital health, the use of mobile health apps is increasing, which not only allows patients to be more actively involved in their health management and treatment but also significantly improves the efficiency of healthcare professionals. Yet despite the success of mHealth apps in a large portion of the field, there is room for improvement thrown in the field of pelvic organ prolapse (POP). Pelvic Health Place (PHPlace) is an example of a new mHealth app designed specifically for POP. It aims to improve patient comprehension and healthcare provider efficiency. These features include engaging animated presentations, a groundbreaking algorithm-based scoring system to measure the severity of a condition and versatile medical information management tools. In addition, by effectively localising the application, PHPlace transcends geographic constraints and extends healthcare services globally. Initial user feedback shows an impressive 90% improvement in users' understanding of their POP condition and its associated treatments, signalling the success of the design implementation. This paper's in-depth exploration of PHPlace provides a strategic blueprint for the design and development of future mHealth applications, setting a new standard for digital healthcare platforms.

Keywords: Pelvic Organ Prolapse · mHealth · Medical animation · Questionnaire system

This publication has emanated from research conducted with the financial support of Science Foundation Ireland under Grant number 18/CRT/6223.

A. Cunha et al. (Eds.): MobiHealth 2023, LNICST 578, pp. 386–399, 2024.
https://doi.org/10.1007/978-3-031-60665-6_29

1   Introduction

As technology continues to advance, mobile health applications have become a major force for change in healthcare. These apps are profoundly changing the way we understand, diagnose, and treat disease, as well as reshaping the way patients interact with healthcare professionals [1]. The unique innovation of mHealth applications lies in their ability to cleverly blend knowledge and technology from computer science, data science, medicine, and health care. With real-time health monitoring and personalised disease prevention information, patients are able to more actively engage and manage their health status, potentially improving treatment outcomes and quality of life. At the same time, these apps provide an integrated platform for healthcare professionals to more efficiently manage patient information, monitor patient health status and provide timely feedback and interventions, which not only enhances the quality of healthcare delivery but also helps to reduce the workload of healthcare professionals [2]. However, while mHealth applications have made significant progress in most areas, there are still many challenges in the area of Pelvic Organ Prolapse (POP).

POP is a common gynecological condition that refers to the prolapse of pelvic organs from their original position in the pelvis and includes Bladder prolapse, Rectal prolapse, Small bowel prolapse, Urethral prolapse, Uterine prolapse, and Vault prolapse [3]. It is a widespread public health problem, a phenomenon that has a major impact on women's physical health worldwide, as well as a profound impact on the quality of life of those affected. Numerous scientific studies have reported that approximately half of all women worldwide will suffer from POP during their lifetime [4]. POP not only causes physical problems, but can also lead to a range of complications, including sexual life disorders, mental health problems, and dysfunction related to activities of daily living [5]. The effects extend far beyond the realm of physical health and reach into the mental life and social activities of the patient, thus causing a serious impact on their quality of life.

In the medical field, despite the considerable efforts that have been invested in the research and treatment of POP [6], many problems remain. One of the most prominent of these problems is the complexity and subjectivity of disease assessment. As current disease assessment relies mainly on the patient's self-report and the doctor's clinical judgment, this approach is susceptible to a number of factors, such as the patient's memory and ability to express themselves, and the doctor's professional experience and judgment, which may lead to biased assessment results [7]. Another issue is the diversity of treatment options. treatment options for POP often involve multiple modalities, such as surgery, medication, and physiotherapy, which makes it difficult for patients to understand and remember information about the condition and treatment to ensure compliance [8]. In addition, workflow optimisation for healthcare professionals is an important challenge. Current working practices often require physicians to perform extensive manual data recording, analysis, and sharing, which is not only inefficient but can also lead to missed or misunderstood information [9]. In addition, it is a major challenge for healthcare to better serve and manage patients from different language and cultural backgrounds on a global scale, and to provide the same quality of service to patients worldwide.

In response to these issues, we have designed and implemented Pelvic Health Place (PHPlace), a mobile health application for POP (see Fig. 1). PHPlace is an innovative medical software that presents symptoms and treatment processes in a visual and animated format, allowing patients to better understand their condition and treatment plan, thus improving adherence to treatment. In addition, it automates the management of patient records and the scoring of diseases, which is extremely helpful for doctors in terms of improving efficiency, optimising workflow, and improving the quality and efficiency of care. Moreover, the software is also localised to accommodate different languages and cultures, thus increasing the accessibility of healthcare services worldwide. We expect PHPlace to drive digital transformation in healthcare and have a real impact on improving the quality of life for women around the world.

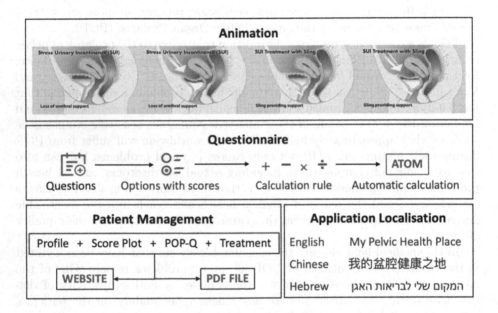

Fig. 1. Pelvic Health Place features

2   Methods

We initiated the development of the PHPlace app with a qualitative study, involving 20 in-depth interviews with patients who have experienced pelvic organ prolapse (POP) and 15 consultations with healthcare professionals specializing in urogynecology. The thematic analysis of these interviews highlighted a significant communication gap and identified specific areas where technology could intervene. The patients expressed a need for visual and interactive content to better understand their condition, while professionals emphasized the importance of personalized and dynamic information sharing to enhance patient engagement and compliance.

To convert these insights into app features, we employed a co-design approach. Five workshops were conducted with the participation of both patients and professionals to brainstorm, prioritize, and validate the initial feature set of PHPlace. PHPlace incorporates integrated mobile technology and automation tools to greatly enhance the efficiency of POP disease management. To foster a better understanding of POP disease in patients, animated presentations detailing disease symptoms and treatments are designed and implemented. Disease assessment is further automated through the creation of questionnaires and automated scoring systems. Optimisation of the medical information management process also takes place for both doctors and patients, encompassing the generation of PDF files and patient management functions. Localised design of the application is implemented to heighten the accessibility of healthcare services. Further discussion will delve into the process of designing, implementing and optimising these key features.

2.1   General Architecture

Designing an application that can effectively manage the POP disease treatment process requires consideration of various usage environments and user roles. Therefore, a decentralised, multi-sided architecture was adopted, comprising a server side, a doctor side, and a patient-side, each working independently and in collaboration with the other.

The server side is responsible for processing and managing the data and is developed in Go, a language whose strength lies in its excellent concurrency and performance, enabling it to process large volumes of requests quickly and ensure real-time data accuracy. Data security and privacy protection are taken into account when handling sensitive medical information of patients. The server side is responsible for processing and managing the data, and advanced encryption algorithms and Secure Sockets Layer/Transport Layer Security (SSL/TLS) technology are introduced for encrypted data transmission to ensure data security during transmission and storage [10]. At the same time, the stored data is hashed and salted, making it difficult to crack even if the data is compromised. In addition, the system ensures that only authorised users and systems can access sensitive information, thus protecting patient privacy.

The doctor and patient sides are designed and developed with the needs of doctors and patients in mind, with the user interface (UI) and user experience (UX) in mind. The doctor side uses the React framework, based on its rich component library and flexible state management [11]. Its interface is designed to provide intuitive and easy-to-use operations based on the doctors' daily workflow and habits and offers rich interactive elements to optimise the doctors' working experience. The patient side uses the Flutter framework and its ability to develop cross-platform applications ensures a consistent and high-quality user experience for both iOS and Android users [12]. The interface was designed with a particular focus on making it simple and easy to understand and suitable for patients of all ages. The use of large fonts, clear instructions, and a simplified flow of operations make it easier for patients to understand and use.

2.2   Animation of Symptoms and Treatment

There is a clear correlation between the effectiveness of treatment for POP diseases and the level of understanding of the disease and treatment modalities by the patient. With this in mind, a set of symptom and treatment animations was developed specifically to help patients gain a deeper understanding of the disease and its treatment.

The 2D animation capabilities of Unity3D were used in depth in the construction of this animation system, resulting in a practical application of computer graphics and programming to the visualisation of diseases and the presentation of treatment options [13]. The animation system first generates a series of accurate 2D vector graphics that accurately depict the morphology of biological structures associated with POP, such as the urethra, bladder, rectum and other organs. These graphics are shown in detail in a healthy state as well as in the morphology of POP in its different disease states. In the Unity3D environment, these graphics are further transformed into manipulable objects or sprites. Skeletal and skinning techniques are then applied to the dynamic manipulation of these 2D objects.

In order to give the patient a better visualisation of the condition, the animation system shows the changes in the position of the pelvic organs in different states of Pelvic Organ Prolapse Quantification System(POP-Q). For example, the degree of prolapse or prolapse of the organ position is shown in detail in the animation, thus enabling the patient to better understand the specific impact of POP on quality of life, such as difficulty in urination, and pelvic pressure.

In the treatment animation section, the animation system shows changes in the position of the pelvic organs before and after treatment, and how treatment can improve the symptoms of POP. For example, in the animation on surgical treatment, it is shown in detail how the surgery repairs damaged ligaments and muscles to restore the pelvic organs to their normal position.

Finally, through parametric design, the animation system can generate corresponding animation effects based on different POP-Q parameter values. The POP-Q system contains several parameters, such as Aa, Ba, Ap, Bp, C, D, TVL, GH, PB, which represent the position of organs in different parts of the pelvis. When the value of each parameter changes, the animation system is designed to present the corresponding animation effect. For example, when the value of C (the maximum distance from the cervix or vaginal tip to the external anal opening) changes, the animation system shows the corresponding change in the position of the cervix or vaginal tip (see Fig. 2). In this way, both for the patient and the doctor, the pathological changes of the disease and the treatment process can be understood more visually.

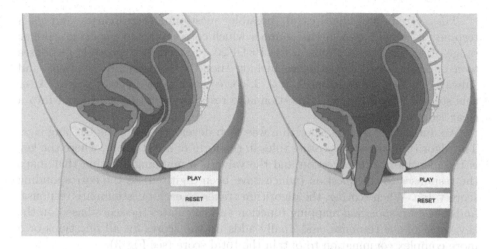

Fig. 2. The first and last frames of the animation

2.3   Questionnaire Design and Automated Scoring System

Questionnaire assessment is an important part of POP disease management. Commonly used assessment questionnaires include the Patient Global Impression of Improvement (PGI), the Pelvic Floor Distress Inventory-20 (PFDI-20) and the Pelvic Floor Impact Questionnaire-7 (PFIQ- 7) (see Table 1 for more information). We collaborated with ten senior urogynecologists to ensure the clinical relevance and accuracy of these tools within the app. Each questionnaire was reviewed, and its scoring algorithm was adapted to the app's interactive and dynamic interface. Traditional assessment methods are time-consuming for both physicians and patients, and the scoring can be subjective due to the human factors involved. To improve the efficiency and accuracy of assessments, PHPlace has developed an automated questionnaire scoring system.

Table 1. Questionnaires for POP

Questionnaires	Cite
Pelvic Floor Distress Inventory-20 (PFDI-20)	[14]
Pelvic Floor Impact Questionnaire-7 (PFIQ-7)	[14]
Pelvic Organ Prolapse/Urinary Incontinence Sexual Function Questionnaire (PISQ-12)	[15]
The Questionnaire for female Urinary Incontinence Diagnosis (QUID)	[16]
Female sexual function index scoring (FSFI)	[17]
Patient Global Impression of Improvement (PGI)	[18]
King's Health Questionnaire(KHQ)	[19]
International Consultation on Incontinence Questionnaire-Urinary Incontinence Short Form(ICIQ-UI)	[20]

The system first digitises all possible questionnaire responses and each response is coded into a specific number which corresponds to a specific score or range of scores. For example, in the PFDI-20 questionnaire, possible responses to a question about incontinence include "none", "occasionally", "often" and "always", which are coded as 0, 1, 2, 3, corresponding to different scores. After this step of processing, each questionnaire response could be translated into a clear score or range of scores.

An automated scoring algorithm was then developed using the Go language. The algorithm stores the scoring rules in the form of a dictionary, where the key is the identifier of the question and the value is a mapping function that maps the responses to the question (which have been digitised) to the corresponding score value. When scoring, the algorithm traverses each questionnaire response, finds the corresponding mapping function and calculates the score based on the key value of the response, and finally adds up the scores for all questions or a more complex combination to obtain the total score (see Fig. 3).

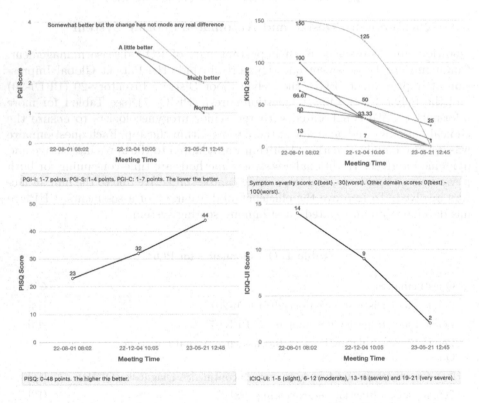

Fig. 3. Multiple questionnaire score visualisation chart

In addition, the automated scoring system takes into account all possible exceptions. Missing questionnaire responses are treated as invalid input and excluded from the final scoring. For specific borderline cases, such as questions on the impact of sexuality in the PFIQ-7 questionnaire, the system sets up specific conditional judgement logic so that responses to these questions are only included in the final score if the patient indicates that he or she has a sexual life.

Finally, to verify the accuracy and stability of this automated scoring system, the consistency of the system's scoring rules and manual scoring was verified by comparing the system's automated scoring results with historical manual scoring data.

This automated questionnaire scoring system has greatly improved the efficiency of the POP disease assessment, while ensuring accuracy through accurate calculations and comprehensive exception handling.

2.4 PDF Generation and Patient Management

Effective medical information processing, access and management is essential in POP disease management. To address this, PHPlace has developed two key features: a file PDF generation function and a patient management function.

The file PDF generation function uses react-pdf, an open source PDF library based on React.js, to enable the centralised visualisation of patient medical information. Specific PDF templates were developed which followed the design standards of the healthcare industry and were designed with HTML/CSS to ensure their readability and user-friendliness. The template covers various sections such as basic patient information, disease assessment questionnaire, questionnaire scores, POPQ scores, surgical recommendations and medication information. Each section is designed with a separate visual presentation module to improve the clarity and ease of printing the information (see Fig. 4). The system is able to automatically update PDF files when new medical information is generated or when existing information changes, and in this way provides up-to-date and accurate medical information.

For the patient management function, a doctor-side web application has been developed to provide a unified and convenient interface for doctors to manage their patients' medical information. The application accepts the POP-Q scores entered by the doctor and calls the back-end API to translate the scores into parametric animations. The animations are rendered directly in Canvas via WebGL technology, ensuring smoothness and adaptability to different devices and resolutions. After the animation has been generated, the system inserts specific frames of the animation into the patient's profile PDF, enabling doctors and patients to understand the disease status more visually. In addition to this, the application also allows doctors to view and manage basic patient information, questionnaire details, and questionnaire scores (see Fig. 5). The app allows doctors to access real-time, accurate medical information, which in turn improves the efficiency of diagnosis and treatment.

These two features have been designed and implemented to not only improve the efficiency of medical information management, but also to improve the under-

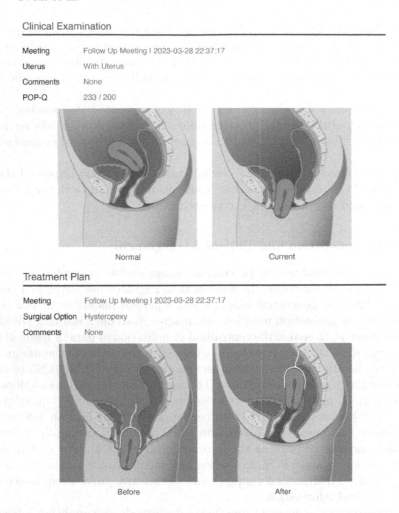

Fig. 4. Example of the generated pdf showing the visualisation of the animation

standing of disease status for both doctors and patients through the visual presentation of information.

2.5   Application Localisation

In PHPlace, particular attention was paid to the localised design of the application in order to improve the experience of patients and doctors in different parts of the world, involving two key components: internationalisation (i18n) and localisation (l10n) [21].

In terms of internationalisation, the application leverages the internationalisation support of the React and Flutter frameworks. Specifically, by collecting all the string information that needs to be displayed and storing them in a

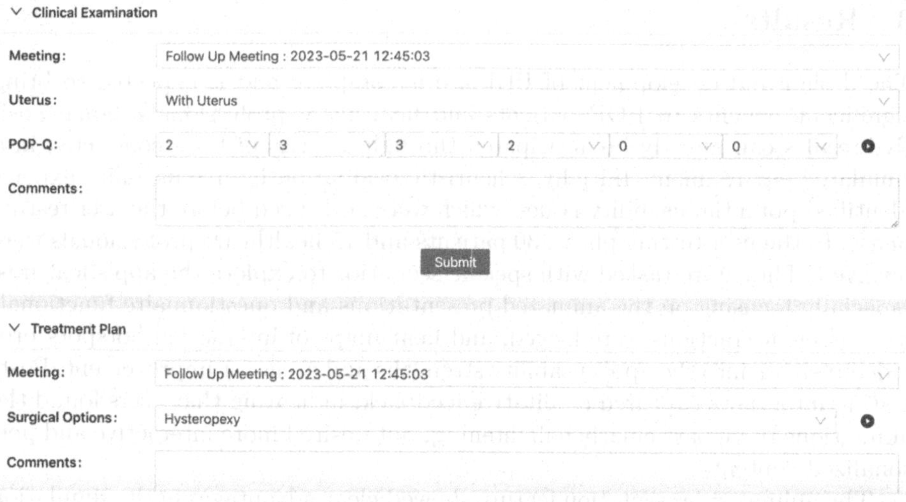

∨ Clinical Examination

Meeting:	Follow Up Meeting : 2023-05-21 12:45:03
Uterus:	With Uterus
POP-Q:	2 3 3 2 0 0
Comments:	

Submit

∨ Treatment Plan

Meeting:	Follow Up Meeting : 2023-05-21 12:45:03
Surgical Options:	Hysteropexy
Comments:	

Fig. 5. Patient management user interface

separate language file. This string information is then translated into different language versions depending on the language needs of the target user group. When patients or doctors use the application, depending on their language preference, the system automatically loads the file in the corresponding language, thus providing an interface adapted to the user's language environment. As for dynamic content that may be updated frequently, such as questions and answers of the questionnaire, when this information is returned by the server, the api of Google translate is called for machine translation according to the corresponding language tokens, returning the questionnaire in the corresponding language version.

In terms of localisation, emphasis is placed on the specific details and habits of different cultures and regions. This includes date and time presentation formats, currency units, and units of measure. Localisation tools for React and Flutter make this process much easier. These tools automatically recognise the user's language and locale settings and then provide the corresponding date, time, number and currency formats based on these settings. This way, users get a localised presentation that matches their habits, no matter what region they are from.

This careful design and implementation enables the application to provide a more user-friendly and personalised service to users around the world, effectively improving the accessibility and user experience of healthcare services. This localised design not only enhances the global reach of POP Disease Management, but also allows more patients and doctors to access and understand medical information more accurately and easily in a language and format they are familiar with.

3   Results

The design and development of PHPlace is complete and is expected to bring significant benefits to POP patients and healthcare professionals. Some positive results can already be anticipated through a series of tests conducted in a simulated environment. Initially, a heuristic evaluation by five usability experts identified potential usability issues, which were addressed before the user testing phase. In the user testing phase, 30 patients and 15 healthcare professionals were involved. They were tasked with specific scenarios to explore the app's features, especially focusing on the animated presentations and questionnaire functionalities. User interactions were logged, and heat maps of interaction hotspots provided insights into the app's usability strengths and areas for improvement. Post-testing interviews captured qualitative feedback, indicating that users found the animations to be particularly enlightening, but desired more interactive and personalized content.

The animated presentation feature showed clear advantages in the simulation tests. These tests covered 45 simulation users worldwide, including patients with POP disease and medical staff. Test results showed that 93.3% of users reported that the animated presentation enhanced their understanding of POP disease and treatment options. This clear visual presentation is expected to improve patient adherence to treatment. The superiority of the animated presentations was evident not only in the users' subjective feedback but also in objective measures. We introduced a comprehension test post-interaction, consisting of 20 questions designed to assess the users' understanding of POP and its treatments. The group exposed to animated presentations scored, on average, 75% higher than the control group, who were provided with traditional text-based information.

In a simulated environment, PHPlace's automated scoring system showcased significant efficiency and accuracy. A comparative analysis, involving 100 questionnaires, revealed a drastic reduction in scoring time from an average of 5 min per questionnaire in traditional manual methods to 1.2 s with PHPlace, marking a 99.6% improvement. However, the system's merit isn't confined to its speed. A concordance correlation coefficient of 0.98, obtained from comparing the automated scores with expert manual assessments, attests to the system's accuracy and consistency, ensuring that the rapidity of assessments doesn't undermine their quality. Furthermore, PHPlace is equipped with a feature to automatically generate PDF reports. This addition enhances the ease and precision in recording and sharing scores, promising to further elevate the efficiency and reliability of clinical assessments in real-world applications.

Also in the simulation test, the questionnaire scoring function demonstrated good ease of use. 84.4% of the simulated users reported that they could easily complete the questionnaire scoring and quickly understand and record the results.

PHPlace has also shown significant potential for healthcare information management. Clinicians in our team reported that they were 60% more efficient at processing patient information using PHPlace than without it. This is backed by a detailed time-motion study. The study observed clinicians during their consultation sessions, measuring the time taken to explain the POP conditions and treatments to the patients. With PHPlace, the explanation time reduced from an average of 15 min to 6 min per session without compromising the quality of information shared, as affirmed by the patients' feedback.

The localization features were further evaluated in terms of the accuracy of translation and cultural appropriateness of the content. A separate evaluation involving 30 non-English speaking users from five different countries was conducted. Feedback indicated not just ease of use, but also a high level of satisfaction with the accuracy and relevance of the translated content.

Overall, PHPlace demonstrates significant potential in terms of educational effectiveness, scoring efficiency, ease of use, and information management efficiency, and is expected to provide significant benefits to POP patients and healthcare professionals. All of these tests and studies were conducted by a team of experienced healthcare professionals and data scientists to ensure their impartiality and accuracy. In the future, expect further real-world application testing to validate these expected results and enable PHPlace to better serve POP patients and physicians through ongoing optimisation.

4   Discusstion and Outlook

Today's healthcare environment is being rapidly transformed by digital tools and apps, particularly those focused on disease management and patient education. For example, apps such as MyChart provide a convenient way for patients to view their medical records, communicate with their doctors and even perform some basic health education in one centralised place [22]. However, these apps tend to take a more traditional and text-heavy approach to education, especially for those complex medical concepts such as POP, which can lead to patients struggling to understand their condition and treatment plan.

PHPlace introduces an animated presentation approach to present these complex medical concepts in a more visual and vivid manner. This approach is expected to improve patients' understanding of their condition and treatment plan, thereby increasing their adherence to treatment. Such anticipated effects may play an important role in reducing relapse and deterioration of the condition. However, whether these effects can be validated in practice will need to be determined through additional clinical studies and patient feedback. Long-term follow-up and research may reveal the specific impact of this educational approach on improving patient adherence to treatment and quality of life.

On the flip side, PHPlace also attempts to address some common problems that physicians face in disease management. Specifically, it integrates a range of automated tools, such as automated questionnaire scoring and information management systems, to improve the efficiency of doctors in POP management. This innovation may help doctors save a lot of time relative to existing applications, allowing them to focus more on caring for their patients' conditions and improving the quality of care. However, the actual effectiveness of PHPlace in improving doctors' efficiency needs to be further tested and validated in a real-world environment.

While the innovation and functionality of the app are encouraging, there are limitations that need to be recognised. The app is somewhat dependent on the digital skills of the user, which may pose a challenge for some patients, especially older patients or those with weaker digital skills. In addition, privacy and security issues in handling personal health data must be adequately addressed. These issues will need to be addressed by future research and improvements.

Overall, the development of PHPlace demonstrates the potential for positive impact through innovative approaches to integrating mobile technology and automated tools into disease management. The design and expected results of PHPlace contribute to the digital transformation of the healthcare sector and provide new ideas for POP management. However, in order to achieve these expected results, more practical research and clinical testing are needed to address the issues and challenges and to continuously optimise the functionality and performance of the application.

5 Conclusion

The study highlights the potential of a new mobile app to optimise POP disease management. PHPlace demonstrates the key role of digital technology in enhancing the efficiency and accessibility of healthcare delivery through a blend of intuitive animations, automated disease assessment, efficient healthcare information management, and a localised design adapted to multiple cultures.

The innovation of PHPlace is reflected in its new approach, which aims to improve patients' understanding of diseases and treatments, save doctors' assessment time, standardise the assessment process and provide easy management of medical information. Particularly noteworthy is the localised design that significantly improves the accessibility of healthcare services to meet diverse global needs.

While work in this area still needs to be deepened, PHPlace has provided a viable pathway towards digitising healthcare services and offers valuable lessons and insights for future research. With more such research and further refinement of the application, it is expected that digitisation and automation of healthcare services will be achieved in a wider range of areas to provide more efficient and accurate healthcare services.

References

1. Rowland, S.P., Fitzgerald, J.E., Holme, T., Powell, J., McGregor, A.: What is the clinical value of mHealth for patients? NPJ Dig. Med. **3**(1), 4 (2020)
2. World Health Organization. mHealth: new horizons for health through mobile technologies (2011)
3. Jelovsek, J.E., Maher, C., Barber, M.D.: Pelvic organ prolapse. Lancet **369**(9566), 1027–1038 (2007)

4. Wilkins, M.F., Wu, J.M.: Epidemiology of pelvic organ prolapse. Curr. Obstetr. Gynecol. Rep. **5**, 119–123 (2016)
5. Iglesia, C.B., Smithling, K.R.: Pelvic organ prolapse. Am. Fam. Physician **96**(3), 179–185 (2017)
6. American College of Obstetricians and Gynecologists: Pelvic organ prolapse. Urogynecology **25**(6), 397–408 (2019)
7. Raju, R., Linder, B.J.: Evaluation and management of pelvic organ prolapse. In: Mayo Clinic Proceedings, vol. 96, no. 12, pp. 3122–3129. Elsevier (2021)
8. Weintraub, A.Y., Glinter, H., Marcus-Braun, N.: Narrative review of the epidemiology, diagnosis and pathophysiology of pelvic organ prolapse. Int. Braz. J. Urol. **46**, 5–14 (2019)
9. Grimes, C.L., et al.: Collaborative research in pelvic surgery consortium: correlation of electronic (web-based and smartphone) administration of measures of pelvic floor dysfunction: a randomized controlled trial. Urogynecology **26**(6), 396–400 (2020)
10. Naylor, D., et al.: The cost of the "s" in https. In: Proceedings of the 10th ACM International on Conference on emerging Networking Experiments and Technologies, pp. 133–140 (2014)
11. Gackenheimer, C.: Introduction to React. Apress, Berkeley (2015)
12. Tashildar, A., Shah, N., Gala, R., Giri, T., Chavhan, P.: Application development using flutter. Int. Re. J. Modern. Eng. Technol. Sci. **2**(8), 1262–1266 (2020)
13. Thorn, A.: Unity Animation Essentials. Packt Publishing Ltd., Birmingham (2015)
14. Teleman, P.I.A., Stenzelius, K., Iorizzo, L., Jakobsson, U.L.F.: Validation of the Swedish short forms of the pelvic floor impact questionnaire (PFIQ-7), pelvic floor distress inventory (PFDI-20) and pelvic organ prolapse/urinary incontinence sexual questionnaire (PISQ-12). Acta Obstet. Gynecol. Scand. **90**(5), 483–487 (2011)
15. Rogers, R.G., Coates, K.W., Kammerer-Doak, D., Khalsa, S., Qualls, C.: A short form of the pelvic organ prolapse/urinary incontinence sexual questionnaire (PISQ-12). Int. Urogynecol. J. **14**, 164–168 (2003)
16. Bradley, C.S., et al.: The questionnaire for urinary incontinence diagnosis (QUID): validity and responsiveness to change in women undergoing non-surgical therapies for treatment of stress predominant urinary incontinence. Neurourol. Urodyn. **29**(5), 727–734 (2010)
17. Sen, I., et al.: The impact of urinary incontinence on female sexual function. Adv. Ther. **23**, 999–1008 (2006)
18. Srikrishna, S., Robinson, D., Cardozo, L.: Validation of the patient global impression of improvement (PGI-I) for urogenital prolapse. Int. Urogynecol. J. **21**, 523–528 (2010)
19. Hebbar, S., Pandey, H., Chawla, A.: Understanding King's Health Questionnaire (KHQ) in assessment of female urinary incontinence. Int. J. Res. Med. Sci. **3**(3), 531–8 (2015)
20. Klovning, A., Avery, K., Sandvik, H., Hunskaar, S.: Comparison of two questionnaires for assessing the severity of urinary incontinence: the ICIQ-UI SF versus the incontinence severity index. Neurourol. Urodyn. Off. J. Int. Contin. Soc. **28**(5), 411–415 (2009)
21. de Couto, M.R.L., Miranda, B.: Towards improving automation support for internationalization and localization testing. In: Anais Estendidos do XXI Simpósio Brasileiro de Qualidade de Software, pp. 9–14. SBC (2022)
22. Milani, R.V., Lavie, C.J., Bober, R.M., Milani, A.R., Ventura, H.O.: Improving hypertension control and patient engagement using digital tools. Am. J. Med. **130**(1), 14–20 (2017)

Behavioural Changes Using mHealth: An Experimental Case Study

Zahra Mungloo-Dilmohamud$^{(\boxtimes)}$ ⓘ, Abha Jodheea-Jutton, Kavi Khedo,
Sudha Cheerkoot-Jalim, Leckraj Nagowah, Soulakshmee Nagowah,
Abdallah Peerally, and Shakuntala Baichoo

University of Mauritius, Reduit, Mauritius
z.mungloo@uom.ac.mu

Abstract. Mauritius has a very high prevalence of diabetes, hypertension and cardiovascular diseases, which are often linked to bad eating habits. The use of mHealth applications to bring about positive behavioural changes is practically non-existent in Mauritius since the local unique culinary scene makes it difficult to use such existing applications. The primary objective of this study is to create a customized mHealth application that caters for the peculiarities of the eclectic Mauritian cuisine. *MauLifeStyle*, a web-based application that caters for calorific content of different types of Mauritian foods and typical activities of the Mauritian population, has been developed and tested using recruited participants. The *MauLifeStyle* application has been evaluated based on different criteria of MoHTAM, which is a refined technology acceptance model for smart mobile phones. The clinical outcomes were not statistically significant following three months of monitoring. However, the participant feedback supports the demand for digitally mediated self-education for motivated individuals. The developed mHealth application comprises four main functionalities: *Blood Glucose Monitoring*, *Food Intake*, *Health and Fitness*, and *Calorie Monitor*. It is anticipated that over time, *MauLifeStyle* has the potential to reduce the prevalence of Diabetes in Mauritius and consequently alleviate the financial burden on the healthcare system through the application of preventive medicine.

Keywords: self-management · type 2 diabetes · mobile app · mHealth · self-monitoring

1 Introduction

Diabetes mellitus (DM) presents a significant global health challenge due to its high incidence, its serious impact on health and the substantial burden it places on healthcare systems. The global prevalence of diabetes has reached hundreds of millions with a trend of continued increase. Besides, it is found to be among the top 10 causes of death [1]. In Mauritius the prevalence of DM is alarming, with the figures in 2021 showing around 20% of the population being affected according to the Mauritius Non Communicable Diseases Survey 2021.[1]

---

[1] https://www.afro.who.int/.

A. Cunha et al. (Eds.): MobiHealth 2023, LNICST 578, pp. 400–416, 2024.
https://doi.org/10.1007/978-3-031-60665-6_30

DM leads to several complications, which results in a heavy financial burden on the Mauritian healthcare system. In 2019, 16.9% of the total health expenditure was allocated to the disease [1]. However, patients' self-management of DM, particularly Type 2, can lead to a significant reduction in the complications associated with the disease, thus alleviating the financial load on the healthcare system. Proper education about self-monitoring of food-intake in lower glycemic levels by pre-diabetes patients can prevent them from developing diabetes in the long run. Patients' self-management requires behavioural changes in terms of regular physical activities and dietary control leading to weight-loss and improvement in metabolism.

Lately, there has been a growing recognition of the substantial impact that digital technologies, particularly mobile applications, can make on the behavioural changes of patients dealing with various medical conditions. This awareness has led to the development of many self-management applications for behavioural changes, which may reduce dependence on medications. Self-management applications for lifestyle management can help patients record their daily food intake and level of physical activities, and provide feedback on the correlation between the variation of their glucose and cholesterol levels and other parameters.

Internet access (including mobile technologies) by households in Mauritius, for years 2016 and 2018, has increased from 63% to 70%.[2] Leveraging on this high penetration of mobile and internet technologies, we have developed an innovative mHealth application, adapted to the Mauritian context, that can help people monitor their food intake and physical activities, based on calorific content of different types of Mauritian foods and typical activities of the Mauritian population. The aim of this application is to assist individuals living with pre-diabetes revert to normal (non-diabetic) state, while also helping those without diabetes to prevent developing diabetic conditions. The rest of the paper is organized as follows: Sect. 2 offers pertinent background information. Section 3 describes the proposed mobile application. Section 4 describes the methodology adopted to evaluate *MauLifeStyle*. Section 5 discusses the results obtained and Sect. 6 concludes the paper.

2 Background

This section presents the related works, mHealth for behavioural changes and health monitoring methods.

2.1 Related Works

Mobile devices provide a gamut of facilities and services in our contemporary society including the healthcare domain. The number of mobile health (mHealth) applications has witnessed an unprecedented growth to approximately 325, 000 in 2017 [2]. Their utilization has great potential in healthcare support in terms of quick access to healthcare information, patient empowerment and inclusion of people who have very limited access

---

[2] http://statsmauritius.govmu.org/English/Publications/Documents/2019/EI1464/ICT_Yr18. pdf.

to healthcare services [3]. Thousands of such applications are used for disease prevention and healthy lifestyles [4]. According to Larson [5], researchers have characterized four general categories of mHealth applications: (I) information applications, which depict information to the public; (II) diagnostic applications, which take patient information as input and assist to guide the physician to a diagnosis; (III) control applications, which enable remote control of medical equipment such as glucose analysers; and (IV) adapter applications, which convert a smartphone into a mobile medical device.

2.2 mHealth for Behavioural Changes

mHealth applications have been widely used for weight management. They can be useful to monitor behaviour and user self-management, leading to lifestyle changes in the long run [6]. The risk of obesity and chronic diseases like diabetes, hypertension and cardiovascular diseases is therefore mitigated. Features, which are usually favoured in mHealth applications are self-monitoring, goal setting, physical activity, professional feedback and calorie counting. Essential requirements for such applications include security and privacy concerns, clinical guidance, usability issues and proper laboratory testing [6]. In their study on user acceptance for mHealth applications, Smahel et al. [4] reported that the most adopted features by users were those related to weight monitoring including BMI monitoring, calorie usage and calorie intake.

Direito et al. [7] conducted an mHealth programme to compare the effectiveness of mHealth interventions to foster physical activity (PA) and curb sedentary behaviour (SB) in free-living adolescents and adults with a comparator exposed to usual care/minimal intervention. SB decreased more following mHealth interventions than after usual care. As a result, the mHealth interventions have small effects on the physical activities and sedentary behaviour. Likewise, a study was set up to determine the presence/absence of behaviour change techniques (BCTs) in the top 20 free and top 20 paid physical activity and dietary applications from App Store [8]. It was found that the presence of BCTs varied by application type and price; nevertheless, BCTs related to increased intervention effectiveness were generally in paid applications.

Vandelanotte et al. [9] provide an overview of the state of evidence for the use of eHealth and mHealth in improving physical activity and nutrition behaviours among a group of people due to the prevalence of inadequate physical activity and poor diets. Investigations revealed that health and fitness applications accessible on iTunes and Google Play barely or did not use BCTs and rarely integrated evidence-based recommendations. Moreover, it is unclear how the BCTs are implemented, and hence it cannot be concluded whether they are as effective as face-to-face interventions. It was also found that most commercially available applications are not designed with the partnership of behavioural experts, thus leading to a scarcity of engagement techniques.

Various mHealth applications for behavioural changes have been analysed and a summary of their features is shown in Table 1. Most of the analysed applications keep track of food intake and physical activities. They all adopt different BCTs namely social media support, personalized feedback and notifications, gamifications, tailored messages and visualizations among others to provide a healthier lifestyle to users. However, evidence of achieving weight loss is missing for applications like Noom, HAPPY ME and Bant II. MyFitnessPal reported minimal weight change after a period of 6 months while

Weight Management Mentor reported substantial weight loss over a period of 8 weeks. Visual presentations of patient progress are available in a few applications. More efficient strategies to improve the logging mechanism and increase patient engagement such as personalized recommendations based on users' eating habits and physical activities are required.

2.3 Health Monitoring Methods

Several tools, such as pedometers, glucometers, blood pressure monitors and electrocardiograms (ECG/EKG) [21], are embedded in mobile phones, smartwatches and fitness devices, to monitor the health of individuals. The Apple Watch, for example, has helped to save lives in numerous occasions [22]. It has an ECG/EKG feature which can detect atrial fibrillation within 30 s [23] and a fall detection technology which can detect if the user is unconscious and 911 is called automatically [24].

Body Mass Index (BMI) is a measure which can be used for calculation of calories and facilitate weight management. The BMI is calculated as per the Europe World Health Organization [25] formula and the nutritional status as per BMI range is listed in Table 2.

According to several studies, there is a strong association between excess weight and an increased risk of Type 2 Diabetes [26]. When a person is trying to lose weight, s/he wants to know how much to fuel his/her body after a workout or how many calories s/he has burnt during any exercise. The following methods can be used to estimate the calorie expenditure by using a simple calculator/equation:

- **Calorie burned from pedometer.** Regular exercising plays an important role in maintaining an ideal weight. The easiest form of exercising is walking, with a minimum number of steps. The pedometer or step-counter can be used to count the number of steps a person has walked during a certain amount of time. Pedometers are being integrated more and more into mobile phones, smart watches and fitness device [27]. The calorie burned for a certain number of steps is computed using an unofficial formula from a physical fitness stack exchange [28]. Nonetheless, the equation is subsequently validated with weight, height and step count data from a partner of The Cleveland Clinic, *Verywell Fit*, to ensure that the equation accurately calculates calorie expenditure [29].
- **Calorie burned for specific exercises.** The calories burned for any exercise is calculated using the respective metabolic equivalent (MET) for each exercise [30] and the calorie expenditure formula by Roland [31].
- **Basal Metabolic Rate (BMR).** The Mifflin - St Jeor formulas by Hazell [32] are used to calculate the BMR for male and female respectively. BMR is the amount of energy required by the human body to function at rest.
- **Calorie to gram conversion**. The formula proposed by Haponiuk and Díez [33] is used for the calorie to gram conversion.

3 *MauLifeStyle* App

Mauritius features a diverse population characterized by Indo-Mauritians (of Indian origin), Creole (mixed African and European heritage), Sino-Mauritians (of Chinese origin) and others primarily of European descent. This plethora of cultures and religious

Table 1. Summary of mHealth Applications for Behavioural Changes.

Application	Open-Source/Paid	Target Audience	Features	Behaviour Change Techniques (BCT)	Areas of Improvement
Noom [10]	Paid	Adults	Individual food logging, Recommend daily calorie intake, Deliver relevant articles on health and nutrition	Social support - groups similar users so that they can interact together	Social support encouraged logging behaviour, but still needs to accomplish weight loss
MyBehavior [11]	Paid	Adults	Track physical activity, user location and food, Analyse activity and food logs	Personalized suggestions based on user's environment and previous behaviour	Addition of more human control over the suggestions, Provide easier logging mechanisms for food and exercise
Accupedo-Pro Pedometer [12]	Open-Source	Adults	Measure daily step counts, Feedback on distance, time, speed and calories burned	Automatic feedback, Visually appealing graphic display, Goal-setting, Goal-achievement feedback	Include objective measures of fitness like heart rate
NutriWalking [13]	Open-Source	Adults	Help users build healthy eating habits, Encourage users to adopt exercise habits	Personalized goals, Peer support	Adaptive features for personalizing daily nutrition goals based on behavioural adherence
DietApp [14]	N/A	Adults	Feedback on total energy balance based on food intake, Indication on calorie intake and burnt	Personalized suggestions according to illness. Attractively designed	Put nutritionists or endocrinologists in contact with patients for more personalized care

(continued)

Table 1. (*continued*)

Application	Open-Source/Paid	Target Audience	Features	Behaviour Change Techniques (BCT)	Areas of Improvement
Bant II [15]	Open-Source	Adults	Recording of food intake photos and weight, Body-worn activity monitors to count steps	Real-time feedback, Report trends in lifestyle against glycaemic control	Social support to facilitate connections among patients across geographical areas
Application	**Open-Source / Paid**	**Target Audience**	**Features**	**Behaviour Change Techniques (BCT)**	**Areas of Improvement**
Few Touch Application (FTA) [16]	Open-Source	Adults	Register eating habits, Automatic Step Counter	Feedback, Goal setting, Ease of use, Monitoring of lifestyle and progress by healthcare providers	Use sensors elements for other use cases apart from motivated healthy patients
Weight Management Mentor [17]	N/A	Adults	Collect food intake and weight data	Visualizations, Virtual rewards such as ribbons and trophies, Motivating feedback, Tailored textual messages of praise and support	Perform live user studies
HAPPY ME [18]	N/A	Children	Self-monitoring tool for preventing obesity, Collect data regarding dietary habits and physical performance, Step count used to measure activity	Tailored messages, Use of gamification and self-monitoring strategies	Perform randomized controlled trials, Develop gender-specific programs for preventing obesity
MyFitnessPal [19]	Open-Source	Adults	Track nutritional values of diets, Include exercise functions	Automatic notifications, Goal-setting, Social Support- Share progress with friends on social media, Visualizations	Develop a streamlined interface for entering food details, Sensitize users about the importance of self-monitoring prior to using the application
CarpeDiem [20]	N/A	All	Self-monitoring tool for preventing obesity, Collect data regarding food group intake, Gamification and rewards, Recommender system	Feedback, Goal setting, Ease of use, Use of gamification and self-monitoring strategies	Some information like physical exercise is collected using questionnaires and not through the app

Note: N/A means information not available

Table 2. Nutritional Status based on BMI range

BMI	Nutritional Status
Below 18.5	Underweight
18.5–24.5	Normal weight
25.0–29.9	Pre-obesity
30.0–34.9	Obesity class I
35.0–39.9	Obesity class II
Above 40	Obesity class III

beliefs is reflected in Mauritian cuisine, which is usually a combination of the ethnic favorites. The local foods include the dholl-puri (roti), curried rolls, noodles, gateau piment (a fried snack), Biryani and Boulettes (meatballs) amongst many others. This unique culinary scene makes it difficult to use existing applications to monitor the food intake of the participants. It is therefore vital for any application to take into consideration the peculiarities of the eclectic Mauritian cuisine.

MauLifeStyle is a responsive web-based application designed to be compatible with both desktop and mobile web browsers irrespective of operating systems and thus offers the inherent advantage of reaching out to a larger number of users. Figures 1 and 2 both show the main menu of *MauLifeStyle* with Fig. 1 representing the mobile view and Fig. 2 representing the desktop view. The mHealth application comprises the following four main functionalities: Blood Glucose Monitoring, Food Intake, Health and Fitness, and Calorie Monitor, are further described in the following subsections. The application incorporates the health monitoring formula discussed in Sect. 4.

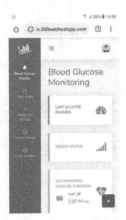

Fig. 1. Main Menu - Mobile View

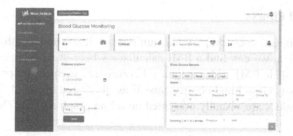

Fig. 2. Main Menu - Desktop View

3.1 Self-Blood Glucose Monitoring

Blood sugar readings are important parameters used by doctors for effective diabetes management. These can also be used by individuals to self-monitor their blood sugar levels pre and post meals. *MauLifeStyle* allows for the recording of these readings before and after breakfast, lunch, afternoon snack and dinner. It also provides an option for downloading these readings in CSV, Excel or PDF formats which may then be shared with treating doctors for monitoring purposes. Additionally, a print option is provided.

3.2 Food Intake

MauLifeStyle may become a useful tool for making healthy lifestyle changes. It is therefore vital that the users of the application record the food items that they are taking during each meal. The food intake functionality has also been carefully designed to suit the Mauritian context. There is a cultural habit in the country to eat locally prepared delicacies commonly known as 'Gâteaux De L'huile' (translated as *oily snacks*) during either breakfast or teatime. These local foodstuffs, currently unavailable in similar existing applications, have been included in the *MauLifeStyle* as shown in Fig. 3. Like the blood glucose monitoring, the food intake details may be downloaded or printed.

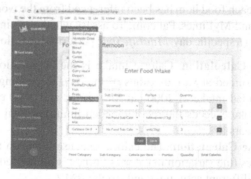

Fig. 3. Food Intake including local foodstuffs

3.3 Health and Fitness

MauLifeStyle application encompasses a multitude of fitness and health monitoring features among which, we can find a BMI calculator where users input their weight and height to obtain their BMI with customized comments such as underweight, normal, pre-obesity, obesity class I and obesity class II as illustrated in Fig. 4. The saved input and calculated values are visually presented on a line graph and bar chart as shown in Fig. 5.

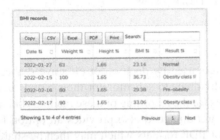

Fig. 4. BMI Recordings   **Fig. 5.** Graph of BMI over time

Additionally, the mobile version of *MauLifeStyle* comprises a pedometer that works with the accelerometer sensor of the mobile phone and automatically records the number of steps that a user takes daily. However, users of the web version must manually enter the number of steps on the *MauLifeStyle* platform. *MauLifeStyle* also entails an exercise section where the user enters one or multiple physical activities undertaken during the day or week and their respective durations. *MauLifeStyle* automatically calculates the approximate number of calories burned during those respective activities.

3.4 Calorie Monitor

MauLifeStyle has a diet-tracking feature that estimates the number of calories per food item. The calorie of each food item has been referenced from the world's largest verified nutrition database[3] and MyFitnessPal.com. To assess whether an individual has gained or lost calories during a specific day, *MauLifeStyle* performs the following computations:

(i) **Calorie Intake Calculation**: Calorie intake is the aggregation of calorie values from meals consumed at various times of the day. Depending on gender (with a daily recommended intake of 2000 cal for women and 2500 cal for men[4]), if the daily calorie intake exceeds the recommended limit, the total is displayed in red; otherwise it appears in green.

(ii) **Calorie Expense Calculation**: The calorie expense relies on two key factors: (a) physical activities (the variation in calories burned is influenced by the MET values associated with different activities) and (b) the BMR.

---

[3] https://www.nutritionix.com/.

[4] https://health.gov/our-work/food-nutrition/2015-2020-dietary-guidelines/guidelines/.

The calorie gain or loss at the end of a person's journey is approximated into grams. *MauLifeStyle* also saves the calorie intake and expenditure over time and these may also be downloaded or printed. The calorie gain/loss is converted to grams through the formula proposed by Haponiuk and Díez [32].

4 Methods

A study was designed to assess the receptiveness of an mHealth application, investigate the behavioural changes resulting from its use, measure the change in selected biomarkers following a 3 months intervention and determine the change in clinical outcomes before and after the intervention among individuals at risk of developing diabetes mellitus. The pilot study was conducted over 12 weeks. Ethical clearance was received by the University of Mauritius Research Ethics Committee prior to the recruitment of participants for the study. All procedures were in line with the Helsinki declaration.[5] All participants signed an informed consent prior to enrolment. Participants were recruited from the University of Mauritius and neighbouring institutions. All interested participants were screened for the inclusion and exclusion criteria. The inclusion and exclusion criteria for the selection of participants are as follows:

Inclusion Criteria

- Participants aged 18 years and above
- Participants with a predisposition for developing DM by meeting at least one of the following criteria: (1) One or more member of the family being diagnosed with Type 2 Diabetes Mellitus (2) Participants who have a BMI of 25 kg/m^2 and above
- Participants with known pre-diabetes conditions diagnosed by repeated fasting blood sugar, HbA1c or oral glucose tolerance test
- Participants with previous history of gestational diabetes

Exclusion Criteria

- Any pregnant or lactating women
- Participants with diabetes mellitus or current gestational diabetes
- Participants on anti-lipid agents
- Participants on specific diets

All baseline and demographic information were retrieved through face-to-face sessions, which consisted of an interview to capture all information concerning their medical history, past medical history, family history, medications, smoking and drinking habits and lifestyle practices such as eating and exercise. A standard template was used to facilitate this process. An informative session on how to use the application was conducted, during which participants were introduced to the use of *MauLifeStyle*.

---

[5] https://www.wma.net/what-we-do/medical-ethics/declaration-of-helsinki/doh-sept1989/

Twenty-five(25) participants attended the screening session. All participants had their clinical indicators such as height, weight and blood pressure measured at baseline following the debriefing session and 3 months after the intervention to determine any changes following the use of the application. Measurement of blood sugar levels: fasting blood glucose and fasting lipid levels were undertaken using clinical biochemistry testing, at baseline and after 3 months of using *MauLifeStyle*.

During the debriefing session, the *MauLifeStyle* app was installed on the participants smartphones. Participants were further advised to record their daily food intake and daily duration of exercise on the application. During the 3 months of the study, the participants were contacted regularly for follow up and to offer any technical support needed. By the end of the 3 months, a survey was undertaken to assess the acceptability of the application using a validated MARS (Medication Adherence Report Scale) questionnaire. The MARS scale is used to assess the quality of mobile apps that are used in health promotion. It is an objective tool that measures acceptability of the application.

A participant survey was conducted to capture the participants' experience while using *MauLifeStyle* during the study period. The details of the user evaluation were categorized according to different criteria of the refined technology acceptance model for smart mobile phones (MoHTAM) [34]. All data were analyzed using Microsoft Excel. All categorical data were presented in percentages, while continuous data were presented in means, standard deviations and confidence intervals. Confidence intervals were set at 95% and a P-value of less than 0.05 was considered as significant.

5 Results and Discussions

Of the participants who attended the screening workshop, 28% were excluded as they did not satisfy the eligibility criteria. There were 36% male and 36% female participants and the mean age of participants was 38.68 ± 8.41 (CI 34.2–43.2). Table 3 shows the participants profile information.

5.1 Primary Outcomes

The primary outcomes of the participant survey are presented here.

A. Perceived Ease of Use
Given the target audience, it was imperative to consider HCI issues in the design of the application. Participants were therefore requested to give feedback on the user interface. Concerning usability features, participants stated that the application was good in terms of performance (78%), ease of use (78%), navigation (56%), gestural design (67%) and interactive features (78%). 78% of the participants found that the layout was well-designed and that the graphics were of high quality and resolution. 44% of the participants found the overall visual appeal as pleasant and beautiful while the remaining found it average.

B. Perceived Usefulness of mHealth
The findings indicate that the application has had a positive impact on participants.

Table 3. Participants Profile

Participants (Total, N)	18
Gender (n: male, n: Female)	9,9
Mean age (SD, CI)	38.68 ± 8.41 (CI 34.2 - 43.2)
Mean BMI (Baseline)/Kg/m²	27.06
Medical History • Healthy • Major comorbidity • Minor comorbidity	6 participants had minor problems (Low platelets white blood cells, Asthma, Blood Pressure, Hypertension, Knee pain)
Medications	Amlodipine, Zyloric, Atorvastatin, Ventolin, Astrix
Smoking	2 participants: 6–10 cigarettes / day
Alcohol	None
Baseline Fasting blood glucose (mmol/L)	4.84 ± 0.35 (CI 4.64 - 5.04)
Baseline total cholesterol (mmol/L)	4.48 ± 0.91 (CI 3.95- 5.00)
Baseline HDL (mmol/L)	1.18 ± 0.25 (CI 1.04 -1.33)
Baseline Triglycerides (mmol/L)	1.19 ± 0.84 (CI 0.71 - 1.68)
Baseline LDL (mmol/L)	2.75 ± 0.72 (CI 2.33 - 3.17)

Notably, 78% of the participants reported an increase in awareness while 89% noted an improvement in their knowledge regarding the importance of their health behaviour. 78% of the participants confirmed that their attitudes and motivation towards their health behaviour have improved and that the application motivates them to seek further help regarding their health. 67% of participants agreed that usage of the application indeed helped them in achieving positive behavioural changes.

C. Intention to Use mHealth
The responses were quite positive and it was encouraging to learn that all participants were willing to continue using the application even after the study. Most of them also stated that they would recommend the application to other people. All the participants (100%) found that the quality of information presented as well as visuals used in the application were correct, comprehensive, concise and relevant to the topic. They also agreed that the information provided in the application comes from credible sources. 75% of the participants stated that they would surely recommend the application to others while 25% stated that they would probably recommend it to users who might need it. 62.5% mentioned that they intended to use the application 2–3 times a week while 37.5% mentioned that they would use the application daily. However, only 12.5% of participants were agreeable to pay for the application. The participants were quite satisfied with the application as 37.5% rated it as average and 62.5% rated it as above average.

D. Technological Factors (Technology Design & mHealth)
A significant portion of the participants, 67%, found the application to be engaging and capable of holding their interest for an extended time. While some participants believed that the application was not really customisable to their individual preferences, 78% of them agreed that it provided interactivity through the user input functions and the personalised feedback. Furthermore, all participants unanimously agreed that the application content (visuals, language, design) was well-suited for the intended target audience.

E. Socio-Cultural Factors
Socio-cultural factors have been taken in consideration while designing the application. The inclusion of food items relevant to the country's culture has contributed to the perceived ease of use (78%) by the participants, since they found that the selection of food items for each of their meals was straightforward, thus facilitating data entry. Approximately 55.5% of the participants affirmed that the application offers customisation options and all participants concurred that *MauLifeStyle* has been well-designed for the intended users. The information session at the start of the study reassured participants that their data would be kept confidential and anonymised, thus building trust in the application.

5.2 Secondary Outcomes

Of the 18 participants who were registered in the study, 50% regularly used the *MauLifeStyle* application. Among those who used the application regularly, the mean calorie intake was 2119 ± 253.83 (CI 2047.7–2190.5). Additionally, the average carbohydrate intake was 274.6 ± 32.9 (CI 265.4- 283.9) daily. The mean exercise duration was 34 ± 7.90 (CI 32.08–36.67, which notably increased from 27.5 ± 3.78 (CI 37.34–30.66) minutes to 34.2 ± 7.32 (CI 27.5–41.1) minutes daily by week 6. The exercises consisted of essentially walking and cycling. It was found that there is no major difference in these outcomes between the start of the use of the intervention and towards the end of the intervention. The calorie and carbohydrate intake was the same throughout the use of the intervention for up to 60 days.

Secondary outcomes included change in weight, BMI, waist circumference and lipid levels after a minimum of three months of using *MauLifeStyle*. As per our findings, there were no significant differences in secondary outcomes in the baseline and post intervention groups. There were also no remarkable baseline differences between the group of participants who used the *MauLifeStyle* application and the group of participants who did not use the application.

5.3 Limitations of the Study

This pilot study has tested the feasibility of implementing mHealth for positive behavioural changes in Mauritius. A small sample of working adults were enrolled in this study. The enrolment was driven essentially by the participant's motivation to adopt a change in behaviour that might delay a diagnosis of diabetes mellitus. Participants who have at least one risk factor of diabetes mellitus, such as being overweight, having a family history of diabetes or experiencing pre-diabetic conditions, were invited to participate in the study. Following the Covid-19 pandemic, staff at the university are working in a hybrid mode. Hence, not all staff were on campus during the study and this may have impacted on the recruitment of participants.

Minimal differences in the biomarker and the anthropological measurements were noted but none were statistically significant. This observation can be justified by a small group sample. We had only 18 participants and out of them, only 9 used the mobile application regularly. Due to the small sample, it might be difficult to draw conclusions as to the efficacy of the mobile application as a tool that can be used to delay the development of diabetes mellitus or adopt healthy lifestyle behaviours. Further, rigorous longitudinal studies might be required to determine the efficacy of *MauLifeStyle*.

5.4 Evaluation of *MauLifeStyle*

Several mHealth applications which aim at bringing about behavioural changes in individuals in terms of food intake and physical exercise have been analysed and summarised in Table 1. However, none of these is appropriate for use in the Mauritian context, given the peculiarities of the Mauritian cuisine. Entering data in the "Food Intake" functionality of *MauLifeStyle* is very quick and efficient due to the comprehensive list of food items which include all specific Mauritian meals. However, *MauLifeStyle* does not cater for scanning of store-bought foods and drinks using barcode as compared to *MyFitnessPal* and does not allow the capture of meal photos using the mobile phone's camera like *Bant II*.

Applications like *DietApp* also have a calorie counter, however, the counter may not be appropriate for the local context. For example, "Fried Rice" in the Mauritian context may be different from the general "Fried Rice" and may have different calorie values, therefore giving a wrong estimation of the calorie intake. The design of *MauLifeStyle* included a careful computation of calorie values of different meals, based on the cooking habits of Mauritian people. Apart from *DietApp*, applications like *Noom* and *Accupedo-Pro Pedometer*, only computed either the calorie intake or calorie expense. On the other hand, the Calorie Monitor of *MauLifeStyle* computes the total calorie gain or loss at the end of the day from the calorie intake and calorie expense. Based on the calorie computation, a personalized message is displayed to the user. This feature is not available in most applications.

The *Few Touch Application* has considered only three exercise activities namely walking, stairs and jogging motions as compared to *MauLifeStyle* which considers eighteen activities namely badminton, basketball, cycling, dancing, football, hiking, jogging, karate, swimming, muscle strengthening, rope skipping, stair climbing, running, stretching, tai chi, slow walking, moderate walking, brisk pace walking and yoga.

Weight Management Mentor provides virtual rewards such as ribbons and trophies for positive behaviour. This feature can be included in *MauLifeStyle* in the future to encourage users to improve their health behaviour. Additionally, a social-networking feature that enables users to find friends and share their progress can be included in *MauLifeStyle* like in *MyFitnessPal*. Furthermore, *MauLifeStyle* presently allows recording of blood glucose pre and post breakfast and pre and post dinner as compared to *Bant II*, which considers recording of blood glucose pre and post lunch in addition to breakfast and dinner. This feature can be considered in future to enhance the application. Additionally, like *MyFitnessPal*, *MauLifeStyle* can include automatic notifications or reminders when the application is left unused to motivate users.

6 Conclusion

This paper discusses the development and evaluation of the *MauLifeStyle* application which aims at promoting positive behavioural changes in the lifestyle among the people of Mauritius. The *MauLifeStyle* application comprises four main functionalities: blood glucose monitoring, food intake monitoring, fitness activity tracking, and calorie monitoring. It has been tailored specifically for the local context, providing information on the calorie content of Mauritian foods and the typical activities of the Mauritian population.

Individuals who have at least one risk factor of diabetes mellitus were invited to participate in the study. A screening session was conducted to outline the objectives of the study and attracted 44 potential participants. Unfortunately, given that the participants were recruited on University premises through investigators contacts and staff were still working from home in a hybrid format, we were not able to recruit a larger number of participants. Ultimately, 25 participants chose to participate in the 6-week study; however 28% of them were excluded as they did not satisfy the eligibility criteria. 50% of the participants were classified as regular users of the *MauLifeStyle* application while the others did not use the application regularly. Among the participants who used the applications regularly, the mean calorie intake was 2119 and the average carbohydrate intake was 274.6 daily. An increase in the mean daily duration of exercises, from 27.5 min to 34.2 min, was observed by the end of the study.

Post-study changes in the biomarker (lipid profiles and Fasting blood glucose) and the anthropological measurements did not reach statistical significance. This outcome could be attributed to the small number of participants who actively used the *MauLifeStyle* application. Therefore, it may currently be too early to draw any definitive conclusions on the effectiveness of the application within the local context.

In the future, more diverse participants can be recruited. With the situation returning to normality, we plan to embark on a new study with more number of people, both with pre-diabetic conditions and those who are not pre-diabetic but have the problem of obesity, and measure the impact of this application on their lifestyle. Additionally, it is known that gamification techniques can improve the experience of application users in m-health. Hence, we also plan to improve the application using gamification techniques. Eventually, we plan to propose this application to the Mauritian Ministry of Health to be used alongside other health campaigns in view of promoting a healthy lifestyle among Mauritians.

References

1. IDF Diabetes Atlas. International Diabetes Federation. 9th edn (2019). https://www.diabetesatlas.org/en/. Accessed 05 Sept 2023
2. Pohl, M.: 325,000 mobile health apps available in 2017. Berlin: Research2Guidance (2017). https://research2guidance.com/325000-mobile-health-apps-available-in-2017/. Accessed 05 Sept 2023

3. Messner, E.-M., Probst, T., O'Rourke, T., Stoyanov, S., Baumeister, H.: mHealth applications: potentials, limitations, current quality and future directions. Stud. Neurosci. Psychol. Behav. Econ. 235–248 (2019)

4. Smahel, D., Elavsky, S., Machackova, H.: Functions of mHealth applications: a user's perspective. Health Inform. J. **25**(3), 1065–1075 (2017)

5. Larson, R.S.: A path to better-quality mHealth Apps. JMIR Mhealth Uhealth **6**(7), e10414 (2018)

6. Vlahu-Gjorgievskam, E., Mulakaparambil Unnikrishnan, S., Win, K.T.: MHealth applications: a tool for behaviour change in weight management. Stud. Health Technol. Inform. **252**, 158–163 (2018)

7. Direito, A., Carraça, E., Rawstorn, J., Whittaker, R., Maddison, R.: MHealth technologies to influence physical activity and sedentary behaviors: behavior change techniques, systematic review and meta-analysis of randomized controlled trials. Ann. Behav. Med. **51**(2), 226–239 (2017)

8. Direito, A., Dale, L.P., Shields, E., Dobson, R., Whittaker, R., Maddison, R.: Do physical activity and dietary smartphone applications incorporate evidence-based behaviour change techniques? BMC Public Health **14**, 646 (2014)

9. Vandelanotte, C., Müller, A.M., Short, C.E., Hingle, M., Nathan, N., Williams, S.L., et al.: Past, present, and future of ehealth and mhealth research to improve physical activity and dietary behaviors. J. Nutr. Educ. Behav. **48**(3), 219-228.e1 (2016)

10. Kim, H., Faw, M., Michaelides, A.: Mobile but connected: harnessing the power of self-efficacy and group support for weight loss success through mHealth intervention. J. Health Commun. **22**(5), 395–402 (2017)

11. Rabbi, M., Pfammatter, A., Zhang, M., Spring, B., Choudhury, T.: Automated personalized feedback for physical activity and dietary behavior change with mobile phones: a randomized controlled trial on adults. JMIR Mhealth Uhealth **3**(2), e42 (2015)

12. Walsh, J.C., Corbett, T., Hogan, M., Duggan, J., McNamara, A.: An mHealth intervention using a smartphone app to increase walking behavior in young adults: a pilot study. JMIR Mhealth Uhealth **4**(3), e109 (2016)

13. Hartzler, A.L., et al.: Acceptability of a team-based mobile health (mHealth) application for lifestyle self-management in individuals with chronic illnesses. In: Conference on Proceedings of IEEE Engineering in Medicine and Biology Society (EMBC), pp. 3277–3281 (2016)

14. De la Torre Díez, I., Garcia-Zapirain, B., López-Coronado, M., Rodrigues, J.J.P.C., Del Pozo Vegas, C.: A new mHealth App for monitoring and awareness of healthy eating: development and user evaluation by Spanish users. J. Med. Syst. **41**(7), 109 (2017)

15. Goyal, S., Morita, P., Lewis, G.F., Yu, C., Seto, E., Cafazzo, J.A.: The systematic design of a behavioural mobile health application for the self-management of Type 2 diabetes. Can. J. Diabetes **40**(1), 95–104 (2016)

16. Arsand, E., Tatara, N., Østengen, G., Hartvigsen, G.: Mobile phone-based self-management tools for type 2 diabetes: the few touch application. J. Diabetes Sci. Technol. **4**(2), 328–336 (2010)

17. Freyne, J., Brindal, E., Hendrie, G., Berkovsky, S., Coombe, M.: Mobile applications to support dietary change: Highlighting the importance of evaluation context. In: Proceedings of the 2012 ACM annual conference extended abstracts on Human Factors in Computing Systems Extended Abstracts - CHI EA 2012, p. 1781. ACM Press, New York (2012)

18. Yang, H.J., et al.: Interventions for preventing childhood obesity with smartphones and wearable device: a protocol for a non-randomized controlled trial. Int. J. Environ. Res. Public Health **14**(2) (2017)

19. Laing, B.Y., et al.: Effectiveness of a smartphone application for weight loss compared with usual care in overweight primary care patients: a randomized, controlled trial. Ann. Int. Med. **161**(10 Suppl.), S5–12 (2014)

20. Orte, S., Migliorelli, C., Sistach-Bosch, L., Gómez-Martínez, M., Boqué, N.: A tailored and engaging mHealth gamified framework for nutritional behaviour change. Nutrients **15**, 1950 (2023)
21. Cho, D.J.: Editoral commentary: beyond the early adopter: the smartwatch ECG goes mainstream. Trends Cardiovasc. Med. **30**(7), 449–450 (2020)
22. Apple Watch saves life: Washington man credits Apple Watch's fall detection feature for saving father after falling - CBS News. https://www.cbsnews.com/news/apple-watch-saves-life-hard-fall-apple-watch-series-4-falling-emergency-bob-burdett/. Accessed 05 Sept 2023
23. Isakadze, N., Martin, S.S.: How, useful is the smartwatch ECG? Trends Cardiovasc. Med. **30**(7), 442–448 (2020)
24. Watch – Apple. https://www.apple.com/watch/. Accessed 05 Sept 2023
25. WHO/Europe—Nutrition - Body mass index – BMI. https://www.euro.who.int/en/health-topics/disease-prevention/nutrition/a-healthy-lifestyle/body-mass-index-bmi. Accessed 05 Sept 2023
26. Ganz, M.L., Wintfeld, N., Li, Q., Alas, V., Langer, J., Hammer, M.: The association of body mass index with the risk of type 2 diabetes: a case-control study nested in an electronic health records system in the United States. Diabetol. Metab. Syndr. **6**(1), 50 (2014)
27. Van der Weegen, S., Verwey, R., Spreeuwenberg, M., Tange, H., van der Weijden, T., de Witte, L.: The development of a mobile monitoring and feedback tool to stimulate physical activity of people with a chronic disease in primary care: a user-centered design. JMIR Mhealth Uhealth **1**(2), e8 (2013)
28. Walking - how to calculate calorie from pedometer? - Physical Fitness Stack Exchange. https://fitness.stackexchange.com/questions/25472/how-to-calculate-calorie-from-pedometer. Accessed 05 Sept 2023
29. Bumgardner, W.: Pedometer Steps to Calories Converter. verywellfit (2020). https://www.verywellfit.com/pedometer-steps-to-calories-converter-3882595. Accessed 05 Sept 2023
30. Ainsworth, B.E., Haskell, W.L., Herrmann, S.D., Meckes, N., Bassett, D.R., Tudor-Locke, C., et al.: 2011 Compendium of physical activities: a second update of codes and MET values. Med. Sci. Sports Exer. **43**(8), 1575–1581 (2011)
31. Roland, J.: What Are METs, and How Are They Calculated? https://www.healthline.com/health/what-are-mets. Accessed 05 Sept 2023
32. Hazell, A.: BMR Formula (Basal Metabolic Rate). https://www.thecalculatorsite.com/articles/health/bmr-formula.php. Accessed 05 Sept 2023
33. Haponiuk, B., Díez, Á,, Miszewska, D.: Calories Burned Calculator—Exercise, Fitness, Sex. https://www.omnicalculator.com/sports/calories-burned. Accessed 05 Sept 2023
34. Mohamed, A.H.H., Tawfik, H., Al-Jumeily, D., Norton, L.: MoHTAM: a technology acceptance model for mobile health applications. In: 2011 Developments in E-systems Engineering. IEEE, pp. 13–18 (2011)

Gym at Home - A Proof-of-Concept

Nuno Almeida[✉], Ana Patrícia Rocha, Adalberto Rosário, Pompeu Costa,
Rafael Amorim, Rafael Pinto, Tiago Alves, and António Teixeira

Institute for Electronics and Informatics Engineering of Aveiro (IEETA), Intelligent
Systems Associate Laboratory (LASI), Department of Electronic,
Telecommunications, and Informatics (DETI), University of Aveiro, Aveiro, Portugal
{nunoalmeida,aprocha,adalberto.rosario,pompeu,
rafael.amorim,rafaelpbpinto,tiagojba9,ajst}@ua.pt

Abstract. The average life expectancy has increased in the last decades,
but it is still necessary to promote a healthy and active aging. Although
older people need to have more caution when doing exercise, it is an
important aspect to maintain a healthy and active life. Access to facilities
by older people to do exercises in groups and having someone guiding
them in the execution of the exercises usually poses challenges for them,
due to transportation-related limitations. Our goal is to enable older
people to do exercises in their homes, allowing them to have exercise
plans that meet their needs. Group exercises with their friends is also
an important feature to motivate them to exercise more often. In this
paper, we propose a proof-of-concept of a smart gym at home system
based on defined scenarios and its installation in a near-real scenario.
The proof-of-concept provides a guide to a given exercise plan, with
video demonstrations of each exercise. The interaction of the system was
carefully thought, since older people are typically not comfortable with
technologies. The main interaction method in this proof-of-concept is
speech, since the users are distant from the system's devices while doing
the exercises.

Keywords: Active aging · Physical exercise · Health at home ·
Virtual gym · Speech interaction

1 Introduction

According to the Eurostat, between 2019 and 2050, the median age is projected
to increase by 4.5 in Europe [1]. The aging of the population began a few decades
ago and is mainly due to the increase in average life expectancy and low birth
rate. Due to this factor, it is more important than ever to look for ways to improve
the quality of life of older people, with physical exercise playing a major role in
this improvement [2].

© ICST Institute for Computer Sciences, Social Informatics and Telecommunications Engineering 2024
Published by Springer Nature Switzerland AG 2024. All Rights Reserved
A. Cunha et al. (Eds.): MobiHealth 2023, LNICST 578, pp. 417–431, 2024.
https://doi.org/10.1007/978-3-031-60665-6_31

Unfortunately, older people are more prone to suffer certain types of injuries due to a lack of knowledge about the most correct posture while performing some exercises [3] with bad postures can result in more serious injuries, resulting in longer and more difficult treatment. To prevent this problem, it is necessary that older people are properly instructed on how to perform certain exercises.

Aging and the need for health care for older people have been increasing [4]. On the other hand, citizens' access to healthcare is decreasing [5]. Therefore, it is essential to invest in prevention, creating conditions for the elderly to stay longer at home and at the same time be more active and healthy, thus improving their quality of life.

For many older people, wellness and health services, namely the gym and physiotherapy, are difficult to access, both due to travel and cost. This makes it impossible for them to take advantage of these services. Probably, in a few decades, it will be possible for anyone to have their own set of equipment at home, capable of helping in the practice of physical exercise. At the same time, a physical therapist would be receiving the same information regarding the execution of the exercise plan and monitor progress, providing suggestions and an exercise plan appropriate for each person.

The goal of the "Casa da Saúde" or "Health Home" project is to provide autonomy, control of own life, and better living conditions to older adults staying at home. To achieve this goal, a real home was designed, as illustrated in Fig. 1, and is being built especially for the project. This home will integrate a variety of novel solutions to monitor and support an older person living in it.

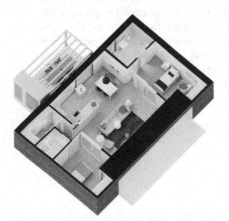
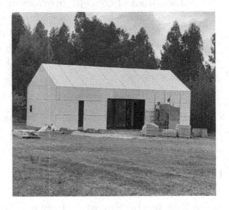

Fig. 1. On the left figure, the 3D model of the house of the "Health Home" project ("Casa da Saúde" in Portuguese) being built at Rovisco Pais Rehabilitation Center in Portugal (https://www.roviscopais.pt). The house consists of a large and central living room connected to the kitchen, a main bedroom with private WC (right side in the left figure) and a guest room and WC (left side). In the right figure, the construction of the house.

For the first phase of the project, in 2022–2023, there are three main objectives that were selected as the most important to be addressed:

1. Support of inhabitant's activities, that is, the exploration of technological solutions that facilitate certain aspects of the person's daily activities (e.g., checking food validity);
2. Global health state monitoring, installing systems that allow the monitoring of the person's health in a non-intrusive way;
3. Prevention and rehabilitation, by the introduction of systems that allow the prevention of certain occurrences associated with age and clinical conditions or rehabilitation following these occurrences.

The main goal of this work is to develop a smart gym system that motivates the elderly to stay active at home. To do this, we will make use of new technologies to support traditional approaches, in order to support the execution of physical exercises through demonstrative videos. The goal is that the user will not feel alone while exercising, so that he or she will feel more motivated, that is, he or she can interact with other users who are also practicing exercise.

2 Related Work

To find related work, a query was carried out on Google Scholar. Several keywords were used to query for literature, namely: (1) home gym old adults; (2) personal healthcare in gym; (3) interactive elder assistant. From all the results obtained in the query, a smaller list of recent papers were selected based on the similarities and functionalities of the envisioned system. They are briefly presented next.

Martinho et al. [6] proposed a prototype for an intelligent coach application "CoaFEld" with the goal of reducing the impact of aging in terms of physical, cognitive, social, and emotional deterioration. This allows for motivational strategies to persuade older people to be healthier and to stay connected to these systems. The application was developed using a cognitive virtual assistant to interact directly with the users, which plays and communicates with them through different emotions. It is also able to adapt to each user, aware that each person has their own personal characteristics, and will consequently react differently to each one. Information technology was developed following a microservice-oriented architecture. The system is composed of three main components: a user web application, an API (Application Programming Interface) gateway, and a set of microservices.

Another recent application, GymCentral, was proposed by Báez et al. [7]. It explores the design and validation of a virtual fitness environment focused on older people. From a tablet, users can access a virtual room and connect with others to do group exercises online. The app consists of two interfaces, one for the people doing the exercise and one for the trainers who can be in contact with doctors or physiotherapists. Users have access to different rooms and features within the app such as reception, locker room, classroom, schedule, messages, and progress report, just like in a real gym. The progress of users can be monitored manually or automatically with sensors placed at the place of exercise.

Vigorous, long and exhausting exercise can cause major long-term health problems, such as heart disease, kidney failure, and high blood pressure, especially in people with a weak immune system. Ahanger et al. [8] developed a smart treadmill with the capability to find health vulnerabilities of the user.

More oriented to virtual assistants, Basanta et al. [9] proposed a system allowing older people to control home appliances using voice and gestures. This system was designed so that the users, even with their health problems, can easily do their routines, for example, open/close blinds or turn on/off heaters without major problems.

Khaghani-Far [10] conducted a study on the use of home training applications (fitness apps) for older adults. To this end, a total of 200 apps for mobile devices, consoles and computers were explored. The study analyzed five aspects:

- Type of app - training apps, tracking apps (they do not offer training but are important to detect physical aspects in the user such as heartbeat, breathing, etc.), training games (training in the context of games).
- Interaction - technology used during training and for interactions with the app.
- Monitoring - mechanisms used to measure the user's performance in relation to the exercise.
- Coaching and tailoring - types of instructions and feedback given during training.
- Motivation - defines how the apps motivate the users to start and continue exercising.

A summary of Khaghani-Far results, comparing the applications in different aspects, is present in Table 1.

Although not all papers describe a home gym for older people, Table 2 identifies some of the aspects present in each paper. Information in the table makes clear that the creation of systems for performing exercises at home has a large margin for improvement and inclusion of several innovative features with the potential of benefiting their older users. For example, voice-based interaction or video are not commonly adopted.

3   Method: User-Centered Development

To design and develop of the smart gym at home for older people, a methodology based on a user-centered design was used [11,12]. The first step begins with understanding the target audience and the creation of a Persona, which are based on the behaviors of real people. This is followed by the creation of scenarios for the persona. The scenarios allow the extraction of the main requirements for the system. This approach is essential to develop a system that is usable and meets the users' needs.

Table 1. Summary of the results of the study on fitness apps, from [10].

Design Dimension	Current Applications	Research Opportunities
Interaction	Mobile and game consoles provide input and output mechanisms that best facilitate interaction. Both platforms have higher adoption of bidirectional and multimodal interfaces.	We need to study how applications use these ingredients to implement usable interfaces.
Monitoring and sensing	Automatic detection of activities are preferable for older adults, especially when it comes to objective measures. Still, self-reporting is widely used as a method for data collection, despite potential effects in adoption and precision of readings.	Because the integration of sensors in fitness applications is limited (with the exception of applications in game consoles that offer motion-tracking capabilities during training), we need to further explore and exploit sensor integration.
Coaching and tailoring	Training programs supervised by an expert human coach are preferable for older adults. However, most of the applications on the outlined markets rely on hybrid solutions (technology and self-coaching), focusing mainly on exercise prescription.	We need to better incorporate expert human coaching support.
Persuasion and motivation	The few studies on persuasion strategies to boost adherence, especially in older adults, show strong evidence of the benefits of using persuasion strategies, and especially social strategies.	Few training applications exploit these features, other than allowing users to reflect on their activities. This presents a clear opportunity for applications that exploit these aspects

3.1   Main Persona

Mrs. Maria is a 73-year-old woman who lives in a house in a low population density. She has some health problems, such as hypertension, diabetes, memory problems, reduced motor function, and vision problems, requiring health monitoring. In addition, she is not comfortable interacting with modern technologies.

3.2   Example Scenario

One of the defined scenarios addresses the execution of an exercise plan, presented next. Integrated in the scenario description are shown, inside square brackets, the requirements related to each passage. They are classified as functional (F) or non functional (NF).

Table 2. Comparing features described in the different works

Papers	[9]	[6]	[10]	[7]	[8]
Year	2017	2022	2016	2017	2022
Home	✓		✓	✓	
Elder	✓	✓	✓	✓	
Info Exercise		✓		✓	✓
Video					✓
Voice Interaction	✓	✓			
Gestures	✓				
Simulation	✓	✓	✓	✓	✓
Monitoring	✓	✓	✓	✓	✓

Mrs. Maria wants to **perform the exercise plan that her physical therapist made for her** for today. She turns the system on by using the voice command "Call" [voice interaction - F] or by using the system's remote control [interaction via control - F].

The interface is projected on the wall [interface projection - F].

The system asks Mrs. Maria "What do you want to do today?" [voice interaction - F] [system initiative - F] [system timely response - NF]. She is presented with two options [give few options - NF]:

- a specific exercise plan made by the physiotherapist accompanying Mrs. Maria [having exercise plans - F] [physiotherapists can add exercise plans - F].
- all exercise plans available in the system [list of exercise plans - F].

Mrs. Maria selects the exercise plan option made by the physiotherapist [select exercise plan made by the physiotherapist - F] who accompanies her by saying "Physiotherapist plan" [voice interaction - F] [timely response of the voice recognition system - NF] [interaction through the control - F], a short description of what is to be done is displayed on the wall [exercise plan description - F].

The system says/shows "When you are ready say Start" [system initiative - F] [practical and simple interactions - NF]. Mrs. Maria prepares everything in the room and says/selects "Start" [voice interaction - F] [interaction via control - F].

The exercise is then showed to her using a video with a demonstration [show demonstration video of the exercise - F].

Each time Mrs. Maria wants to do the next exercise, she tells the system "I finished the exercise, you can move on to the next one" [voice interaction - F].

At the end of the exercises, Mrs. Maria loved the plan and so she gives a positive evaluation by saying "Rate" and "4 stars" [voice interaction - F] [self-evaluation of performed exercises - F] [practical and simple interaction - NF].

3.3   Requirements

The set of defined scenarios enabled the extraction of requirements for the system, which were divided into the functional and non-functional requirements listed below.

Functional Requirements

- A large part of the system functionalities must be voice-controlled
- Display exercise plan information consisting of text, image and/or video
- Display a video demonstrating the exercise to be carried out
- Capture and stream video of the user doing the exercises
- Receive video of other users of the system doing the exercises
- Allow the person to choose if they want to share their exercise session with other users or not
- Allow the person to choose which users they want to see doing their exercises
- Allow physical therapists to add exercise plans
- Ability to follow the person using a camera with PTZ (Pan-Tilt-Zoom) capabilities
- Self-evaluation by the user of a exercise plan
- Ability to monitor exercises
- Ability to recognize if the person did the exercise correctly
- Interaction by gestures

Non-Functional Requirements

- Simple and intuitive interface
- Interactions with the system must be practical and simple
- Timely feedback from voice recognition system
- Give few options to interact with the system at a time
- Processing must be local
- The processing units in which the modules run should be small in size and low in cost
- The video system module must be capable of High quality video
- Web Connection must be always available
- Microphones that pick up sound at a distance

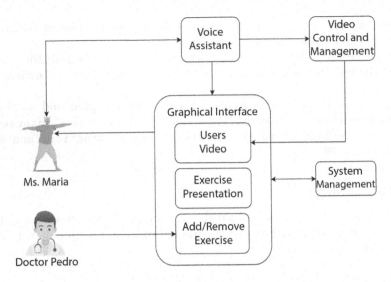

Fig. 2. General Architecture, composed by the main modules: System Management; Voice Assistant; Graphical Interface; and Video Control and Management.

4   Architecture

The architecture of the system follows a decoupled approach, as illustrated in Fig. 2, consisting of four modules: graphical interface, voice assistant, system manager, and video management and control. The system has two types of user: the older person and the physical therapist.

The older person is the main user, who interacts with the system mainly by voice. The user can choose and control which exercises he wants to do and also control the video camera. Additionally, the user can also move forward, restart, and pause the videos of the exercises. The physical therapist is the user who adds and/or removes exercises from the system's database. Using a web interface, the physical therapist can add exercises with name and description, as well as add a demo video or a demo image for each exercise.

The voice assistant module receives audio from the user and interprets what was said. If it recognizes that an action has been requested, a message is published so that other modules can receive it and process the request. The assistant also interacts with the user, giving feedback on what was understood. The graphical interface module encompasses everything that is displayed in the user interface and is subdivided into three sub modules: user video, exercise presentation, and add/remove exercises. The video management and control module sends video to the graphical user interface (GUI) and can receive messages from the voice assistant to change the camera orientation. The system manager module controls the storage of exercise data and exercise plans and provides the exercise information to the GUI module.

5   Implementation

The implementation of our prototype followed a decoupled approach. Modules are implemented separately to facilitate future updates or addition of new modules to the system. To allow the communication between most of the decoupled modules of the system, the MQTT protocol was used. MQTT is a message exchange protocol that follows the publisher subscriber model, where a broker is responsible for receiving and delivering the messages. In addition to this communication method, a REST service was created to manage the information in the database regarding the users and exercises.

Voice Assistant – One of the main challenges of this work was to create an accessible and easy way for the older users to interact with the system. To enable this, a virtual assistant capable of understanding natural language was developed using the following three tools:

– RASA[1] - used to develop virtual assistants. Composed of two main parts: Rasa NLU (Natural Language Understanding) and Rasa Core. Rasa NLU is responsible for understanding the user's intention from text and extracting the important information. Rasa Core is responsible for defining the flow of the conversation and what responses are to be given by the assistant.
– Vosk[2] - enables the development of applications with local speech recognition.
– Pyttsx3[3] - allows for speech synthesis.

A new model was trained for RASA to support the interaction for our system in Portuguese. The module is capable of providing feedback but also publishing the intent to other modules, namely the interface and video modules.

User Interface – The GUI was implemented in C#, using WinUI3[4]. The interface focuses on giving the user the information of the plan and exercises and presenting the videos of the different users. In order to facilitate the use of the system, it is possible to interact with the system by voice. There are features associated with commands, i.e., when the assistant sends a command, the associated function will be automatically executed (only when the command is known). The available functions include: view exercise; choose exercise/plan; play video.

User and Exercise Service – This service handles all the persistent information regarding of our system. It was implemented as a REST service using Flask[5] and SQLite[6]. The service offers methods to retrieve the list of exercises, user sessions, and add/remove exercises.

---

[1] https://rasa.com/.
[2] https://github.com/alphacep/vosk-api.
[3] https://github.com/nateshmbhat/pyttsx3.
[4] https://learn.microsoft.com/en-us/windows/apps/winui/winui3/.
[5] https://flask.palletsprojects.com/en/2.3.x/.
[6] https://www.sqlite.org/index.html.

Video Service – One of the objectives of our project is to make the older users feel accompanied. The camera module presents a solution for capturing and transmitting video to friends, in real time, of him performing the exercises. The Reolink E1 Zoom camera[7] was used for this purpose, which offers PTZ capabilities, allowing more control. The user can change the direction of the camera or move the focus closer or further away. The camera provides an API which enables our system to control it programmatically. The YouTube platform[8] was used to stream the videos to other users.

6   First Results

Considering the development stage (proof-of-concept), this section presents information regarding results of the development, focusing on the user interface (graphical and Conversational Assistant) and an initial deployment demonstration.

6.1   User Interface

The GUI consists of a series of specialized screens that enable the selection of plan/exercises, present rich information regarding each exercise, such as the visualization of a video, and allow the visualization of video of friends doing the same exercise plan.

The first screen, shown in Fig. 3 A), allows the user to navigate to the exercise plan or see the list of all exercises, as presented in Fig. 3 B). In the next screen, the user selects the exercise, after clicking on `Start`. The video screen will appear and the video will start playing automatically.

The essential screen, seen in Fig. 3 C), sequentially presents information regarding each exercise integrating the selected plan. This screen features the name of the exercise at the top, the video guide of the exercise at the bottom, and the video stream of the user's friends doing the same exercises on the right. At the end of the video, the interface asks if the user wants to move on to the next video or, if there are no more exercises, if he/she wants to end the plan.

6.2   Conversational Assistant

The assistant enables the interaction with the system using natural language. To activate voice recognition, the user must use the wake-up sequence "Olá Maria" (portuguese for *Hi Maria*). After that, the user can speak with the system to: navigate the user interface; start/pause the video; go to the next or previous exercise; and control the camera.

---

[7] https://reolink.com/product/e1-zoom/.
[8] https://www.youtube.com/howyoutubeworks/product-features/live/.

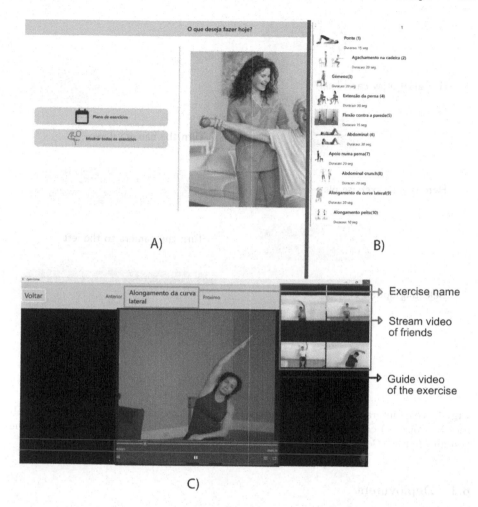

Fig. 3. Screens with different parts of the user interface in Portuguese: A) Main screen; B) Screen with the list of exercises; C) Presentation of the exercise and the video from other users.

As a representative example of navigation in the User interface by voice, Fig. 4 shows a possible conversation between a user (Rafael) and the assistant (Maria). In Fig. 4 a) the user wants to start a plan from the beginning and in b) the user adjusts the focus of the camera.

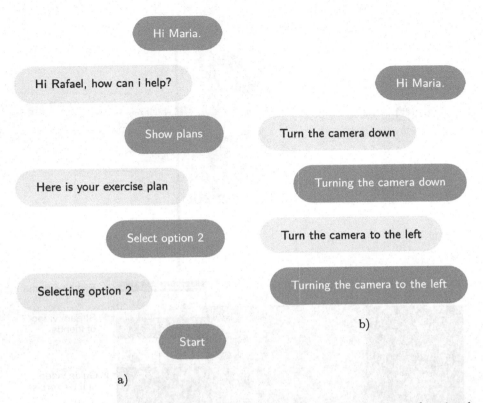

Fig. 4. Voice interaction example, demonstrating: a) navigation in system functionalities by voice; b) controlling the camera. The user dialog is in green bubbles and the system in gray. (Color figure online)

6.3 Deployment

To enable the demonstration of the proof-of-concept and its potential, an initial deployment was made in an environment approximating the real scenario. One of our institute research labs, dedicated to Ambient Assisted Living research, with some of the usual furniture we can encounter at home (e.g., a bed) and the dimensions of spacious living room, was selected. The deployment, shown in Fig 5, uses a mini-computer running the system, a router to provide connectivity, a mic/speaker ready for meetings, a wireless camera with PTZ capabilities, and a video projector.

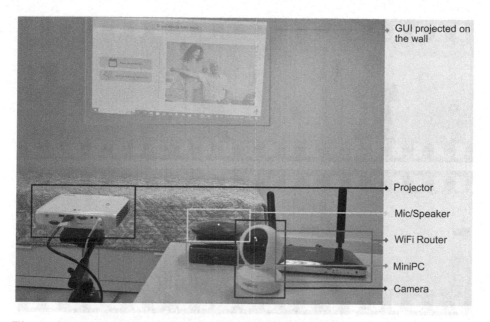

Fig. 5. All the hardware components used in the deployment of the proof-of-concept developed.

6.4   Initial Demonstrations

The deployment allowed us to test and demonstrate the system in a near reality scenario. One of the public demonstrations already performed was based on one of the scenarios defined to derive the system's requirements. In the scenario, Ms. Maria wants to perform the exercise plan that her physical therapist prescribed for her. She carries out the steps needed to select the plan but, before she starts, she needs to adjust the camera to focus on her position.

Figure 6 shows images from the video recorded during the demonstration[9] using the deployed gym system proof-of-concept. The first image presents the main screen, the second and third the steps to select the exercise, fourth and fifth the control of the camera position, and sixth making the exercise.

---

[9] https://www.youtube.com/watch?v=AxsVyO-H1ss.

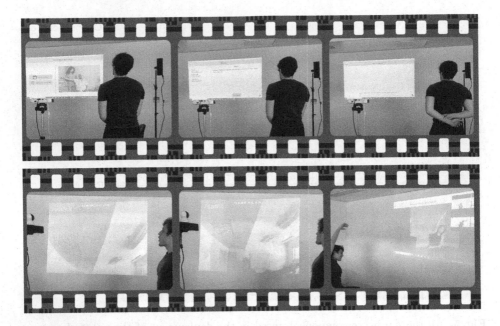

Fig. 6. Screenshots from the video demonstrating the use of the system, illustrating the navigation from the main screen to the exercise screen. Video in Portuguese can be accessed at https://www.youtube.com/watch?v=AxsVyO-H1ss.

7   Conclusion

With the aging of the world population, it is necessary to develop health systems capable of supporting the older people in their daily lives and to promote active and healthy aging. Thus, it is important to define strategies to persuade and motivate older people to make and maintain positive behavioral changes.

In this project, "Casa da Saúde", we implemented a system targeted at older people that enables them to exercise in the community from the comfort of their homes. We believe that the system developed has the potential to improve the quality of life of older people by increasing their physical and, consequently, mental well-being.

The goal to create a proof-of-concept system to guide older users to motivate and do exercise was reached. The system is able to provide information about the exercise performed and can also show the video of other users. Additionally, the system is easy to use, with the virtual assistant supporting natural interaction by listening to the user's speech.

Future Work

This proof-of-concept demonstrated the importance of this work, but improvements can be made, namely: improving the responsiveness of the conversational voice assistant, making the interaction with the assistant more natural, and improving the feedback of the graphical interface (e.g., having a caption showing what the assistant understood). Also, the decoupled nature of the architecture enables easy addition of new modules or features, such as a module that enables the camera to follow the user and monitor exercise execution and a module providing gesture interaction. Finally, the deployment of the future house will allow the evaluation with real people in real scenarios.

Acknowledgement. This Research Unit is funded by National Funds through the FCT - Foundation for Science and Technology, in the context of the project UIDB/00127/2020.

References

1. Eurostat: Ageing europe - statistics on population developments - statistics explained (2020). https://ec.europa.eu/eurostat/statistics-explained/index.php?title=Ageing_Europe_-_statistics_on_population_developments, accessed 08/08/2023
2. Shaikh, A.A., Dandekar, S.P.: Perceived benefits and barriers to exercise among physically active and non-active elderly people. Disabil. CBR Incl. Dev. **30**, 73–83 (2019)
3. Izquierdo, M., et al.: International exercise recommendations in older adults (ICFSR): expert consensus guidelines. J. Nutr. Health Aging **25**, 824–853 (2021)
4. Helwig, A.: Challenges in healthcare for the elderly | rti health advance (2007). https://healthcare.rti.org/insights/chronic-disease-healthcare-for-the-elderly
5. Barros, P.P., Costa, E.: Acesso a cuidados de saúde, 2022 as escolhas dos cidadãos no pós-pandemia (2022)
6. Martinho, D., Crista, V., Carneiro, J., Corchado, J.M., Marreiros, G.: An intelligent coaching prototype for elderly care. Electronics **11**, 460 (2022)
7. Báez, M., Ibarra, F., Far, I.K., Ferron, M., Casati, F.: Online group-exercises for older adults of different physical abilities. In: 2016 International Conference on Collaboration Technologies and Systems (CTS), pp. 524–533 (2016)
8. Ahanger, T.A.: IoT inspired smart environment for personal healthcare in gym. Neural Comput. Appl. **35**, 23007–23023 (2022)
9. Basanta, H., Huang, Y.P., Lee, T.T.: Assistive design for elderly living ambient using voice and gesture recognition system. In: 2017 IEEE International Conference on Systems, Man, and Cybernetics, SMC 2017 2017-January, pp. 840–845 (2017)
10. Khaghani-Far, I., Nikitina, S., Báez, M., Taran, E.A., Casati, F.: Fitness applications for home-based training. IEEE Perv. Comput. **15**, 56–65 (2016)
11. Cooper, A., Reimann, R., Cronin, D.: About Face 3: The Essentials of Interaction Design. Wiley, Hoboken (2007)
12. Teixeira, A., et al.: Design and development of medication assistant: older adults centred design to go beyond simple medication reminders. Univ. Access Inf. Soc. **16**(3), 545–560 (2017). https://doi.org/10.1007/s10209-016-0487-7

Automatic Food Labels Reading System

Diogo Pires[1], Vítor Filipe[1,2], Lio Gonçalves[1,2], and António Sousa[1,2(✉)]

[1] School of Sciences and Technology, University of Trás-os-Montes and Alto Douro (UTAD),
5000-811 Vila Real, Portugal
`a164273@alunos.utad.pt`, `{vfilipe,lgoncalv,amrs}@utad.pt`
[2] INESC Technology and Science (INESC-TEC), 4200-465 Porto, Portugal

Abstract. Growing obesity has been a worldwide issue for several years. This is the outcome of common nutritional disorders which results in obese individuals who are prone to many diseases. Managing diet while simultaneously dealing with the obligations of a working adult can be difficult. Today, people have a very fast-paced life and sometimes neglect food choices. In order to simplify the interpretation of the Nutri-score labeling this paper proposes a method capable of automatically reading food labels with this format. This method is intended to support users when choosing the products to buy based on the letter identification of the label. For this purpose, a dataset was created, and a prototype mobile application was developed using a deep learning network to recognize the Nutri-score information. Although the final solution is still in progress, the reading module, which includes the proposed method, achieved an encouraging and promising accuracy (above 90%). The upcoming developments of the model include information to the user about the nutritional value of the analyzed product combining it's Nutri-score label and composition.

Keywords: Nutri-Score · Digital Image Processing · Artificial intelligence · Deep Learning · Image Classification

1 Introduction

Obesity is a worldwide issue that accounts for 8% of global deaths annually [1]. People with obesity are at higher risk for many serious diseases and health conditions, including high blood pressure, diabetes, cardiac arrest, and an overall low quality of life. Dietary intake is one of the major causes of excess weight and fat accumulation. Sometimes the problem is not the quantity of food ingested but the quality: the nutritional balance. The Nutri-Score is an alternative label that consists in a food product rating system which was initially created and implemented in the food market in France and is now applied to many food labels in Europe. The system classifies foods by the nutritional balance. In general, it shows the 'macro' balance between nutrients/ingredients that must be privileged and nutrients/ingredients that must be avoided. The problem is that many people don't pay attention to the score or do not know how to interpret it. Usually, the consumer doesn't know why a certain food has a better classification than other, when apparently is not correct. Although the classification is correct.

A. Cunha et al. (Eds.): MobiHealth 2023, LNICST 578, pp. 432–444, 2024.
https://doi.org/10.1007/978-3-031-60665-6_32

Nowadays deep leaning is being applied in several fields including food industry. Various architectures of convolutional neural networks (CNNs) such as LeNet, VGGNet, GoogleNet, and AlexNet have also been used for "food recognition". The structure of CNNs was inspired by neurons in human and animal brains. The CNN simulated the complex sequence of cells that forms the visual cortex [2]. Their filters and other components are used to read the main image features and learn from them. This is image-based recognition which uses computer vision techniques to analyze images and identify their contents, detecting features such as color, texture, and shape. In general, CNN networks tend to present high performance for image analysis [3].

At the time of writing of this paper and, to authors knowledge, there are no related work in the literature proposing the automatic extraction and evaluation of products nutritional value from their packaging. The main purpose of this paper is to develop an image classification model that can be implemented on a mobile application for future daily use to support user's choices when buying products.

This paper is divided in 5 sections. In Sect. 2, the research work is presented which includes detailed information related to Nutri-score labeling system. Next, in Sect. 3 the materials and methodology used during this work are described focusing on the dataset building and the development of the proposed model. In Sect. 4, the model evaluation is performed including the presentation and discussion of the obtained results and the developed mobile app prototype. Finally, in Sect. 5 the conclusions are shown with some final remarks and future work.

2 Research Work

The Nutri-score is based on official rules defined by regulatory authorities. The labeling consists in a set of rules used to generate new labels with algorithms.

2.1 European Union Food Labeling Laws

Firstly, some of the topics contained in the official regulations of the competent authorities developed for labeling are reviewed. The use of different information sources allows one to have a different perspective of the topic to get the most correct idea about this theme.

The regulation of an appropriate system for food labeling is a method of health safety and safeguarding the interests of consumers. This regulation governs the labeling of all types of foods (solid, liquid, or processed) in all the countries that integrate the European Union. In addition, it may be supplemented by rules to be defined by each country for application to the national system. For that, it requires the examination by the European committee deliberated for this purpose.

These are some of the general rules which define the parameters that must be displayed on a food label [4]: the name of the food; the list of ingredients; any ingredient or processing aid listed or derived from a substance or product causing allergies or intolerances used in the manufacture or preparation of a food and still present in the finished product, even if in an altered form; the quantity of certain ingredients or categories of ingredients; the net quantity of the food; the date of minimum durability or the "use by" date; any special storage conditions and/or conditions of use; the name or business name and address of the food business operator; the country of origin or place of provenance; instructions for use where it would be difficult to make appropriate use of the food in the absence of such instructions; with respect to beverages containing more than 1.2 (%) by volume of alcohol, the actual alcoholic strength by volume; a nutrition declaration.

Nutritional Declaration

Nutritional declaration incorporates some information about the nutrient compositions in a product. The percentage of nutrients in 100 g or 100 ml of food must be presented. Sometimes the values can be shown per portion or the consumption unit.

These are the nutritional elements that must be integrated into the Nutritional declaration: energy value; the amounts of fat, saturates, and carbohydrates; the amounts of sugars, protein, and salt.

2.2 Nutri-Score

As seen earlier the amount of information presented to the consumer can be overwhelming. In turn, the diversity of information can have a negative effect in the consumer capability of choosing the most adequate product. This section exposes the fundamentals at the base of the Nutri-Score classification system.

As mentioned earlier, the Nutri-Score is based in a food components balance. Components that must be privileged by this system are: fiber, protein, vegetables, fruits, legumes, nuts, olive oils, rapeseed, and walnut oils. On the other hand, the components to avoid are: energy, saturated acids, sugar, and salt. In accordance with the balance, the aliment can be classified into 5 categories (good to bad, respectively): A (dark green); B (light green); C (yellow); D (light orange); E (dark orange/red) as seen in Fig. 1.

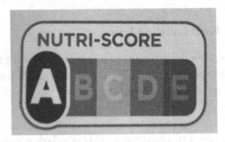

Fig. 1. The Nutri-Score label (Color figure online)

The Nutri-Score Main Algorithm

The classification of the food is based on the calculation of the final score. The score results from the sum of negative and positive points. The negative points (Table 1) are assigned according to the composition of the components to be avoided (per 100 g). The positive points are assigned by the quantity (per 100 g) of good components that exist on aliments. The algorithm regulates three different types of categories: The main algorithm general aliments; fats, oils, nuts and seeds category and beverages [5].

Table 1. Negative points attribution [6]

Points	Energy(KJ/100 g)	Sugars (g/100 g)	Saturates (g/100 g)	Salt (g/100 g)
0	≤335	≤3.4	≤1	≤0.2
1	>335	>3.4	>1	>0.2
2	>670	>6.8	>2	>0.4
3	>1005	>10	>3	>0.6
4	>1340	>14	>4	>0.8
5	>1675	>17	>5	>1
6	>2010	>20	>6	>1.2
7	>2345	>24	>7	>1.4
8	>2680	>27	>8	>1.6
9	>3015	>31	>9	>1.8
10	>3350	>34	>10	>2
11		>37		>2.2
12		>41		>2.4
13		>44		>2.6
14		>48		>2.8
15		>51		>3
16				>3.2
17				>3.4
18				>3.6
19				>3.8
20				>4

The main algorithm will be explained in detail. The other groups follow the same logic but different reference values and calculation algorithms [6]. For the general aliments, it is necessary to reference Table 1and Table 2.

The aliment's label must be analyzed, and the values of the different components must be retrieved. Then the tables must be consulted and added the corresponding points to each parameter. For example, if the protein quantity in the food was 10 g per 100 g, is added 4 points to a positive score according to Table 2. It is necessary to do the same for all positive parameters. For negative parameters, for example, if the amount of sugar is 2 g per 100 g, it isn't added negative points to a negative score. Is the same logic used for the good points. At the end of the process, exist a positive point score and a negative point score.

With the final score calculated, it is necessary to attribute the corresponding letter following Table 3.

Table 2. Positive points attribution [6]

Points	Proteins (g/100 g)	Fibers (g/100 g)	Fruit, vegetables and legumes (%)
0	≤2.4	≤3.0	≤40
1	>2.4	>3.0	>40
2	>4.8	>4.1	>60
3	>7.2	>5.2	
4	>9.6	>6.3	
5	>12	>7.4	>80
6	>14		
7	>17		

Table 3. Final Nutri-score thresholds points attribution [6]

Final NScore Points	Class/category	Colour
Min to 0	A	Dark Green
1 to 2	B	Light Green
3 to 10	C	Yellow
11 to 19	D	Light Orange
19 to max	E	Dark Orange or Red

Nutri-Score Other Algorithms

As referred previously, the main algorithm has some variances that must be adjusted to different groups like beverages and other specific aliments. The tables are different for the fats, oils, nuts, and seeds category [6] and beverages [5]. The conditions to calculate the final score are also different. For fats, oils, nuts, and seeds category: a) if previous negative points sum ≥7, so the final score is (negative points - (fruit, legumes, and vegetables)); b) if previous negative points sum <7, so the final score is (negative points - total positive points).

For beverages, the algorithm is equal to the main algorithm but is necessary to adjust the sugar parameter (add 1.5 g/100 g at each tabled level) and energy (add 30 kJ/100 g at each tabled level) [5]. The final score is calculated by subtraction of positive points to negative points. Note that the classification ranges are different between the different categories, depending on whether it is food in general, beverages, or another group mentioned.

3 Materials and Methodology

To run the code, a laptop with the following main specs was used: AMD Ryzen 5, 8 GB RAM, and Nvidia Geforce RTX 2 GB. The laptop programs employed and fundamental to the project are the latest Matlab version Matlab 2023a, Python, Flutter Dart, and Visual Studio Code.

Matlab 2023a was used to treat the dataset and to create the deep learning model. Flutter used for the mobile application development. For app development, an Android smartphone was used to receive and test the depurated app.

3.1 Dataset

Image Capture

An iPhone 13 camera with 12 megapixels and an f/1.2 lens opening was used to capture the dataset images. These were captured in 3024 × 3024 × 3 format. Processing technologies already incorporated in the smartphone were used. The main technologies are active rapid capture prioritization that intelligently adapts image quality to shutter press speed. Furthermore, the smartphone has an active lens correction that corrects lens distortion on the front camera and an ultra-wide-angle camera. The image capture quality can be optimized by considering lighting conditions, capture angle, and other relevant factors like the camera specs, for example. It's important to focus the camera on the scale of letters and capture the minimum objects/details in the background.

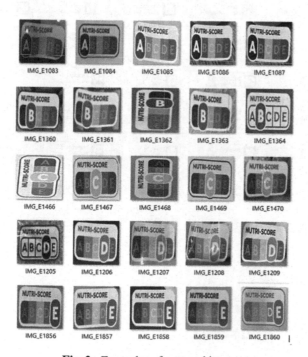

Fig. 2. Examples of captured images

Random products chosen in a hypermarket were captured resulting in 500 Nutri-score images (100 images for each category A, B, C, D, E). Figure 2 shows some examples of the captured images.

Image Pre-processing and Data Augmentation
In order to increase the number of images in the dataset, data augmentation was performed. To perform this procedure, the "imageDataAugmenter" function from Matlab [7] was used. The code allows the generation of new dataset images from the original images. The new images are generated by applying rotation and scaling transformations to the original images and applied randomly. This procedure resulted in a dataset with a total number of 5000 images (1000 images for each category). Due to GPU's limited performance images resizing to $512 \times 512 \times 3$ was applied.

3.2 Model Development

Dataset Division
The dataset was divided into train/validation set (4000 images): 560 images for each category (70% of the total) to train and 240 images for each category (30% of the total) to validate the model. The test set was constituted by the remaining 1000 images.

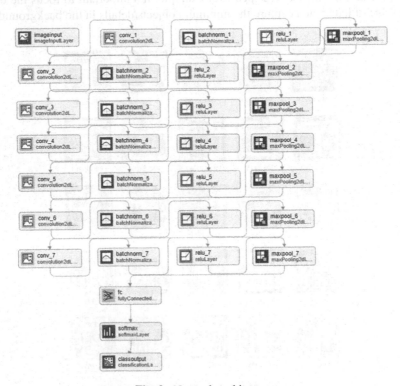

Fig. 3. Network architecture

Neural Network Architecture

The proposed neural network architecture (Fig. 3) was obtained thru experimentation and finetuning based on a simple image classification network using deep network designer available in Matlab. The model is composed by the input layer which receives the image and then, has six convolution layers with 3×3 filters. The number of filters in each one of the convolutional layers are 8, 16, 32, 64, 128, 512 respectively. After applying a convolution layer, the model always has a batch normalization layer, a Relu layer, and a max pooling layer (pool size 2, and stride 2). The last layer is composed by a fully connected layer, a softmax layer and a classification layer that classifies the images in one of the 5 classes.

Training Options

Relatively to the parametrizations of the training process, the hyperparameter values were obtained heuristically based on experimentation. It was established that the initial learning rate was 0.01 and the train epochs were 15. The minibatch size was 16 which means 16 images were shown to the model each time. Additionally, an Adam optimizer was applied since it obtained better results than similar optimizers (sgdm for example).

4   Results and Discussion

The model performance in the dataset was evaluated using several metrics. To integrate the proposed Nutri-Score classification method, for assisting the consumer, a mobile application was developed.

4.1   Model Evaluation

Performance Metrics

To analyze the performance the accuracy, confusion matrix, recall, precision, and F1-score were used, applying the following equations for each of the categories.

$$Precision = \frac{TP}{TP + FP} \tag{1}$$

$$Recall = \frac{TP}{TP + FN} \tag{2}$$

$$F1\text{-}Score = 2 * \left(\frac{Precision * Recall}{Precision + Recall} \right) \tag{3}$$

$$Accuracy = \frac{TP + TN}{TP + FN + FP + TN} \tag{4}$$

P represent true positive cases; FN represent false negative cases; FP represent false positive cases and TN represent false negative cases.

Evaluation Results

Figure 4 shows the graphic of accuracy during the train and loss of accuracy to validation data. In the graph, it is possible to see the existence of a curve of high growth in an initial phase. After a specific moment, the graphic growth stabilizes, originating a horizontal approximately straight line. The graph showed few oscillations, which indicates that the training process was stable. Accuracy was 97.25% to the train/validation dataset, and 95.00% to the test dataset. When the model was applied to the test dataset, a drop of two percentage points was denoted.

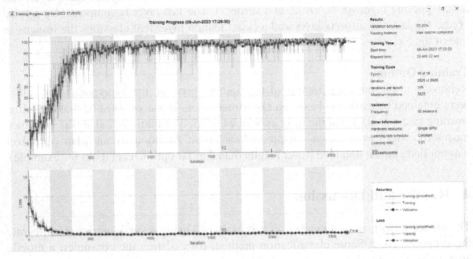

Fig. 4. Model Performance

Evaluation Metrics

Performance metrics were analyzed for two different situations: when the model was applied to training and validation data and when it was applied to test data (never seen before by the neural network). Confusion matrices (Fig. 5) show a comparison between true results and model results. They are commonly used to identify true positives (TP), false negatives (FN), false positives (FP), and true negatives (TN). For model performance purposes, it is more relevant to observe the performance metrics and confusion matrix regarding the test data. This is because the test dataset are images never seen by the model before and, therefore, it shows the real performance of the model comparable to a real-world scenario using images captured and processed using a mobile app.

The model's performance was evaluated using the metrics precision, F1-score, and recall which were calculated for each of the categories. On the training set (Table 4), all the average values of the performance metrics are all greater than 97%, which translates into a good performance of model for training the letter classification.

When the model was evaluated on the test dataset (Table 5), a drop of two percentage points was registered for each of the average values of the metrics, approximately. The drop is natural because the test dataset is compounded by images that were not seen before to the model. So, in this case, is normal to observe a small performance reduction.

These metrics have been calculated in accordance with the confusion matrices as shown in Fig. 5, applying the metric formulas.

Confusion matrix

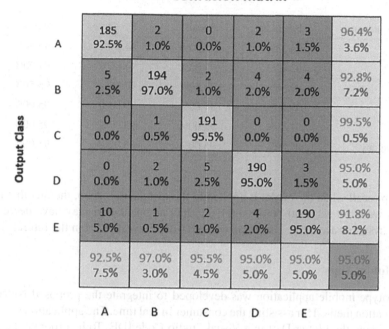

Fig. 5. Confusion Matrix calculated for testset

Table 4. Performance metrics to train and validation dataset

Class (Category)	Precision	Recall	F1-Score	Accuracy
A	97.84%	94.58%	96.19%	94.60%
B	96.71%	97.92%	97.31%	97.90%
C	100.00%	99.58%	99.79%	99.60%
D	97.85%	95.00%	96.41%	95.00%
E	94.07%	99.17%	96.55%	99.20%
Mean values	97.29%	97.25%	97.25%	97.25%

Analyzing each of the performance metrics it was found that the accuracy, recall, and F1-score values are around 95%. Individually, it is worth notice that there were some values below average. It is the case of the precision calculated for category E or the F1-score or accuracy of the same category. These lower values observed for category E may have resulted from the lack of sharpness of the calculated images and the presence of some noise in the images. Everything indicates that the problem could be with the images because this was the group with the lowest values. The same was verified for

Table 5. Performance metrics to test dataset

Class (Category)	Precision	Recall	F1-Score	Accuracy
A	96.35%	92.50%	94.39%	92.50%
B	92.82%	97.00%	94.87%	97.00%
C	99.48%	95.50%	97.45%	95.50%
D	95.00%	95.00%	95.00%	95.00%
E	91.79%	95.00%	93.37%	95.00%
Mean values	95.09%	95.00%	95.02%	95.00%

A group recall when the model is applied to the test dataset. Also, the fact that the test images were not set apart before applying data augmentation may have decrease the overall system's accuracy. This issue will be further investigated in the future.

4.2 Mobile App

A prototype mobile application was developed to integrate the proposed Nutri-Score classification method for assisting the consumer in real time. The application was implemented using the Flutter Dart in a Visual Studio Code IDE. To incorporate the trained model it was necessary to convert it to a ".tflite" file format. First, the original format ".mat" was converted to a Tensorflow model using the "Deep Learning Toolbox Converter for TensorFlow Models" [8], after installing the add-on, a code was created to convert the format model. Finally, in the Spyder-Python environment, a new code was developed to convert the TensorFlow model into a ".tflite" file ready to be incorporated into an Android app.

The application has a simple interface. The user must touch a button to open the camera and, then it is possible to capture the images. Furthermore, it was introduced a space delimiter to help the user to capture just the relevant objects (Nutri-score label). The captured image with the camera has $512 \times 512 \times 3$ default dimensions. The Android app interface can be shown in Fig. 6. This is a prototype of an Android application to implement the trained model. Although not fully functional the mobile app allows the user to capture images at a predefined size. Despite the attempts it was not possible, at this stage of development, to incorporate the model fully functional due to problems with the "dart.io" packages.

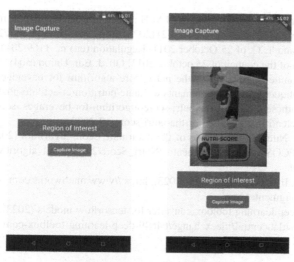

Fig. 6. Mobile app interface

5 Conclusions

In this work a method capable of automatically reading food Nutri-Score labels to simplify its interpretation was proposed. This method was intended to support users when choosing the products to buy based on the letter identification of the label. To accomplish this, a dataset was created, and a prototype mobile application was developed incorporating a deep learning model. The proposed method achieved good accuracy (above 90%). The obtained results were encouraging and are a great incentive to improve the model and the functionalities of the mobile application.

As a future work, it is possible to try to improve the model performance even further by adjusting parameters in the network architecture or increasing the training dataset. Also, the test images will be set apart before applying data augmentation to evaluate the overall system's accuracy improvement. It is also intended to improve the mobile prototype application to present to the user the general scientific information. The upcoming developments include information about the nutritional value of the analyzed product combining it's Nutri-score label and composition to advise the user to consume or not the analyzed product. That will help inform the consumer about the macro nutritional composition of the food, within reach of a photograph, with real impact on consumers health.

References

1. Okunogbe, A., Nugent, R., Spencer, G., Powis, J., Ralston, J., Wilding, J.: Economic impacts of overweight and obesity: current and future estimates for 161 countries. BMJ Glob. Health 7(9), e009773 (2022)
2. Alzubaidi, L., et al.: Review of deep learning: Concepts, CNN architectures, challenges, applications, future directions. J. Big Data 8, 1–74 (2021)

3. Nadeem, M., Shen, H., Choy, L., Barakat, J.M.H.: Smart diet diary: real-time mobile application for food recognition. Appl. Syst. Innov. **6**(2) (2023). https://www.mdpi.com/2571-5577/6/2/53

4. E. Parliament and T. C. of 25 October 2011. Regulation (eu) no 1169/2011 of the European parliament and of the council of 25 october 2011. Off. J. Eur. Union (304), 18–63 (2011)

5. T. N.-S. S. Comite. V2-update of the nutri-score algorithm for beverages (2022). https://www.santepubliquefrance.fr/determinants-de-sante/nutrition-et-activite-physique/documents/rapport-synthese/update-of-the-nutri-score-algorithm-for-beverages.-second-update-report-from-the-scientific-committee-of-the-nutri-score-v2-2023

6. T. S. C. of the Nutri-Score. Update of the main nutri-score algorithm (2023). https://www.asan.gob.es/AECOSAN/docs/documentos/Nutri_Score/2022_main_algorithm_report_update_FINAL.pdf

7. MATWORKS. Imagedataaugmenter (2023). https://www.mathworks.com/help/deeplearning/ref/imagedataaugmenter.html

8. Helper, M.: Deep learning toolbox converter for tensorflow models (2023). https://www.mathworks.com/matlabcentral/fileexchange/64649-deep-learning-toolbox-converter-for-tensorflow-models

Transfer Learning to Detect COVID-19 Coughs with Incremental Addition of Patient Coughs to Healthy People's Cough Detection Models

Sudip Vhaduri[1]($\boxtimes$), Seungyeon Paik[1], and Jessica E. Huber[2,3]

[1] Computer and Information Technology Department, Purdue University,
West Lafayette, IN 47907, USA
{svhaduri,paiks}@purdue.edu

[2] Speech, Language, and Hearing Sciences Department, Purdue University,
West Lafayette, IN 47907, USA
jhuber@purdue.edu

[3] Communicative Disorders and Sciences Department, University at Buffalo, Buffalo,
NY 14214, USA
jehuber@buffalo.edu

Abstract. Millions of people have died worldwide from COVID-19. In addition to its high death toll, COVID-19 has led to unbearable suffering for individuals and a huge global burden to the healthcare sector. Therefore, researchers have been trying to develop tools to detect symptoms of this human-transmissible disease remotely to control its rapid spread. Coughing is one of the common symptoms that researchers have been trying to detect objectively from smartphone microphone-sensing. While most of the approaches to detect and track cough symptoms rely on machine learning models developed from a large amount of patient data, this is not possible at the early stage of an outbreak. In this work, we present an incremental transfer learning approach that leverages the relationship between healthy peoples' coughs and COVID-19 patients' coughs to detect COVID-19 coughs with reasonable accuracy using a pre-trained healthy cough detection model and a relatively small set of patient coughs, reducing the need for large patient dataset to train the model. This type of model can be a game changer in detecting the onset of a novel respiratory virus.

Keywords: transfer learning · COVID-19 · Cough detection

© ICST Institute for Computer Sciences, Social Informatics and Telecommunications Engineering 2024
Published by Springer Nature Switzerland AG 2024. All Rights Reserved
A. Cunha et al. (Eds.): MobiHealth 2023, LNICST 578, pp. 445–459, 2024.
https://doi.org/10.1007/978-3-031-60665-6_33

1 Introduction

1.1 Motivation

Coronavirus and other human-transmissible respiratory viruses have become prevalent and have led to human suffering and a large number of deaths in recent times. According to the World Health Organization (WHO), the novel coronavirus SARS-CoV-2 (COVID-19) has so far caused a total of over 771 million infections and over 6.9 million deaths globally [8]. Even after the development of a vaccine, over 300 thousand infections and 1.5 thousand deaths occur a day [8]. Additionally, COVID-19 created a heavy economic burden on the health sectors, e.g., the United States incurred a total of $163.4 billion in direct medical expenses during the pandemic [40]. Early onset detection can help prevent the rapid spread and its adverse consequences. But, traditional diagnosis approaches are slow and require resources, such as viral tests (based on samples from the nose and mouth) or antibody tests [3], chest X-ray or spirometry tests [4], blood tests, pulse oximetry, and sputum tests [1,7]. These resources are not readily available in peoples' homes or at healthcare access points, such as primary care or urgent care. Therefore, there is a need for an approach that can be easily deployed to quickly detect the onset and control disease spread.

1.2 Related Work

Researchers have been trying to develop tools/systems to objectively detect and remotely report typical symptoms of respiratory diseases, such as coughing. Many of these techniques require the use of wearable technology. For example, researchers have detected coughing with 0.82 accuracy using smartwatch accelerometers and audio recordings [31], and 0.94–0.95 sensitivity using ECG, thermistor, chest belt, accelerometer, contact microphone, audio microphone [23] and chest sensor [11]. Some researchers proposed a respiratory monitoring system using a wearable patch sensor [24] and a wearable radio-frequency (RF) cough monitoring system [26]. On the other hand, a group of researchers proposed a COVID-19 symptom tracker utilizing a headset-like sensor [45].

However, we have found that people's adherence to wearables drops significantly over time, compared to smartphone adherence [9,28]. Therefore, some researchers have been trying to detect objective symptoms, such as coughing, using smartphone data [12,13,20,48,56]. One team of researchers proposed machine learning-based COVID-19 cough, breath, and speech detection using smartphone recording files [37,38]. They achieved up to 0.93 area under the curve using the k-nearest neighbor classifiers. Other researchers developed frameworks to diagnose COVID-19 using a smartphone app and built-in sensors in the smartphone [27,30].

However, a major limitation of all these existing cough detection models is the underlying assumption of the availability of a good amount of relevant data, which is not always possible [13]. For example, during the early stage of a new outbreak, there is not much data to develop a reasonably good traditional machine learning model due to the need for a large volume of data. But coughs from healthy people and patients have similarities, which can be utilized to detect COVID-19 coughs using a healthy cough detection model and a relatively small set of coughs from COVID-19 patients, reducing the need for large amounts of COVID-19 patient coughs. This kind of model would be invaluable in the detection of a new novel respiratory disease.

1.3   Contribution

The main contribution of this work is to present a novel approach leveraging similarities between healthy people's coughs and COVID-19 patients' coughs to incrementally transfer healthy cough detection models to COVID-19 cough detection models with smaller batches or folds of COVID-19 coughs. Compared to large data-driven traditional modeling approaches, incremental transfer learning approaches can help detect the onset of a novel respiratory virus early utilizing a relatively small set of cough samples obtained from the first few people infected and a pre-trained healthy people's cough detection model to control the spread of the novel respiratory disease to minimize adverse consequences.

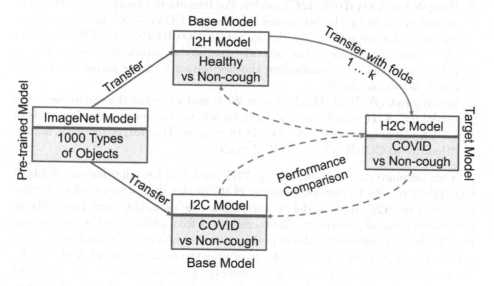

Fig. 1. Proposed modeling approach

2 Methods

In this section, we first present our modeling approach. Next, we discuss cough and non-cough audio recordings obtained from different sources, data processing steps, and neural network architectures and parameters used in this work.

2.1 Modeling Approaches

In Fig. 1, we present our modeling scheme. We start with a pre-trained model [44] developed to detect 1000 objects, i.e., classes from the ImageNet dataset [6]. Next, we use transfer learning to develop two base models and one target model to detect coughs obtained from healthy people and COVID-19 patients using transfer learning.

1. ImageNet to Healthy (**I2H**) model: We transfer our ImageNet 1000 object detection model to a binary model detecting healthy cough versus non-cough. Throughout this manuscript, we name this model as "ImageNet to healthy", i.e., **I2H** model. This is one of the two base models. This model will be later used to develop the target COVID-19 cough detection model incrementally.
2. ImageNet to COVID-19 (**I2C**) model: We transfer the ImageNet 1000 object detection model to a binary model that detects COVID-19 cough versus non-cough, which we refer to as "ImageNet to COVID-19", i.e., **I2C** model in this manuscript. This is the second base model, which will be used as a reference model when comparing the performance of our target COVID-19 cough detection models.
3. Healthy to COVID-19 (**H2C**) model: We transfer the healthy cough detection model, i.e., **I2H** model, incrementally by adding smaller batches, i.e., folds of COVID-19 coughs to detect COVID-19 coughs. This target model is named "Healthy to COVID-19", i.e., **H2C** model.

Our ultimate goal is to utilize the **I2H** model and smaller batches/folds of COVID-19 coughs to develop a target **H2C** model that achieves close performance to the **I2C** base model to investigate the capability and feasibility of incremental transfer learning. The incremental fold addition is the core of our transfer learning approach. Model performance is analyzed to show how the target models improve over time and to determine the minimum number of samples required to identify disease coughs accurately. There may not be a base model for a new disease for the performance comparison, such as the **I2C** model. However, our approach is to demonstrate that incremental transfer learning can be a pathway to get a valid model even when we have few samples of the new disease-specific patient data.

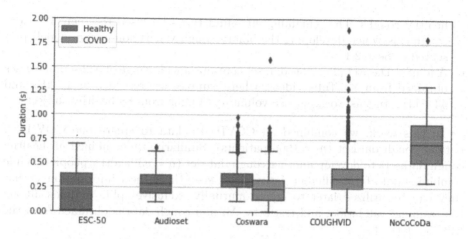

Fig. 2. Distribution of cough duration

2.2 Datasets

This section briefly describes six major datasets used in our experiments, including three COVID-19, two healthy cough datasets, and an image dataset.

1. ImageNet Dataset [6]: This is a publicly available image dataset with a thousand object classes and millions of images. The dataset contains various types of objects types, including geese, balloons, and fruits. We use the ImageNet dataset to develop the pre-trained "ImageNet" model.
2. Coswara Dataset [41]: This crowdsourced dataset consists of breathing, coughing, and voice sound recordings from healthy people and COVID-19 patients. The sampling rate is in the range of 47.82 ± 0.83 kHz. In this work, we use the voluntary coughs obtained from 274 COVID-19-positive patients.
3. COUGHVID Dataset [36]: This crowdsourced dataset contains more than 25,000 cough recordings from COVID-19-positive patients or asymptomatic people of varying ages, genders, and regions. The sampling rate of this dataset is around 44.1 kHz. We use the voluntary coughs obtained from 719 COVID-19-positive patients or asymptomatic people.
4. NoCoCoDa Dataset [17]: This dataset contains natural cough recordings of 13 COVID-19-positive patients collected from public media interviews. Audio recordings are collected at a 44.1 kHz sampling rate.
5. ESC-50 Dataset [39]: The environmental sound classification (i.e., ESC-50) dataset consists of audio recordings from five categories of sounds (i.e., animal, natural soundscapes, human sounds, interior sounds, and exterior noises) with 10 types of sounds per category recorded at a rate of 44.1 kHz. There are 40 audio recordings per type (2,000 recordings in total). We use the voluntary cough recordings from five healthy subjects as the cough class, i.e.,

healthy coughs. The remaining 49 sound types are used to create the non-cough class when developing the binary cough versus non-cough models presented in Sect. 2.1.

6. AudioSet Dataset [25]: This dataset contains a wide range of 632 sound classes obtained from YouTube videos, where samples are recorded at 16 kHz and 44.1 kHz. In this work, we use voluntary coughs from 88 healthy subjects.

In this work, we combined all COVID-19 data to create one COVID-19 patient cough dataset (n = 1006 patients). Similarly, we combined all healthy cough datasets to develop another cough dataset (n = 83 healthy people). While combining data from different datasets, we keep the subject information so that they can be utilized later to create mutually exclusive splits or folds among the training, validation, and test sets. All non-cough data is obtained from the ESC-50 dataset.

2.3 Data Processing

This section presents our cough ground-truth label collection approach from long audio recordings, followed by additional processing steps, including finding an optimal window size, padding, and feature extraction. Finally, we present our cross-validation approach with incremental training to develop **H2C** models from **I2H** model which requires relatively fewer COVID-19 coughs.

Data Cleaning and Ground-Truth Label Collection. Most of the audio data used in this work come from crowd-sourced datasets. Therefore, we first perform a rigorous cleaning process to remove unwanted parts, including quiet, speech, and noises using different audio signal processing libraries and tools, including the Audacity toolbox [2].

After the initial cleaning, we performed data segmentation to extract the ground-truth cough labels from long audio recordings with multiple coughs utilizing the Audacity toolbox. Adapted from our previous work [46,74], we automated the process by developing an energy threshold-based audio segmentation followed by a phase classification approach.

We obtained 144 and 252 healthy coughs from the ESC-50 and AudioSet datasets. Similarly, we obtained 1892, 2690, and 73 COVID-19 coughs from the Coswara, COUGHVID, and NoCoCoDa datasets, respectively. In total, we used 396 healthy coughs and 4655 COVID-19 coughs.

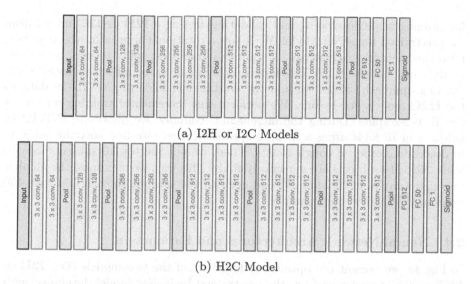

(a) I2H or I2C Models

(b) H2C Model

Fig. 3. Optimal Architecture of different models

Feature Extraction. Since we collected audio recordings from different sources, we first changed all sampling frequencies to 44.1 kHz frequency before additional processing.

Next, we determined a suitable window size before computing features. In Fig. 2, we use boxplots to represent the distribution of cough duration obtained from various datasets. In the figure, we find that 75th percentile of Coswara healthy cough duration, i.e., 0.3917 s, is a suitable choice for window size since most of the other healthy and patient coughs, except the NoCoCoDa coughs, have a duration shorter than that. Compared to other datasets, the NoCoCoDa dataset has relatively fewer samples.

We perform padding (i.e., add 0 s) at the end of coughs shorter than the window size (i.e., 0.3917 s). In the case of longer cough and non-cough audio recordings, we truncate the parts longer than the window size. Finally, we compute the log mel-spectrogram [34] (logmel) and Mel-frequency cepstral coefficient (mfcc) image features from each cough and non-cough audio recording using the Python Librosa library [33].

Training, Validation, and Test Split. First, we uniformly split the cough data into 10 mutually exclusive folds based on subjects. For class balancing, we select the same number of non-cough samples as we have cough samples for the 10 folds. Thereby, we maintain the same number of cough (either healthy or COVID-19) and non-cough instances when training, validating, and testing binary cough (either healthy or COVID-19) versus non-cough detection models presented in Sect. 2.1. Next, we follow a "leave-2-fold-out" for validation and "leave-2-fold-out" for the test approach, where we use the remaining six folds for training while developing and validating/testing a **I2H** or **I2C** model from the pre-trained ImageNet Model. We follow a rotational approach, where we perform this mutually exclusive 6-2-2 train-validation-test split 10 times to develop 10 different models. While developing **H2C** models, we follow an incremental training approach, where we add the six training folds of COVID-19 data to the **H2C** models one-by-one. We perform this incremental training for one of the 10 6-2-2 splits. During the incremental training, we distribute COVID-19 subjects in 10 folds using a snaking approach, where we first sort the subjects in descending order of cough counts. Then, we put the top 10 subjects into 10 folds. Next, 10 subjects are put into 10 folds. This way, we maximize the number of cough samples in 10 folds. We end up with 100 subjects in each fold with 450 random COVID-19 cough samples.

2.4   Neural Network Architectures and Parameters

In Fig. 3a, we present the optimal architecture of the two models (i.e., **I2H** or **I2C** models) transferred from the pre-trained ImageNet model developed with VGG19 [44]. In Fig. 3b, we present the optimal architecture of the **H2C** model transferred from the **I2H** model by adding folds of COVID-19 coughs. In the figure, the sequence and meaning of different parameters in each layer are kernel size and the number of feature maps, i.e., nodes in each layer. The pre-trained ImageNet VGG19 model had fully connected (FC) three layers with 4096, 4096, and 1000 nodes, followed by a softmax layer to classify 1000 objects. We changed the last four layers with FC 512, 50, and 1 node, followed by a sigmoid layer for binary classification of healthy cough versus non-cough (**I2H** model) or COVID-19 cough versus non-cough (**I2C** model). Compared to the **I2H** or **I2C** model, we add four additional convolutional layers and a pooling layer in the case of **H2C** models.

We used TensorFlow and Keras libraries to develop our models. We used the ReLU activation function in the hidden layers and the sigmoid decision function in the final layer for every model. For the loss function, we used binary cross-entropy. We tried Adam and RMSprop optimizer and found Adam achieves 53% higher accuracy than the RMSprop. We also tried batch sizes 16 and 32 and found that batch size 16 is more accurate and has a shorter execution time. The input size used in this work is (320,320). We considered a range of learning rates, including 0.00001, 0.0001, and 0.0005, and epochs ranging from 30 to 200. We found a learning rate of 0.0001 works better for the **I2H** and **I2C** models. Similarly, we found a learning rate of 0.00001 is a good compromise for the **H2C** models. We developed models on Purdue University's Gilbreth GPU server with 8 GPU nodes and 16 cores per node [5]. Each node has 192 GB memory, 100 Gbps Infiniband interconnects, and 2 P100 GPUs.

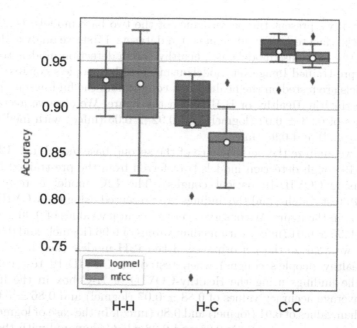

Fig. 4. **I2H** and **I2C** models tested on different coughs (H-H refers to the case when **I2H** models are tested on healthy coughs; similarly, H-C and C-C refer to the cases when **I2H** and **I2C** models are tested on COVID-19 coughs)

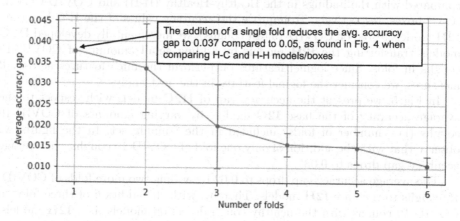

The addition of a single fold reduces the avg. accuracy gap to 0.037 compared to 0.05, as found in Fig. 4 when comparing H-C and H-H models/boxes

Fig. 5. Performance of **H2C** models developed using transfer learning incrementally by adding folds of COVID-19 coughs to **I2H** models

3   Results

Since we use the mutually exclusive folds with the same number of cough and non-cough instances in each fold (Sect. 2.3) when developing binary models, our classes are always balanced, and we use classification accuracy when comparing the performance of different models.

In Fig. 4, we present the performance of the two base models, i.e., **I2H** and **I2C** models when tested on different cough datasets. First, we analyze the performance of the **I2H** base models, i.e., healthy cough detection models transferred from the pre-trained ImageNet models using healthy people's coughs. The **I2H** base models are tested on the healthy test coughs, and the findings are presented using the Healthy-Healthy or H-H box in the figure. We observe average accuracy values of 0.93 ± 0.02 (logmel) and 0.92 ± 0.05 (mfcc) with median values of 0.93 (logmel) and 0.93 (mfcc).

Next, we analyze the performance of the second base model, i.e., **I2C** model (COVID-19 cough detection models transferred from the pre-trained ImageNet models using COVID-19 patient coughs). The **I2C** model is tested on the COVID-19 test coughs, and the findings are presented using the COVID-COVID or C-C box in the figure. We observe average accuracy values of 0.96 ± 0.02 (logmel) and 0.95 ± 0.01 (mfcc) with median values of 0.96 (logmel) and 0.95 (mfcc).

Next, we analyze the performance of the **I2H** models (i.e., base models to detect healthy people's coughs) when tested on COVID-19 test coughs and present the findings using the Healthy-COVID or H-C box in the figure. We observe average accuracy values of 0.88 ± 0.07 (logmel) and 0.86 ± 0.03 (mfcc) with median values of 0.91 (logmel) and 0.86 (mfcc). In the case of logmel feature, the drop in average accuracy is 0.05 and 0.08 when compared with the findings in the Healthy-Healthy (H-H) and COVID-COVID (C-C) boxes, respectively. In the case of mfcc feature, the drop in average accuracy is 0.06 and 0.09 when compared with the findings in the Healthy-Healthy (H-H) and COVID-COVID (C-C) boxes, respectively. To improve the accuracy values of the H-C box (i.e., **I2H** models tested on COVID-19 test coughs), we incrementally developed **H2C** models transferring the **I2H** models by adding small amounts of COVID-19 coughs in folds. Since logmel features outperform the mfcc features across all measures, we consider the logmel features in the next analysis.

In Fig. 5, we present the accuracy gap of **H2C** models with respect to the average accuracy of the base **I2C** models by varying amounts of COVID-19 coughs (i.e., number of folds) included in the training set. In the figure, we observe that with the addition of only one fold of COVID-19 coughs, the average accuracy gap drops to 0.037.

The average accuracy gap drops to 0.02 by adding two more folds of COVID-19 coughs to the base **I2H** models. Thereby, with the addition of three folds of COVID-19 coughs with the healthy cough detection models, i.e., **I2H** models, we can achieve a performance close to that of the base COVID-19 detection model performance.

As we continue adding more folds of COVID-19 coughs to the base **I2H** models, we witness a drop in accuracy gap, and after adding all six folds of COVID-19 patient coughs, the accuracy gap drops to 0.01. Additionally, adding more folds makes the error bar tighter, reflecting more consistent accuracy values. Thereby, using this incremental transfer learning approach, we can develop COVID-19 detection models, such as **H2C** models, from the base healthy people's cough detection models, i.e., **I2H** models and smaller amounts of COVID-19 coughs to achieve very close performance to that of the base COVID-19 detection models, i.e., **I2C** models.

4   Conclusion and Discussion

This work attempts to utilize the power of transfer learning and similarities between two types of coughs, i.e., healthy and COVID-19 coughs, to incrementally develop new models requiring a relatively small set of patient coughs to achieve similar performance to that of the COVID-19 cough detection models trained from a bigger COVID-19 cough dataset. Our findings show the promise of utilizing healthy cough detection models to detect COVID-19 coughs after training with relatively fewer patient coughs.

This model can be useful to detect an early-onset novel respiratory virus with a smaller amount of relevant data. However, before generalizing the findings to similar or other problems, extended studies with a diverse population, diseases, and stages will be needed. While image feature-based transfer learning has been adopted in this feasibility work, in the future, other types of data, e.g., acoustic signals, can be utilized to adapt transfer learning models and can be compared with this feasibility work. This work and findings will also impact other domains of predictive modeling, including place of importance discovery [59, 65, 67, 70, 71], health condition monitoring [14, 42, 43, 57, 66, 72, 73] and well-being tracking [21, 29, 47, 50, 52, 55, 58, 60, 61], securing a user's cyber-physical space [10, 15, 16, 18, 19, 22, 32, 35, 49, 51, 53, 54, 62–64, 68, 69], as it presents the feasibility of developing predictive models with relatively small datasets to alternate the traditional approaches requiring large-scale datasets.

Acknowledgement. The authors would like to thank the Clifford B. Kinley Trust for funding this research.

References

1. Asthma: Steps in testing and diagnosis - Mayo Clinic. https://mayocl.in/3vPs3J7. Accessed Jan 2023
2. Audacity: Free, open source, cross-platform audio software. https://www.audacityteam.org/. Accessed Jan 2023
3. CDC: COVID-19 Testing. https://bit.ly/3nRjYOM. Accessed Jan 2023
4. COPD Symptoms and Diagnosis | American Lung Association. https://bit.ly/3hefi2f. Accessed Jan 2023
5. Gilbreth. https://www.rcac.purdue.edu/compute/gilbreth. Accessed Jan 2023
6. ImageNet. https://image-net.org/download.php/. Accessed Jan 2023
7. Pneumonia | Disease or Condition of the Week | CDC. https://bit.ly/35aOE7Q. Accessed Jan 2023
8. WHO Coronavirus (COVID-19) Dashboard. https://covid19.who.int/. Accessed Jan 2023
9. Aditi Pai: Survey: One third of wearable device owners stopped using them within six months. https://bit.ly/3yjuzrC. Accessed Jan 2023

10. Al Amin, M.T., Barua, S., Vhaduri, S., Rahman, A.: Load aware broadcast in mobile ad hoc networks. In: IEEE International Conference on Communications (ICC) (2009)
11. Amoh, J., Odame, K.: Deepcough: a deep convolutional neural network in a wearable cough detection system. In: 2015 IEEE Biomedical Circuits and Systems Conference (BioCAS), pp. 1–4. IEEE (2015)
12. Cai, J., Vhaduri, S., Luo, X.: Discovering covid-19 coughing and breathing patterns from unlabeled data using contrastive learning with varying pre-training domains. In: INTERSPEECH (2023)
13. Chang, Y., Jing, X., Ren, Z., Schuller, B.W.: Covnet: a transfer learning framework for automatic covid-19 detection from crowd-sourced cough sounds. Front. Digit. Health **3**, 799067 (2022)
14. Chen, C.Y., Vhaduri, S., Poellabauer, C.: Estimating sleep duration from temporal factors, daily activities, and smartphone use. In: IEEE Computer Society Computers, Software, and Applications Conference (COMPSAC) (2020)
15. Cheung, W., Vhaduri, S.: Context-dependent implicit authentication for wearable device users. In: IEEE International Symposium on Personal, Indoor, and Mobile Radio Communications (PIMRC) (2020)
16. Cheung, W., Vhaduri, S.: Continuous authentication of wearable device users from heart rate, gait, and breathing data. In: IEEE RAS & EMBS International Conference on Biomedical Robotics and Biomechatronics (BioRob) (2020)
17. Cohen-McFarlane, M., Goubran, R., Knoefel, F.: Novel coronavirus cough database: Nococoda. IEEE Access **8**, 154087–154094 (2020)
18. Dibbo, S.V.: SoK: model inversion attack landscape: taxonomy, challenges, and future roadmap. In: 2023 IEEE 36th Computer Security Foundations Symposium (CSF), pp. 439–456. IEEE (2023)
19. Dibbo, S.V., Cheung, W., Vhaduri, S.: On-phone CNN model-based implicit authentication to secure IoT wearables. In: EAI International Conference on Safety and Security in Internet of Things (SaSeIoT) (2021)
20. Dibbo, S.V., Kim, Y., Vhaduri, S.: Effect of noise on generic cough models. In: IEEE International Conference on Wearable and Implantable Body Sensor Networks (BSN) (2021)
21. Dibbo, S.V., Kim, Y., Vhaduri, S., Poellabauer, C.: Visualizing college students' geo-temporal context-varying significant phone call patterns. In: 2021 IEEE 9th International Conference on Healthcare Informatics (ICHI), pp. 381–385. IEEE (2021)
22. Dibbo, S.V., Moore, J.S., Kenyon, G.T., Teti, M.A.: Lcanets++: robust audio classification using multi-layer neural networks with lateral competition. arXiv preprint arXiv:2308.12882 (2023)
23. Drugman, T., et al.: Objective study of sensor relevance for automatic cough detection. IEEE J. Biomed. Health Inform. **17**(3), 699–707 (2013)
24. Elfaramawy, T., Fall, C.L., Arab, S., Morissette, M., Lellouche, F., Gosselin, B.: A wireless respiratory monitoring system using a wearable patch sensor network. IEEE Sens. J. **19**(2), 650–657 (2018)
25. Gemmeke, J.F., et al.: Audio set: an ontology and human-labeled dataset for audio events. In: 2017 IEEE International Conference on Acoustics, Speech and Signal Processing (ICASSP), pp. 776–780. IEEE (2017)
26. Hui, X., Zhou, J., Sharma, P., Conroy, T.B., Zhang, Z., Kan, E.C.: Wearable RF near-field cough monitoring by frequency-time deep learning. IEEE Trans. Biomed. Circuits Syst. **15**(4), 756–764 (2021)

27. Imran, A., et al.: Ai4covid-19: AI enabled preliminary diagnosis for covid-19 from cough samples via an app. Inform. Med. Unlocked **20**, 100378 (2020)

28. Kamei, T., Kanamori, T., Yamamoto, Y., Edirippulige, S.: The use of wearable devices in chronic disease management to enhance adherence and improve tele-health outcomes: a systematic review and meta-analysis. J. Telemed. Telecare **28**(5), 342–359 (2022)

29. Kim, Y., Vhaduri, S., Poellabauer, C.: Understanding college students' phone call behaviors towards a sustainable mobile health and wellbeing solution. In: International Conference on Systems Engineering (2020)

30. Laguarta, J., Hueto, F., Subirana, B.: Covid-19 artificial intelligence diagnosis using only cough recordings. IEEE Open J. Eng. Med. Biol. **1**, 275–281 (2020)

31. Liaqat, D., et al.: Coughwatch: real-world cough detection using smartwatches. In: ICASSP 2021-2021 IEEE International Conference on Acoustics, Speech and Signal Processing (ICASSP), pp. 8333–8337. IEEE (2021)

32. Lien, C.W., Vhaduri, S.: Challenges and opportunities of biometric user authentication in the age of IoT: a survey. ACM Comput. Surv. **55**(12), 1–39 (2023)

33. McFee, B., et al.: Librosa: audio and music signal analysis in python. In: Proceedings of the 14th Python in Science Conference, vol. 8, pp. 18–25 (2015)

34. Meng, H., Yan, T., Yuan, F., Wei, H.: Speech emotion recognition from 3D log-mel spectrograms with deep learning network. IEEE Access **7**, 125868–125881 (2019)

35. Muratyan, A., Cheung, W., Dibbo, S.V., Vhaduri, S.: Opportunistic multi-modal user authentication for health-tracking IoT wearables. In: EAI International Conference on Safety and Security in Internet of Things (SaSeIoT) (2021)

36. Orlandic, L., Teijeiro, T., Atienza, D.: The coughvid crowdsourcing dataset, a corpus for the study of large-scale cough analysis algorithms. Sci. Data **8**(1), 1–10 (2021)

37. Pahar, M., Klopper, M., Warren, R., Niesler, T.: Covid-19 cough classification using machine learning and global smartphone recordings. Comput. Biol. Med. **135**, 104572 (2021)

38. Pahar, M., Niesler, T.: Machine learning based covid-19 detection from smartphone recordings: cough, breath and speech. arXiv pre-print (2021)

39. Piczak, K.J.: ESC: dataset for environmental sound classification. In: Proceedings of the 23rd ACM International Conference on Multimedia, pp. 1015–1018 (2015)

40. Richards, F., et al.: Economic burden of covid-19: a systematic review. ClinicoEconomics Outcomes Res. CEOR **14**, 293 (2022)

41. Sharma, N., et al.: Coswara–a database of breathing, cough, and voice sounds for covid-19 diagnosis. arXiv preprint arXiv:2005.10548 (2020)

42. Sharmin, M., et al.: Visualization of time-series sensor data to inform the design of just-in-time adaptive stress interventions. In: Proceedings of the 2015 ACM International Joint Conference on Pervasive and Ubiquitous Computing, pp. 505–516 (2015)

43. Simhadri, S., Vhaduri, S.: Understanding user trust in different recommenders and smartphone applications. In: EAI International Conference on Wireless Mobile Communication and Healthcare (MobiHealth) (2022)

44. Simonyan, K., Zisserman, A.: Very deep convolutional networks for large-scale image recognition. arXiv preprint arXiv:1409.1556 (2014)

45. Stojanović, R., Škraba, A., Lutovac, B.: A headset like wearable device to track covid-19 symptoms. In: 2020 9th Mediterranean Conference on Embedded Computing (MECO), pp. 1–4. IEEE (2020)

46. Vhaduri, S.: Nocturnal cough and snore detection using smartphones in presence of multiple background-noises. In: ACM SIGCAS Conference on Computing and Sustainable Societies (COMPASS) (2020)

47. Vhaduri, S., Ali, A., Sharmin, M., Hovsepian, K., Kumar, S.: Estimating drivers' stress from GPS traces. In: International Conference on Automotive User Interfaces and Interactive Vehicular Applications (AutomotiveUI) (2014)

48. Vhaduri, S., Brunschwiler, T.: Towards automatic cough and snore detection. In: IEEE International Conference on Healthcare Informatics (ICHI) (2019)

49. Vhaduri, S., Cheung, W., Dibbo, S.V.: Bag of on-phone ANNs to secure IoT objects using wearable and smartphone biometrics. IEEE Trans. Dependable Secure Comput. **20**(3), 1–12 (2023)

50. Vhaduri, S., Cho, J., Meng, K.: Predicting unreliable response patterns in smartphone health surveys: a case study with the mood survey. Smart Health J. **28**, 100398 (2023)

51. Vhaduri, S., Dibbo, S.V., Chen, C.Y.: Predicting a user's demographic identity from leaked samples of health-tracking wearables and understanding associated risks. In: 2022 IEEE 10th International Conference on Healthcare Informatics (ICHI). IEEE (2022)

52. Vhaduri, S., Dibbo, S.V., Chen, C.Y., Poellabauer, C.: Predicting next call duration: a future direction to promote mental health in the age of lockdown. In: IEEE Computer Society Computers, Software, and Applications Conference (COMPSAC) (2021)

53. Vhaduri, S., Dibbo, S.V., Cheung, W.: HIAuth: a hierarchical implicit authentication system for IoT wearables using multiple biometrics. IEEE Access **9**, 116395–116406 (2021)

54. Vhaduri, S., Dibbo, S.V., Cheung, W.: Implicit IoT authentication using on-phone ANN models and breathing data. Internet Things **24** (2023)

55. Vhaduri, S., Dibbo, S.V., Kim, Y.: Deriving college students' phone call patterns to improve student life. IEEE Access **9**, 96453–96465 (2021)

56. Vhaduri, S., Dibbo, S.V., Kim, Y.: Environment knowledge-driven generic models to detect coughs from audio recordings. IEEE Open J. Eng. Med. Biol. **4**, 1–12 (2023)

57. Vhaduri, S., Munch, A., Poellabauer, C.: Assessing health trends of college students using smartphones. In: IEEE Healthcare Innovation Point-of-Care Technologies Conference (HI-POCT) (2016)

58. Vhaduri, S., Poellabauer, C.: Design and implementation of a remotely configurable and manageable well-being study. In: EAI SWIT-Health (2015)

59. Vhaduri, S., Poellabauer, C.: Cooperative discovery of personal places from location traces. In: International Conference on Computer Communication and Networks (ICCCN) (2016)

60. Vhaduri, S., Poellabauer, C.: Human factors in the design of longitudinal smartphone-based wellness surveys. In: IEEE International Conference on Healthcare Informatics (ICHI) (2016)

61. Vhaduri, S., Poellabauer, C.: Design factors of longitudinal smartphone-based health surveys. J. Healthc. Inform. Res. **1**(1), 52–91 (2017)

62. Vhaduri, S., Poellabauer, C.: Towards reliable wearable-user identification. In: 2017 IEEE International Conference on Healthcare Informatics (ICHI) (2017)

63. Vhaduri, S., Poellabauer, C.: Wearable device user authentication using physiological and behavioral metrics. In: IEEE International Symposium on Personal, Indoor, and Mobile Radio Communications (PIMRC) (2017)

64. Vhaduri, S., Poellabauer, C.: Biometric-based wearable user authentication during sedentary and non-sedentary periods. International Workshop on Security and Privacy for the Internet-of-Things (IoTSec) (2018)

65. Vhaduri, S., Poellabauer, C.: Hierarchical cooperative discovery of personal places from location traces. IEEE Trans. Mob. Comput. **17**(8), 1865–1878 (2018)

66. Vhaduri, S., Poellabauer, C.: Impact of different pre-sleep phone use patterns on sleep quality. In: IEEE International Conference on Wearable and Implantable Body Sensor Networks (BSN) (2018)

67. Vhaduri, S., Poellabauer, C.: Opportunistic discovery of personal places using smartphone and fitness tracker data. In: IEEE International Conference on Healthcare Informatics (ICHI) (2018)

68. Vhaduri, S., Poellabauer, C.: Multi-modal biometric-based implicit authentication of wearable device users. IEEE Trans. Inf. Forensics Secur. **14**(12), 3116–3125 (2019)

69. Vhaduri, S., Poellabauer, C.: Summary: Multi-modal Biometric-based Implicit Authentication of Wearable Device Users. arXiv preprint arXiv:1907.06563 (2019)

70. Vhaduri, S., Poellabauer, C.: Opportunistic discovery of personal places using multi-source sensor data. IEEE Trans. Big Data **7**(2), 383–396 (2021)

71. Vhaduri, S., Poellabauer, C., Striegel, A., Lizardo, O., Hachen, D.: Discovering places of interest using sensor data from smartphones and wearables. In: IEEE Ubiquitous Intelligence & Computing (UIC) (2017)

72. Vhaduri, S., Prioleau, T.: Adherence to personal health devices: a case study in diabetes management. In: EAI International Conference on Pervasive Computing Technologies for Healthcare (PervasiveHealth) (2020)

73. Vhaduri, S., Simhadri, S.: Understanding user concerns and choice of app architectures in designing audio-based mHealth apps. Smart Health J. **26**, 100341 (2022)

74. Vhaduri, S., Van Kessel, T., Ko, B., Wood, D., Wang, S., Brunschwiler, T.: Nocturnal cough and snore detection in noisy environments using smartphone-microphones. In: IEEE International Conference on Healthcare Informatics (ICHI) (2019)

EEG Monitoring in Driving Using Embedded Systems

Rui Alves[1(✉)] and Paulo Matos[2,3]

[1] Instituto Politécnico de Bragança, Bragança, Portugal
rui.alves@ipb.pt
[2] Research Centre in Digitalization and Intelligent Robotics (CeDRI), Instituto
Politécnico de Bragança, Campus de Santa Apolónia, 5300-253 Bragança, Portugal
pmatos@ipb.pt
[3] Laboratório para a Sustentabilidade e Tecnologia em Regiões de Montanha
(SusTEC), Instituto Politécnico de Bragança, Campus de Santa Apolónia,
5300-253 Bragança, Portugal

Abstract. Epilepsy is a disease that can appear in all age groups, where many patients only have their diagnoses confirmed at more advanced ages and at different stages of their life. This disease manifests through partial and/or total seizures. To avoid more drastic consequences, an accurate diagnosis of seizures is essential to provide the correct medication to the patient. Although many patients are able to control seizures using a single drug, others need multiple medications or even complementary measures. In addition, epilepsy can make the quality of life substantially difficult due to seizures, however, it can also reduce the autonomy of patients in day-to-day tasks such as driving - in most countries, after the diagnosis of epilepsy, the patient is inhibited from driving for a period of time. This paper, through a set of chips and sensors, provides a solution to identify seizures through the study of a patient's electroencephalogram (EEG) waves, then applies several safety measures to protect the patient while driving.

Keywords: Epilepsy · Sensors · Driving · IoT · Edge Computing

1 Introduction

Epilepsy [1] is a disease in the brain, which affects both sexes and all ages and is mainly characterized by generating seizures. These seizures [2] have been defined by the International League Against Epilepsy as the transient occurrence of signs and/or symptoms as a result of abnormal, excessive, or synchronous neuronal brain activity. The root cause of these seizures currently isn't totally known, may result from trauma, hereditary disease, or an unknown cause. In this way,

The authors are grateful to the Foundation for Science and Technology (FCT, Portugal) for financial support through national funds FCT/MCTES (PIDDAC) to CeDRI (UIDB/05757/2020 and UIDP/05757/2020) and SusTEC (LA/P/0007/2021).

A. Cunha et al. (Eds.): MobiHealth 2023, LNICST 578, pp. 460–465, 2024.
https://doi.org/10.1007/978-3-031-60665-6_34

in 1989 [3], the International League Against Epilepsy proposed a classification of epilepsies and epileptic syndrome, grouping them by their symptoms (generalized or focal) and by their etiology (idiopathic and symptomatic).

However, regardless of the cause, the consequences [4] of this disease can be quite severe, including, for example, reduced life expectancy, risk of serious bodily injury, among others. There is even evidence that seizures cause brain damage, including neuronal death and physiological dysfunction. Controlling seizures is vital for the patient's quality of life to be impaired as much as possible since seizures potentially pose a serious threat to health and well-being.

One of the leading social consequences of people with epilepsy is severe driving restrictions [5]. An epileptic seizure leads to loss of situational awareness, which can have very serious consequences, particularly if such seizures occur while the patient is driving, putting the patient and other people's lives at risk. Therefore, when this disease is diagnosed, patients cannot, or at least should not, drive. Evidence shows that in the absence of seizures, the risk of accidents and injuries is reduced and tends to be close to that of the general population. However, the variability of published reports on risk led to several regulations, where each country developed its own rules on epilepsy and driving.

This paper, using a set of chips and sensors, provides a possible solution for monitoring people, diagnosed with epilepsy, while they are driving. This monitoring is performed by processing the EEC waves, using intelligent algorithms on the received data. The results of this analysis are mitigation measures in the vehicle to avoid accidents or other injuries.

The remaining of this paper is organized as follows: in Sect. 2 are described the solutions similar to the illustrated; the technical details of the proposed solution are described in Sect. 3; the preliminary results of some tests already performed are described in Sect. 4; in Sect. 5 is detailed the conclusions and directions for future work.

2 Related Work

Some solutions similar to the approach presented in this paper were found in the state of the art. In [6] is described a solution that intends to improve the emergency braking system, using the analysis of the EEG waves, however, the study of this solution makes no reference to the detection of seizures.

In [7], another approach using IoT and EEG waves is described for driver fatigue analysis. The main idea of this approach is to monitor the cerebral waves and heartbeat to identify fatigue while driving.

Adapted from the Automotive Open System Architecture (AUTOSAR) framework, the main idea of this solution [8] focuses on predicting driver performance before starting driving, based on the waves of EEG, however, as in previous solutions, there is no reference to seizures.

In [9] the authors propose an EEG acquisition and emotion classification scheme in a simulated driving environment. The scheme uses vehicle speed as a variable to simulate different danger levels and evaluate driver capability to avoid obstacles under such conditions. The approach does not focus on epileptic seizure but shares the same effort of capturing and processing the EEG signals.

In [10] is presented a review on physiological signal-based emotion recognition, an approach that among other applications, is also used in the implementation of solutions and technologies for safety driving. The review includes emotion models, emotion elicitation methods, emotional physiological datasets, features, classifiers, and emotion recognition based on physiological signals.

A literature review of the state-of-the-art of emotion recognition systems from EEG signals was published by [11]. Besides a summary of definitions and theories, the authors evaluated several deep learning and shallow machine learning approaches, considering methods, classifiers, number of classified emotions, accuracy, and datasets. It is an important work for a broader perception of what has been done recently in this area.

3   Proposed Solution

The proposal is based on a client-server architecture as can be analyzed in Fig. 1. The client component placed inside the car is an IoT module able to communicate using both LTE/NB-IoT and Bluetooth Low Energy (BLE). It also uses NeuroSky EEG biosensors to collect EEG signals, which must be coupled to the driver.

NeuroSky EEG biosensors allow accurate capture of the brain's electrical signals. It is very similar to a pair of headphones, as such, it is portable and not very intrusive, it doesn't constrain the driver's movements, its placement is easily carried out by the driver itself and it is quite affordable (when compared with traditional solutions).

NeuroSky EEG Biosensor collects the brain's EEG signals and transmits them via BLE to the IoT module. This one, using the LTE/NB-IoT sends the collected signals to the cloud through a broker. Once on the cloud, the signals are processed aiming to identify suspicious or alarming patterns. If such patterns are identified, an alert message is sent to the IoT module with the severity of the identified pattern. On the IoT module are evaluated the driving conditions, such as speed, proximity to obstacles, and other parameters may be useful to define the action to be taken. The action may involve warning the driver to stop the vehicle or a direct intervention, for example, reducing the speed or immobilizing the vehicle. It's important to note that the IoT chip must be able to inject instructions into the car controller (e.g. stop instruction).

In addition, alerts may be issued to emergency contacts registered on the platform (cloud) or, if identified by the IoT module, it may request urgent intervention (in case of crash, shock, collision, ...).

The server part, hosted in the cloud, consists of:

- A set of ML algorithms that process the EEG signals coming from the client, aiming to identify possible indications of an epileptic seizure.
- A web platform to monitor and validate the received signals and their results produced by the ML algorithms.

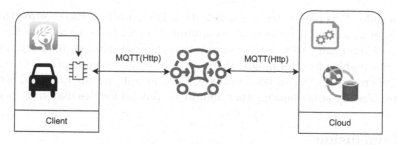

Fig. 1. Architecture of the proposed solution

- An alert system that will inform not only the driver, but also doctors, and possible emergency contacts.

4   Results

In general, the proof of concept was carried out, by collecting the data and sending it to the cloud. A pattern recognition process was simulated in terms of processing time and sending messages to the module. The reason why this was simulated is that we simply do not have data to create the recognition model (that replicates the brain signals we want to identify).

Decision-making by the IoT module on the action to be carried out and the respective action on the vehicle was also not included. This is because there is still work to be done here on what could be the inputs of the decision model, but mainly because we do not have, at least for now, the means to act on the vehicle.

Thus, even considering that there is a lot of work to be done and that some of it will be difficult to complete due to existing constraints, it has nevertheless been possible to validate the architecture operation model and, communication and processing latencies. The initial tests were performed in an ideal scenario, where the NB-IoT signal was strong and stable, minimizing possible impacts caused by data transmission. A latency of about 2% was obtained, however, the scenario used was not close to the real one (with the car in progress), which indicates that this latency can worsen, as the moving car crosses several zones that may have better and/or worse signal for data transmission.

We have no idea whether this latency is, or is not, critical for timely action. The impact of this latency is directly related with the time that goes from the moment that occur the alarm pattern and moment that the driver shouldn't be driving the vehicle. If this is very short, in the order of milliseconds or even a few seconds, than the latency will be very critical. If it take more time, like several seconds or even minutes, the latency might not be relevant. We will only be able to answer this question when we have real data of epilepsies episodes.

In either case, an alternative architecture has already been devised, based on edge computing, in which pattern recognition is carried out directly in the

IoT module. This eliminates communication latencies but also ensures that the solution works, even if there is no communication with the cloud. On the other hand, it is necessary to test which modules (processing units, memory, and the like) are capable of performing this function in a timely manner.

Furthermore, in the authors' opinion, the concept and the idealized architecture are already contributions that should be put up for discussion by peers.

5   Conclusion

This paper presents promising contributions to ensure the solution for patients with epilepsy while driving. The creation of this type of solution enables better control and monitoring of possible crises while driving, allowing one to take mitigation measures to reduce the existing risks of a possible crisis while driving, increasing the safety of the epilepsy patient and the people around him. In addition, as previously mentioned, after the diagnosis of the disease, patients are required by law to comply with a period of driving inhibition. Driving inhibition nowadays easily becomes a problem because it limits and reduces the quality of life of patients with epilepsy since they become dependent on others to perform their daily tasks. Thus, solutions similar to that presented in this paper may contribute to reducing this period of inhibition, or even in some cases cause it to cease to be mandatory.

However, despite the advantages there are still a set of limitations identified during the development process. At the cybersecurity level, a new attack vector is available, as this type of solution needs to inject instructions into the car controller in cases of seizure detection. In addition, it is also necessary to work on the circumstances in which the vehicle is stopped, as an abrupt stop calls into question the safety of other vehicles on the road.

In terms of seizure detection, it should be noted that there is a varied set of epilepsy [12] with very small variations that do not allow ML algorithms to be identified without the help of a health professional. Finally, data transmission is another point that can be problematic since the system is reactive and needs coverage either LTE or NB-IoT [13] to send data and receive responses. Thus, it is necessary to think of a better solution to ensure detection in areas without network coverage in order to ensure a similar level of security or explore the alternative architecture, based on edge computing.

5.1   Future Work

Despite the potential of the solution, the current state of development does not allow to evaluate the solution under real scenarios yet. The following points were left for future work: evaluate the feasibility and adequacy of the distinct communication technologies (LTE/NB-IoT or other); evaluate how far ML algorithms are able to detect the various types of epilepsy; mitigate the attack vector resulting from the need to take control of the car in the event of an epilepsy episode;

study the best approach to immobilize the vehicle, ensuring the safety of everyone - patients, passengers, and other drivers and passersby; and carry out a comparative analysis of the two approached architectures: cloud and edge computing, namely its suitability given cloud access limitations and computational demands of the ML algorithms.

References

1. Beghi, E.: The epidemiology of epilepsy. Neuroepidemiology **54**(2), 185–191 (2020)
2. Manole, A.M., et al.: State of the art and challenges in epilepsy–a narrative review. J. Pers. Med. **13**(4), 623 (2023)
3. Anwar, H., Khan, Q.U., Nadeem, N., Pervaiz, I., Ali, M., Cheema, F.F.: Epileptic seizures. Discoveries (Craiova) **8**(2), e110 (2020)
4. Sperling, M.R.: The consequences of uncontrolled epilepsy. CNS Spectr. **9**(2), 98–109 (2004)
5. Beghi, E., Sander, J.W.: Epilepsy and driving. BMJ **331**(7508), 60–61 (2005)
6. Nguyen, T.-H., Chung, W.-Y.: Detection of driver braking intention using EEG signals during simulated driving. Sensors **19**(13), 2863 (2019)
7. Irsan, M., et al.: A novel prototype for safe driving using embedded smart box system. Sensors **22**(5), 2022 (1907)
8. ElSherif, A., et al.: Monitoring and predicting driving performance using EEG activity. In: 2020 15th International Conference on Computer Engineering and Systems (ICCES), pp. 1–6 (2020)
9. Chen, J., Lin, X., Ma, W., Wang, Y., Tang, W.: EEG-based emotion recognition for road accidents in a simulated driving environment. Biomed. Signal Process. Control **87**, 105411 (2024)
10. Shu, L., et al.: A review of emotion recognition using physiological signals. Sensors **18**(7), 2074 (2018)
11. Islam, M.R., et al.: Emotion recognition from EEG signal focusing on deep learning and shallow learning techniques. IEEE Access **9**, 94601–94624 (2021)
12. Feng, Y.C.A., et al.: Ultra-rare genetic variation in the epilepsies: a whole-exome sequencing study of 17,606 individuals. Am. J. Hum. Genet. **105**(2), 267–282 (2019)
13. Zhang, G., Yao, C., Li, X.: Research on joint planning method of NB-IoT and LTE. Procedia Comput. Sci. **131**, 985–991 (2018)

Complex Systems and Optimal Pandemic Control

Automated Classification of Prostate Cancer Severity Using Pre-trained Models

Sílvia Barros[1], Vitor Filipe[1,2], and Lio Gonçalves[1,2(✉)]

[1] School of Science and Technology, University of Trás-os-Montes e Alto Douro
(UTAD), 5000-811 Vila Real, Portugal
silviab477@outlook.pt, {vfilipe,lgoncalv}@utad.pt
[2] INESC Technology and Science (INESC TEC), 4200-465 Porto, Portugal

Abstract. Prostate cancer is one of the most common types of cancer
in men. The ISUP grade and Gleason Score are terms related to the
classification of this cancer based on the histological characteristics of
the tissues examined in a biopsy. This paper explains an approach that
utilizes and evaluates pre-trained models such as ResNet-50, VGG19, and
InceptionV3, regarding their ability to automatically classify prostate
cancer and its severity based on images and masks annotated with ISUP
grades and Gleason Scores. At the end of the training, the performance
of each trained model is presented, as well as the comparison between
the original and predicted data. This comparison aims to understand if
this approach can indeed be used for a more automated classification of
prostate cancer.

Keywords: ISUP Grading · Gleason Score · Resnet-50 · VGG19 ·
InceptionV3

1 Introduction

Prostate cancer is currently one of the main cancers fought by the male population, being the most common in terms of occurrence and the second leading cause
of death. In Portugal, approximately 6000 cases of prostate cancer are diagnosed
each year, which accounts for twenty one percent of all cancers in males. This
translate to an average of one in six individuals who will be diagnosed with this
cancer in their lifetime, This leads us to conclude that in Portugal, as well as
in other countries, prostate cancer is considered a significant issue. In order to
study this cancer, a methodology was developed by Donald Gleason in 1960 [1].

The Gleason grading system is one of the most important factors in clinical
decision-making for prostate cancer patients [2]. It is entirely based on the classification of tumor growth patterns, and in recent years, it has become clear that
some individual growth patterns have independent prognostic value and can be
used to improve personalized risk stratification. By providing a standardized and
objective classification of tumor growth patterns, this grading system enables

A. Cunha et al. (Eds.): MobiHealth 2023, LNICST 578, pp. 469–482, 2024.
https://doi.org/10.1007/978-3-031-60665-6_35

physicians to assess disease progression and determine the optimal therapeutic approach for each patient, making it an important tool in the field of urology.

The Gleason score is a tissue-based prognostic marker for prostate cancer that suffers from variability, leading to inconsistencies and classification errors. As a result, artificial intelligence (AI) systems based on deep learning have emerged, showing promising results in achieving performance similar to that of pathologists in Gleason grading [4].

Over the years, the Gleason grading system has been enhanced with the use of artificial intelligence (AI). AI has been applied to the analysis of histopathological images from prostate biopsy samples, assisting pathologists in the classification of tumor growth patterns. In this regard, AI algorithms can be trained on large datasets containing histological images previously analyzed by experts. These algorithms can learn to identify and classify the different patterns of prostate cancer growth, providing automated and accurate evaluation. The integration of artificial intelligence into this grading system brings significant benefits, which can reduce inter-observer variability in the interpretation of growth patterns and improve result consistency.

The ISUP (International Society of Urological Pathology) classification is a grading system used to assess prostate cancer based on histological features observed in tissue samples examined by pathologists. This classification was developed by the International Society of Urological Pathology and is widely used to provide prognostic information and assist in treatment planning.

AI systems are trained on large datasets that contain information about tissue characteristics and patterns associated with different disease grades, and they can learn to automatically recognize and extract these patterns. This assists experts in accurately classifying the disease grade. Additionally, AI systems can be used to create prediction models that estimate the risk of disease progression based on Gleason and ISUP grading.

Wouter Bulten et al. [3] evaluated the impact of AI assistance on the diagnostic performance of pathologists in Gleason grading of prostate biopsies. The results showed that AI assistance significantly improved the performance of pathologists, reducing variability and leading to more consistent grading. The AI system outperformed most pathologists in the unassisted read, but the panel's performance surpassed that of the AI system in the assisted read. The study highlights the potential of AI systems to support pathologists in achieving higher accuracy and consistency in Gleason grading, particularly in regions with limited access to specialized pathologists. Further research and validation are needed to fully understand the benefits of AI assistance in clinical practice.

Wouter Bulten et al. [4] created the PANDA challenge. The PANDA challenge aimed to improve the Gleason grading of prostate cancer by using AI algorithms. The challenge organized a global competition and provided a large dataset for algorithm development and validation. The dataset included over 12,000 prostate biopsy images from different sites. Experienced uropathologists established reference standards for the training and validation sets, ensuring consistency across different regions. The competition attracted teams from 65 countries, and the algorithms submitted by the teams were blindly validated on an internal validation set. The top-performing algorithms utilized deep learning methods and demonstrated high agreement with the uropathologists. In the external validation sets, the algorithms showed high agreement with the reference standards, although they had a tendency to overdiagnose benign cases as low-grade cancer. The algorithms performed better than general pathologists in terms of sensitivity but had lower specificity in correctly identifying benign cases. Overall, the AI algorithms achieved pathologist-level concordance and outperformed previous methods. However, the study had limitations, such as a limited number of participating teams and a focus on specific cancer types. Further research is needed for broader evaluation and to address potential errors.

According to Kimmo Kartasalo et al. [5], the use of artificial intelligence (AI) systems for diagnosing and grading prostate cancer in biopsies shows promise in overcoming the variability between pathologists. AI systems have demonstrated high accuracy in cancer detection and Gleason grading, comparable to expert pathologists. However, further validation using diverse and independent datasets is needed before clinical implementation. Challenges include the need for larger and more diverse training datasets, the ability to recognize benign mimics of cancer, and the development of anomaly detection systems for quality control. Future developments may involve training AI algorithms using long-term follow-up data for improved prognostication.

According to Lars Egevad et al. [6] Standardization in pathology grading, particularly for prostate cancer, is crucial for accurate diagnosis and treatment decisions. While the Gleason grading system has been widely used, variability among pathologists and evolving definitions have led to disagreements. Pathology Imagebase and AI technology offer opportunities to overcome these challenges by providing a standardized reference and assisting in grading. Collaborative efforts between experts, AI developers, and pathologists are essential to refine and validate these tools, leading to improved consistency and precision in prostate cancer grading, ultimately benefiting patient care.

Felicia Marginean et al. [7] demonstrates the potential of artificial intelligence (AI) in addressing the challenges of Gleason grading variability in prostate cancer diagnosis. The AI algorithm trained on annotated biopsy scans showed high accuracy and reproducibility in detecting cancer and assigning Gleason grades. These holds promise for improving the consistency and efficiency of diagnostic processes, reducing the burden on pathologists, and potentially enhancing patient outcomes. The findings highlight the importance of leveraging AI and medical image analysis to standardize and optimize diagnostic practices in prostate cancer and pave the way for future advancements in AI-assisted pathology.

Liron Pantanowitz et al. [8] focuses on the development and validation of an AI algorithm for prostate cancer diagnosis and Gleason grading. The algorithm exhibited high accuracy in distinguishing between low-grade (Gleason score 6 or ASAP) and high-grade (Gleason score 7–10) tumors, as well as detecting the presence of Gleason pattern 5. The algorithm's performance surpassed previous studies and addressed the limitations of narrow AI approaches. Its successful deployment in routine clinical practice has the potential to improve diagnostic accuracy, reduce interobserver variability in Gleason grading, and provide valuable insights for treatment planning in prostate cancer.

This paper highlights the training of a network that aims to detect and classify the severity of prostate cancer in images of prostate tissue samples that have been previously analyzed and scored by pathologists according to the Gleason system, which is then converted into an ISUP grade.

Therefore, this paper is divided into sections such as Materials and Methods, Results, Discussion and Conclusion. All sections are written with the aim of providing the reader with a clear explanation of the topic.

2   Material and Methods

2.1   Dataset

To carry out the research, a database provided by the Karolinska Institute and the Radboud University Medical Center was used. It includes:

- A folder containing 10,616 images in TIFF format, with 5,455 images provided by the Karolinska Institute and 5,060 images by the Radboud University Medical Center;
- A folder containing segmentation masks that show which parts of the image contributed to the ISUP grade. Not all training images have label masks, and there may be false positives or false negatives in the masks. These masks are provided to assist in the development of strategies for selecting the most useful image subsets, and their values depend on the data provider; Considering this, the number of images without labeled masks was checked, and a new dataframe was created that removes the rows from the training file where masks are missing.
- A CSV file containing information, such as the ISUP grade and the Gleason Score of each image, corresponding to the training data (train.csv). Their distribution is shown in the Figs. 1.
- A folder with pre-trained models, including ResNet-50, VGG19 and InceptionV3.

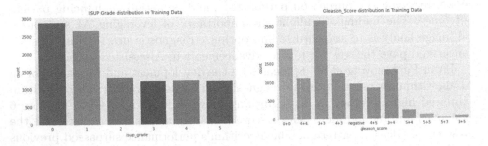

Fig. 1. ISUP Grade and Gleason Score Distribution in Training Data

	isup_grade	image_id
0	0	2873
1	1	2616
2	2	1340
4	4	1245
3	3	1226
5	5	1215

	gleason_score	image_id
1	3+3	2616
0	0+0	1925
2	3+4	1340
4	4+3	1226
5	4+4	1122
10	negative	948
6	4+5	842
8	5+4	248
9	5+5	125
3	3+5	80
7	5+3	43

Fig. 2. Clustering and classification of the data through a color gradient

2.2 Training Images and Masks

As previously described, the masks from the utilized dataset were provided to locate the cancer and aid in understanding each grade of the disease. Thus, the images were displayed along with their corresponding masks. This process is highly useful as it helps visualize the histological patterns present in a tissue sample. The Gleason score and ISUP classification are based on the analysis of these patterns, and the display of images allows for the observation of microscopic details and a better interpretation of tissue characteristics. One training image and corresponding mask is shown in Fig. 3.

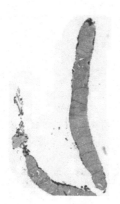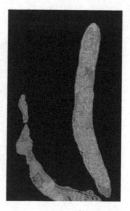

Fig. 3. Image and corresponding mask. Source: Radboud, ISUP:5 and Gleason: 5+4.

2.3   Data Preprocessing

In the Gleason scoring system, there is no ISUP = 2 for a Gleason score of 4+3. Therefore, the existence of images with this classification was verified, and only one was found, which was later removed. After completing this process, the data was clustered to combine the ISUP classification and the Gleason score with the image IDs, as shown in the Fig. 2. The colors present in the tables aim to assist in the analysis and interpretation of the data.

In order to better understand the dataset, the idea arose to replace the "negative" values with "0+0" to have a consistent classification for this value. To achieve this, the data was grouped again, resulting in the graph represented in the Fig. 4. Through analysis, we can observe that the Radboud dataframe does not have "0+0" values, while the Karolinska dataframe does not have "negative" values. Therefore, we conclude that the "negative" values correspond to how Radboud represents "0+0" values. Thus, for the sake of consistency, the "negative" values were replaced with "0+0" (Fig. 5).

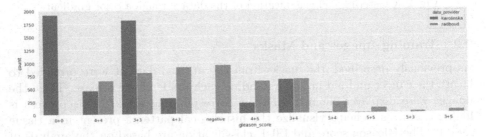

Fig. 4. Count of each Gleason Score value for each data provider institution

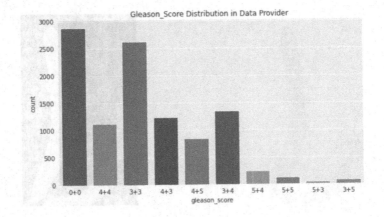

Fig. 5. Gleason Score Distribution after the Replacement

2.4   Gleason Grading and ISUP Classification

The Gleason classification and the ISUP classification are systems used to assess the severity of prostate cancer based on microscopic analysis of tissue samples obtained through biopsy.

The Gleason classification evaluates the appearance of cancer cells in the tissue sample. It consists of a primary Gleason score, which represents the dominant area, and a secondary Gleason score, which represents the second most prevalent area. Both scores range from 1 to 5 and are summed to obtain the total Gleason score, which ranges from 2 to 10. The higher the total Gleason score, the more severe the cancer.

The ISUP classification (International Society of Urological Pathology) is a newer classification system that aims to simplify the interpretation of the Gleason score. It groups Gleason scores into five categories, from 1 to 5. Category 1 corresponds to a Gleason score of 6, category 2 corresponds to Gleason scores of $3+4=7$ or $3+3=6$ with cribriform pattern, category 3 corresponds to Gleason scores of $3+4=7$ or $4+3=7$ without cribriform pattern, category 4 corresponds to Gleason scores of $4+4=8$ or $3+5=8$ or $5+3=8$, and category 5 corresponds to Gleason scores of 9 and 10. The ISUP classification aims to provide a simplified and standardized assessment of the severity of prostate cancer.

The training file in CSV format contains annotations for each image, including both the Gleason and ISUP classifications such as the image ID and the data provider. This can be seen in Fig. 6.

2.5   Resnet-50

The ResNet-50 model is a highly effective approach for image classification tasks, particularly in the field of prostate cancer analysis. By utilizing pre-trained

	image_id	data_provider	isup_grade	gleason_score
0	0005f7aaab2800f6170c399693a96917	karolinska	0	0+0
1	000920ad0b612851f8e01bcc880d9b3d	karolinska	0	0+0
2	0018ae58b01bdadc8e347995b69f99aa	radboud	4	4+4
3	001c62abd11fa4b57bf7a6c603a11bb9	karolinska	4	4+4
4	001d865e65ef5d2579c190a0e0350d8f	karolinska	0	0+0
5	002a4db09dad406c85505a00fb6f6144	karolinska	0	0+0
6	003046e27c8ead3e3db155780dc5498e	karolinska	1	3+3
7	0032bfa835ce0f43a92ae0bbab6871cb	karolinska	1	3+3
8	003a91841da04a5a31f808fb5c21538a	karolinska	1	3+3
9	003d4dd6bd61221ebc0bfb9350db333f	karolinska	1	3+3

Fig. 6. First 10 Lines of the Dataframe of the Training Data

weights from the "imagenet" dataset, the model leverages a wealth of learned visual features. Its deep architecture, with residual connections, allows for the extraction of intricate patterns and improved representation learning. Dropout regularization helps prevent overfitting, while the inclusion of a fully connected layer with ReLU activation enables nonlinear transformations. The RMSprop optimizer and binary cross-entropy loss function ensure efficient training and accurate predictions. Evaluation metrics such as binary accuracy and AUC provide a comprehensive assessment of the model's performance. By saving the trained model and visualizing the training history, researchers can effectively communicate the progress and capabilities of the model.

2.6 VGG19

The VGG19 model implementation in the study leverages the pre-trained weights from the "imagenet" dataset, allowing for the extraction of meaningful features from prostate cancer images. The architecture consists of multiple convolutional layers with 3×3 filters, maximizing feature extraction capabilities. Dropout regularization is applied to reduce overfitting, while dense layers with ReLU activation contribute to the classification process. The model is trained using the binary cross-entropy loss function and RMSprop optimizer, and key evaluation metrics such as accuracy and AUC are monitored. By visualizing the training history, the model's performance can be assessed, providing valuable insights for further research and application in prostate cancer detection.

2.7 InceptionV3

The InceptionV3 model, based on the Inception architecture, is employed in this research. Pre-trained weights from the "imagenet" dataset provide a strong initialization for the model. The architecture utilizes Inception modules with parallel convolutional layers of varying sizes to capture intricate features at different scales. Dropout regularization is incorporated to prevent overfitting, and a fully connected layer with 32 units and ReLU activation is added.

The final output layer utilizes the softmax activation function to produce class probabilities. The model is compiled with binary cross-entropy loss and the RMSprop optimizer, while evaluation metrics such as accuracy and AUC provide insight into its performance. During training, the fit-generator function is employed, allowing for efficient batch processing of the training and validation data. Callbacks for early stopping, model checkpointing, and learning rate scheduling contribute to better training results.

The trained model is saved, and the training history is visualized using plots that depict the loss, AUC, and accuracy curves for both the training and validation sets. This comprehensive implementation of the InceptionV3 model demonstrates its potential for accurate prostate cancer classification and can be a valuable contribution to research studies in the field.

3   Results

With the implementation of the models, three graphs were obtained representing the train and validation Loss, train and validation AUC, and train and validation Accuracy for each of them.

3.1   Performance of Resnet-50 Model

With the implementation of the ResNet-50 model, we were able to characterize its behavior by analyzing the curves of the graphs. The Train Loss curve behaves in a manner considered normal, indicating that the model is learning and reducing its loss during the training process. However, the Validation Loss curve suggests the presence of underfitting during model training. This indicates that the model was unable to sufficiently capture the complexity of the data and may not generalize well to unseen examples.

In the AUC graph, both the validation and training curves show an increasing trend as the model is trained. This indicates that the model is capturing and learning relevant discriminative patterns from the training data.

Analyzing the Accuracy graph, the train accuracy curve shows a positive behavior, indicating a good fit of the model to the training data. However, for a more detailed evaluation, it is necessary to consider the validation accuracy curve. In this case, it suggests that the model initially struggled to generalize well to the validation data but eventually improved its performance by adjusting to the patterns present in that data (Fig. 7).

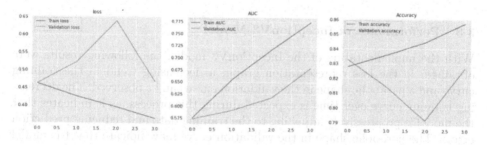

Fig. 7. Graphical Representation of the Metrics for the ResNet-50 model

3.2   Performance of VGG19 Model

With the implementation of the VGG19 model, we were able to analyze its performance using the same metrics. By examining the loss representation, we can observe that the Train Loss curve decreases during training, indicating that the error between the model's predictions and the actual values is decreasing. The

Validation Loss curve also decreases, indicating that the model's performance improves as it learns to make more accurate predictions on unseen data.

In the AUC graph, we can see that both the training and validation curves increase during training, indicating that the model's performance improves on both the training and validation data as it progresses. This means that the model becomes more capable of correctly distinguish between the classes of interest.

In the accuracy graph, we observe a similar behavior to the AUC curves. Both the training and validation curves increase during training, which can be the result of various improvements in the model, such as proper parameter tuning, appropriate feature selection, or regularization. The increasing curves indicate that the model becomes more skilled at making correct predictions and performs good generalization to new data (Fig. 8).

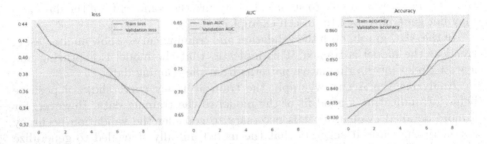

Fig. 8. Graphical Representation of the Metrics for the VGG19 model

3.3 Performance of InceptionV3 Model

With the implementation of the InceptionV3 model, the following results were obtained: in the loss representation graph, a decreasing trend in the training curve and a parabolic shape in the validation curve can be observed. The decreasing training curve over time is expected during this process, as it indicates that the model is progressively adjusting to the training data and reducing prediction errors. The parabolic shape in the validation curve may indicate that the model is reaching a point where it is overfitting to the training data, resulting in higher loss on the validation data.

In the AUC representation, an increase is observed in both the training and validation curves. This can be considered a positive sign, indicating that the model is learning to capture discriminative patterns in the training data and is able to generalize this learning to the validation data.

In the Accuracy representation, the training curve increases over time, while the validation curve initially decreases and then increases, with a slight decrease towards the end. The increasing training curve signifies that the model is fitting more closely to the training data. The shape of the validation curve indicates a common training pattern. The initial decrease suggests that the model is still learning to generalize the patterns from the training data to unseen data. The subsequent increase may represent natural fluctuations in the validation data or the introduction of more challenging training steps. Finally, the slight decrease observed could be a sign of overfitting, indicating that the model may be becoming too specific to the training data and does not generalize well to unseen data (Fig. 9).

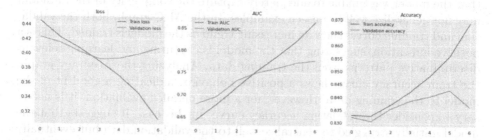

Fig. 9. Graphical Representation of the Metrics for the InceptionV3 model

3.4   Comparison Between the Data and the Predictions

Finally, a comparison was made between the ISUP grade of the original data and the predicted data for the first 40 rows of the validation file. This comparison revealed that the ISUP grade in the original data and the predicted data coincided, as shown in the Fig. 10.

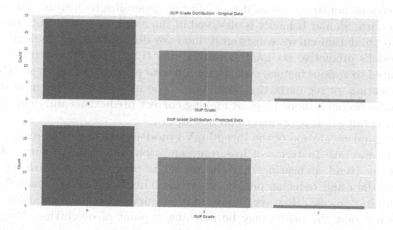

Fig. 10. Comparison between the data and the predictions

4   Discussion

The results obtained with the implementation of the ResNet-50 model show a mixed behavior in terms of the model's performance. On one hand, the Train Loss curve follows an expected trend, gradually decreasing during training, indicating that the model is learning and reducing its error as it is exposed to more data. However, the Validation Loss curve suggests the presence of underfitting, indicating that the model was unable to adequately capture the complexity of the data and may not generalize well to unseen examples. In the AUC graph, both the validation and training curves show an increasing trend as the model is trained. This is a positive indication, suggesting that the model is capturing and learning relevant discriminative patterns from the training data. Analyzing the Accuracy graph, the train accuracy curve shows a positive behavior, indicating a good fit of the model to the training data. However, for a more detailed evaluation, it is necessary to consider the validation accuracy curve. In this case, it suggests that the model initially struggled to generalize well to the validation data but eventually improved its performance by adjusting to the patterns present in that data.

The results obtained with the implementation of the VGG19 model demonstrate positive performance across multiple metrics. In terms of loss, both the Train Loss curve and Validation Loss curve consistently decrease during training. This indicates that the model's predictions are becoming more accurate, as the error between the predicted values and the actual values decreases. This improvement suggests that the model is effectively learning to make accurate predictions on unseen data. The AUC graph further confirms the model's performance improvement. Both the training and validation curves exhibit an increasing trend as the model is trained. This indicates that the model is becoming more proficient at distinguishing between the classes of interest, as it captures and learns relevant discriminative patterns from the training data. The increasing curves demonstrate the model's ability to generalize its learning to new and unseen data. Similar behavior is observed in the accuracy graph. Both the training and validation curves consistently increase during training, indicating that the model's predictive accuracy improves over time. This improvement can be attributed to various factors, such as appropriate parameter tuning, suitable feature selection, or regularization techniques. The increasing curves indicate that the model becomes more adept at making correct predictions and demonstrates good generalization performance on new data.

The implementation of the InceptionV3 model yielded specific results across different metrics. In terms of loss representation, the training curve shows a decreasing trend, indicating that the model is progressively adjusting to the training data and reducing prediction errors. This behavior is expected during the training process. However, the validation curve exhibits a parabolic shape, suggesting that the model may be reaching a point of overfitting. Overfitting occurs when the model becomes too specific to the training data, resulting in higher loss on the validation data. This indicates that the model may struggle to generalize well to unseen data. Moving on to the AUC representation, both the training and validation curves display an increase. This is a positive indication, demonstrating that the model is successfully learning and capturing discriminative patterns from the training data. The ability to generalize this learning to the validation data suggests that the model is effectively identifying and distinguishing between different classes. Examining the accuracy representation, the training curve consistently increases over time. This signifies that the model is fitting more closely to the training data and improving its performance. On the other hand, the validation curve initially decreases and then gradually increases, with a slight decrease observed towards the end. The initial decrease suggests that the model is still in the process of learning to generalize the patterns from the training data to unseen data. The subsequent increase could be attributed to natural fluctuations in the validation data or the introduction of more challenging training steps. However, the slight decrease towards the end may indicate overfitting, implying that the model is becoming too specific to the training data and struggling to generalize well to unseen data.

The alignment observed in the comparison between the ISUP grade of the original and predicted data for the first 40 rows of the validation file indicates that the trained models were able to effectively learn the patterns present in the training data and generalize well to the same data (Fig. 11).

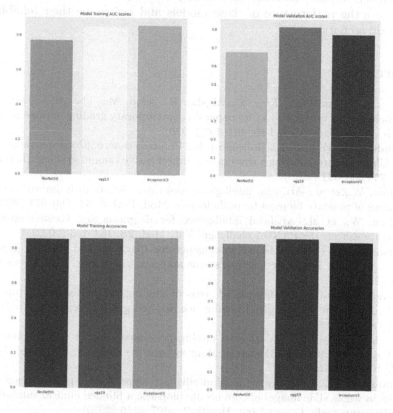

Fig. 11. Graphical representation of Training and Validation for each model

5   Conclusions

Based on these results, it can be concluded that this approach is potentially useful for determining the ISUP grade when provided with training data and masks that have annotated Gleason scores. The ResNet-50, VGG19, and InceptionV3 models demonstrated varying performances in capturing relevant patterns and generalizing to unseen data.

While the ResNet-50 model showed mixed behavior with signs of underfitting, it still captured relevant patterns from the training data. The VGG19 model exhibited positive performance across multiple metrics, indicating accurate predictions and good generalization capabilities. The InceptionV3 model showed potential but struggled with overfitting and generalization to unseen data.

The alignment between the ISUP grade of the original and predicted data for the first 40 rows of the validation file further suggests that the trained models effectively learned the patterns and were able to generalize well to the same data. This indicates that the models have the potential to accurately predict the ISUP grade based on the provided training data and masks with annotated Gleason scores.

However, further evaluation and testing on additional datasets are necessary to validate the performance of these models and determine their reliability in real-world scenarios.

References

1. Epstein, J., Amin, M., Fine, S., Algaba, F., Aron, M.: The 2019 genitourinary pathology society (GUPS) white paper on contemporary grading of prostate cancer. Arch. Pathol. Lab. Med. **145**, 461–493 (2020)
2. Leenders, G., Verhoef, E., Hollemans, E.: Prostate cancer growth patterns beyond the Gleason score: entering a new era of comprehensive tumour grading. Histopathology **77**, 850–861 (2020)
3. Bulten, W., et al.: Artificial intelligence assistance significantly improves Gleason grading of prostate biopsies by pathologists. Mod. Pathol. **34**, 660–671 (2021)
4. Bulten, W., et al.: Artificial intelligence for diagnosis and Gleason grading of prostate cancer: the PANDA challenge. Nat. Med. **28**, 154–163 (2022)
5. Kartasalo, K., et al.: Artificial intelligence for diagnosis and Gleason grading of prostate cancer in biopsies-current status and next steps. Eur. Urol. Focus **7**, 687–691 (2021)
6. Egevad, L., et al.: Identification of areas of grading difficulties in prostate cancer and comparison with artificial intelligence assisted grading. Virchows Archiv **477**, 777–786 (2020)
7. Marginean, F., et al.: An artificial intelligence-based support tool for automation and standardisation of Gleason grading in prostate biopsies. Eur. Urol. Focus **7**, 995–1001 (2021)
8. Pantanowitz, L., et al.: An artificial intelligence algorithm for prostate cancer diagnosis in whole slide images of core needle biopsies: a blinded clinical validation and deployment study. Lancet Digit. Health **2**, e407–e416 (2020)

Author Index

Printed in the United States
by Baker & Taylor Publisher Services